FREE Study Skills Videos/DVD Offer

Dear Customer,

Thank you for your purchase from Mometrix! We consider it an honor and a privilege that you have purchased our product and we want to ensure your satisfaction.

As a way of showing our appreciation and to help us better serve you, we have developed Study Skills Videos that we would like to give you for FREE. These videos cover our *best practices* for getting ready for your exam, from how to use our study materials to how to best prepare for the day of the test.

All that we ask is that you email us with feedback that would describe your experience so far with our product. Good, bad, or indifferent, we want to know what you think!

To get your FREE Study Skills Videos, you can use the **QR code** below, or send us an **email** at studyvideos@mometrix.com with *FREE VIDEOS* in the subject line and the following information in the body of the email:

- The name of the product you purchased.
- Your product rating on a scale of 1-5, with 5 being the highest rating.
- Your feedback. It can be long, short, or anything in between. We just want to know your impressions and experience so far with our product. (Good feedback might include how our study material met your needs and ways we might be able to make it even better. You could highlight features that you found helpful or features that you think we should add.)

If you have any questions or concerns, please don't hesitate to contact me directly.

Thanks again!

Sincerely,

Jay Willis
Vice President
jay.willis@mometrix.com
1-800-673-8175

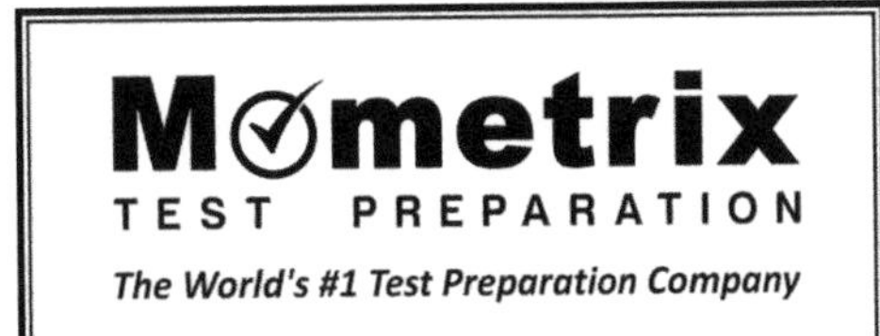

NPTE®

SECRETS

Study Guide

Your Key to Exam Success

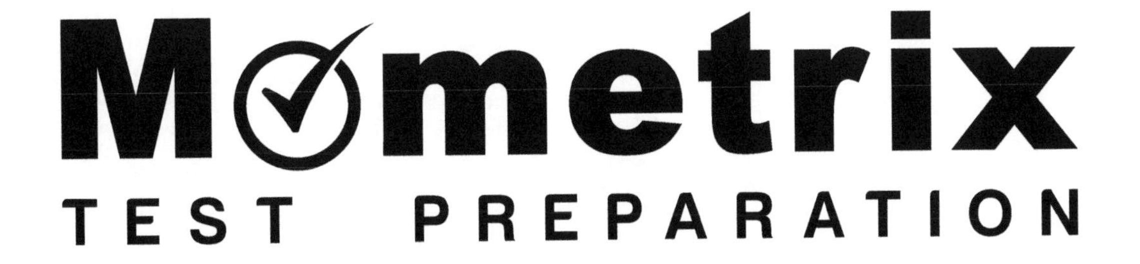

Written and edited by the Mometrix Physical Therapy Certification Test Team

Paperback
ISBN 13: 978-1-61072-317-6
ISBN 10: 1-61072-317-1

Ebook
ISBN 13: 978-1-62120-437-4
ISBN 10: 1-62120-437-5

Hardback
ISBN 13: 978-1-5167-0573-3
ISBN 10: 1-5167-0573-4

Dear Future Exam Success Story

First of all, **THANK YOU** for purchasing Mometrix study materials!

Second, congratulations! You are one of the few determined test-takers who are committed to doing whatever it takes to excel on your exam. **You have come to the right place.** We developed these study materials with one goal in mind: to deliver you the information you need in a format that's concise and easy to use.

In addition to optimizing your guide for the content of the test, we've outlined our recommended steps for breaking down the preparation process into small, attainable goals so you can make sure you stay on track.

We've also analyzed the entire test-taking process, identifying the most common pitfalls and showing how you can overcome them and be ready for any curveball the test throws you.

Standardized testing is one of the biggest obstacles on your road to success, which only increases the importance of doing well in the high-pressure, high-stakes environment of test day. Your results on this test could have a significant impact on your future, and this guide provides the information and practical advice to help you achieve your full potential on test day.

Your success is our success

We would love to hear from you! If you would like to share the story of your exam success or if you have any questions or comments in regard to our products, please contact us at **800-673-8175** or **support@mometrix.com**.

Thanks again for your business and we wish you continued success!

Sincerely,
The Mometrix Test Preparation Team

Need more help? Check out our flashcards at:
http://MometrixFlashcards.com/NPTE

TABLE OF CONTENTS

Introduction

Thank you for purchasing this resource! You have made the choice to prepare yourself for a test that could have a huge impact on your future, and this guide is designed to help you be fully ready for test day. Obviously, it's important to have a solid understanding of the test material, but you also need to be prepared for the unique environment and stressors of the test, so that you can perform to the best of your abilities.

For this purpose, the first section that appears in this guide is the **Secret Keys**. We've devoted countless hours to meticulously researching what works and what doesn't, and we've boiled down our findings to the five most impactful steps you can take to improve your performance on the test. We start at the beginning with study planning and move through the preparation process, all the way to the testing strategies that will help you get the most out of what you know when you're finally sitting in front of the test.

We recommend that you start preparing for your test as far in advance as possible. However, if you've bought this guide as a last-minute study resource and only have a few days before your test, we recommend that you skip over the first two Secret Keys since they address a long-term study plan.

If you struggle with **test anxiety**, we strongly encourage you to check out our recommendations for how you can overcome it. Test anxiety is a formidable foe, but it can be beaten, and we want to make sure you have the tools you need to defeat it.

Secret Key #1 – Plan Big, Study Small

There's a lot riding on your performance. If you want to ace this test, you're going to need to keep your skills sharp and the material fresh in your mind. You need a plan that lets you review everything you need to know while still fitting in your schedule. We'll break this strategy down into three categories.

Information Organization

Start with the information you already have: the official test outline. From this, you can make a complete list of all the concepts you need to cover before the test. Organize these concepts into groups that can be studied together, and create a list of any related vocabulary you need to learn so you can brush up on any difficult terms. You'll want to keep this vocabulary list handy once you actually start studying since you may need to add to it along the way.

Time Management

Once you have your set of study concepts, decide how to spread them out over the time you have left before the test. Break your study plan into small, clear goals so you have a manageable task for each day and know exactly what you're doing. Then just focus on one small step at a time. When you manage your time this way, you don't need to spend hours at a time studying. Studying a small block of content for a short period each day helps you retain information better and avoid stressing over how much you have left to do. You can relax knowing that you have a plan to cover everything in time. In order for this strategy to be effective though, you have to start studying early and stick to your schedule. Avoid the exhaustion and futility that comes from last-minute cramming!

Study Environment

The environment you study in has a big impact on your learning. Studying in a coffee shop, while probably more enjoyable, is not likely to be as fruitful as studying in a quiet room. It's important to keep distractions to a minimum. You're only planning to study for a short block of time, so make the most of it. Don't pause to check your phone or get up to find a snack. It's also important to **avoid multitasking**. Research has consistently shown that multitasking will make your studying dramatically less effective. Your study area should also be comfortable and well-lit so you don't have the distraction of straining your eyes or sitting on an uncomfortable chair.

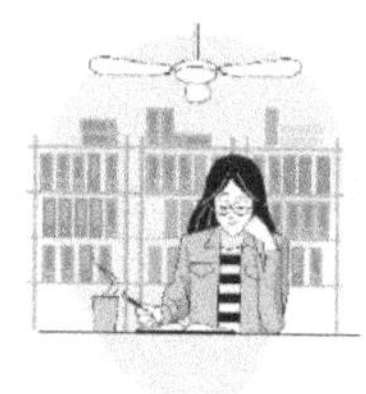

The time of day you study is also important. You want to be rested and alert. Don't wait until just before bedtime. Study when you'll be most likely to comprehend and remember. Even better, if you know what time of day your test will be, set that time aside for study. That way your brain will be used to working on that subject at that specific time and you'll have a better chance of recalling information.

Finally, it can be helpful to team up with others who are studying for the same test. Your actual studying should be done in as isolated an environment as possible, but the work of organizing the information and setting up the study plan can be divided up. In between study sessions, you can discuss with your teammates the concepts that you're all studying and quiz each other on the details. Just be sure that your teammates are as serious about the test as you are. If you find that your study time is being replaced with social time, you might need to find a new team.

Secret Key #2 – Make Your Studying Count

You're devoting a lot of time and effort to preparing for this test, so you want to be absolutely certain it will pay off. This means doing more than just reading the content and hoping you can remember it on test day. It's important to make every minute of study count. There are two main areas you can focus on to make your studying count.

Retention

It doesn't matter how much time you study if you can't remember the material. You need to make sure you are retaining the concepts. To check your retention of the information you're learning, try recalling it at later times with minimal prompting. Try carrying around flashcards and glance at one or two from time to time or ask a friend who's also studying for the test to quiz you.

To enhance your retention, look for ways to put the information into practice so that you can apply it rather than simply recalling it. If you're using the information in practical ways, it will be much easier to remember. Similarly, it helps to solidify a concept in your mind if you're not only reading it to yourself but also explaining it to someone else. Ask a friend to let you teach them about a concept you're a little shaky on (or speak aloud to an imaginary audience if necessary). As you try to summarize, define, give examples, and answer your friend's questions, you'll understand the concepts better and they will stay with you longer. Finally, step back for a big picture view and ask yourself how each piece of information fits with the whole subject. When you link the different concepts together and see them working together as a whole, it's easier to remember the individual components.

Finally, practice showing your work on any multi-step problems, even if you're just studying. Writing out each step you take to solve a problem will help solidify the process in your mind, and you'll be more likely to remember it during the test.

Modality

Modality simply refers to the means or method by which you study. Choosing a study modality that fits your own individual learning style is crucial. No two people learn best in exactly the same way, so it's important to know your strengths and use them to your advantage.

For example, if you learn best by visualization, focus on visualizing a concept in your mind and draw an image or a diagram. Try color-coding your notes, illustrating them, or creating symbols that will trigger your mind to recall a learned concept. If you learn best by hearing or discussing information, find a study partner who learns the same way or read aloud to yourself. Think about how to put the information in your own words. Imagine that you are giving a lecture on the topic and record yourself so you can listen to it later.

For any learning style, flashcards can be helpful. Organize the information so you can take advantage of spare moments to review. Underline key words or phrases. Use different colors for different categories. Mnemonic devices (such as creating a short list in which every item starts with the same letter) can also help with retention. Find what works best for you and use it to store the information in your mind most effectively and easily.

Secret Key #3 – Practice the Right Way

Your success on test day depends not only on how many hours you put into preparing, but also on whether you prepared the right way. It's good to check along the way to see if your studying is paying off. One of the most effective ways to do this is by taking practice tests to evaluate your progress. Practice tests are useful because they show exactly where you need to improve. Every time you take a practice test, pay special attention to these three groups of questions:

- The questions you got wrong
- The questions you had to guess on, even if you guessed right
- The questions you found difficult or slow to work through

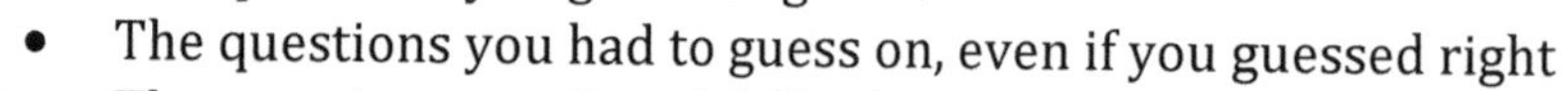

This will show you exactly what your weak areas are, and where you need to devote more study time. Ask yourself why each of these questions gave you trouble. Was it because you didn't understand the material? Was it because you didn't remember the vocabulary? Do you need more repetitions on this type of question to build speed and confidence? Dig into those questions and figure out how you can strengthen your weak areas as you go back to review the material.

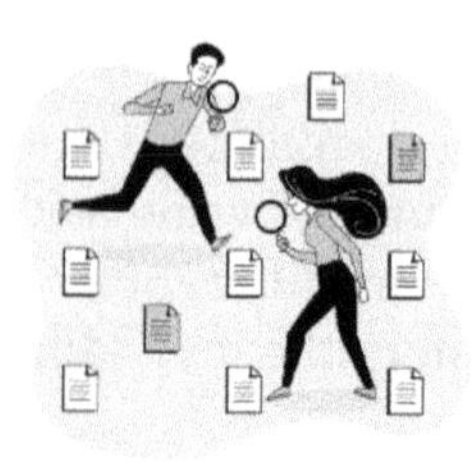

Additionally, many practice tests have a section explaining the answer choices. It can be tempting to read the explanation and think that you now have a good understanding of the concept. However, an explanation likely only covers part of the question's broader context. Even if the explanation makes perfect sense, **go back and investigate** every concept related to the question until you're positive you have a thorough understanding.

As you go along, keep in mind that the practice test is just that: practice. Memorizing these questions and answers will not be very helpful on the actual test because it is unlikely to have any of the same exact questions. If you only know the right answers to the sample questions, you won't be prepared for the real thing. **Study the concepts** until you understand them fully, and then you'll be able to answer any question that shows up on the test.

It's important to wait on the practice tests until you're ready. If you take a test on your first day of study, you may be overwhelmed by the amount of material covered and how much you need to learn. Work up to it gradually.

On test day, you'll need to be prepared for answering questions, managing your time, and using the test-taking strategies you've learned. It's a lot to balance, like a mental marathon that will have a big impact on your future. Like training for a marathon, you'll need to start slowly and work your way up. When test day arrives, you'll be ready.

Start with the strategies you've read in the first two Secret Keys—plan your course and study in the way that works best for you. If you have time, consider using multiple study resources to get different approaches to the same concepts. It can be helpful to see difficult concepts from more than one angle. Then find a good source for practice tests. Many times, the test website will suggest potential study resources or provide sample tests.

Practice Test Strategy

If you're able to find at least three practice tests, we recommend this strategy:

Untimed and Open-Book Practice

Take the first test with no time constraints and with your notes and study guide handy. Take your time and focus on applying the strategies you've learned.

Timed and Open-Book Practice

Take the second practice test open-book as well, but set a timer and practice pacing yourself to finish in time.

Timed and Closed-Book Practice

Take any other practice tests as if it were test day. Set a timer and put away your study materials. Sit at a table or desk in a quiet room, imagine yourself at the testing center, and answer questions as quickly and accurately as possible.

Keep repeating timed and closed-book tests on a regular basis until you run out of practice tests or it's time for the actual test. Your mind will be ready for the schedule and stress of test day, and you'll be able to focus on recalling the material you've learned.

Secret Key #4 – Pace Yourself

Once you're fully prepared for the material on the test, your biggest challenge on test day will be managing your time. Just knowing that the clock is ticking can make you panic even if you have plenty of time left. Work on pacing yourself so you can build confidence against the time constraints of the exam. Pacing is a difficult skill to master, especially in a high-pressure environment, so **practice is vital**.

Set time expectations for your pace based on how much time is available. For example, if a section has 60 questions and the time limit is 30 minutes, you know you have to average 30 seconds or less per question in order to answer them all. Although 30 seconds is the hard limit, set 25 seconds per question as your goal, so you reserve extra time to spend on harder questions. When you budget extra time for the harder questions, you no longer have any reason to stress when those questions take longer to answer.

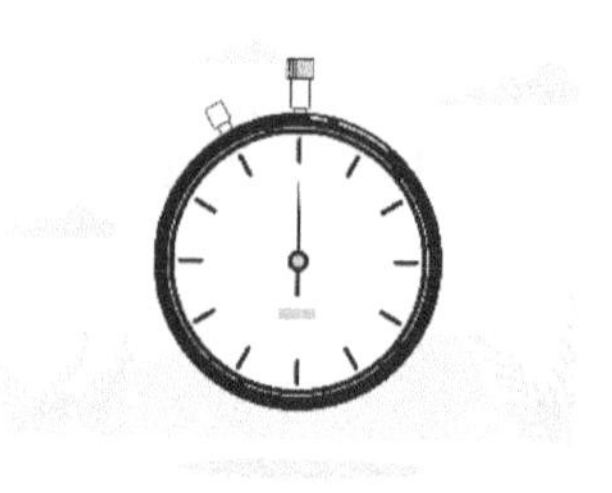

Don't let this time expectation distract you from working through the test at a calm, steady pace, but keep it in mind so you don't spend too much time on any one question. Recognize that taking extra time on one question you don't understand may keep you from answering two that you do understand later in the test. If your time limit for a question is up and you're still not sure of the answer, mark it and move on, and come back to it later if the time and the test format allow. If the testing format doesn't allow you to return to earlier questions, just make an educated guess; then put it out of your mind and move on.

On the easier questions, be careful not to rush. It may seem wise to hurry through them so you have more time for the challenging ones, but it's not worth missing one if you know the concept and just didn't take the time to read the question fully. Work efficiently but make sure you understand the question and have looked at all of the answer choices, since more than one may seem right at first.

Even if you're paying attention to the time, you may find yourself a little behind at some point. You should speed up to get back on track, but do so wisely. Don't panic; just take a few seconds less on each question until you're caught up. Don't guess without thinking, but do look through the answer choices and eliminate any you know are wrong. If you can get down to two choices, it is often worthwhile to guess from those. Once you've chosen an answer, move on and don't dwell on any that you skipped or had to hurry through. If a question was taking too long, chances are it was one of the harder ones, so you weren't as likely to get it right anyway.

On the other hand, if you find yourself getting ahead of schedule, it may be beneficial to slow down a little. The more quickly you work, the more likely you are to make a careless mistake that will affect your score. You've budgeted time for each question, so don't be afraid to spend that time. Practice an efficient but careful pace to get the most out of the time you have.

Secret Key #5 – Have a Plan for Guessing

When you're taking the test, you may find yourself stuck on a question. Some of the answer choices seem better than others, but you don't see the one answer choice that is obviously correct. What do you do?

The scenario described above is very common, yet most test takers have not effectively prepared for it. Developing and practicing a plan for guessing may be one of the single most effective uses of your time as you get ready for the exam.

In developing your plan for guessing, there are three questions to address:

- When should you start the guessing process?
- How should you narrow down the choices?
- Which answer should you choose?

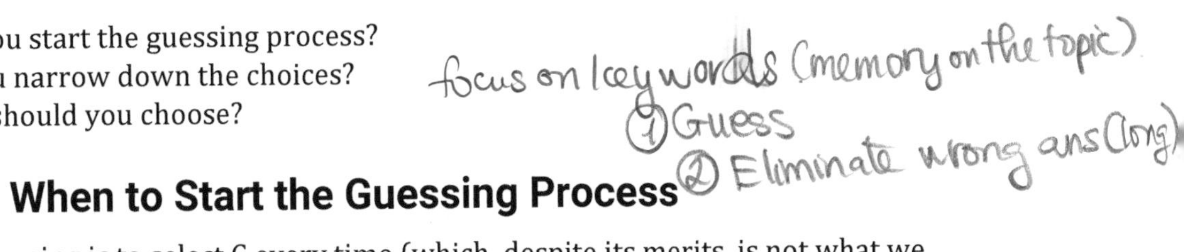

When to Start the Guessing Process

Unless your plan for guessing is to select C every time (which, despite its merits, is not what we recommend), you need to leave yourself enough time to apply your answer elimination strategies. Since you have a limited amount of time for each question, that means that if you're going to give yourself the best shot at guessing correctly, you have to decide quickly whether or not you will guess.

Of course, the best-case scenario is that you don't have to guess at all, so first, see if you can answer the question based on your knowledge of the subject and basic reasoning skills. Focus on the key words in the question and try to jog your memory of related topics. Give yourself a chance to bring the knowledge to mind, but once you realize that you don't have (or you can't access) the knowledge you need to answer the question, it's time to start the guessing process.

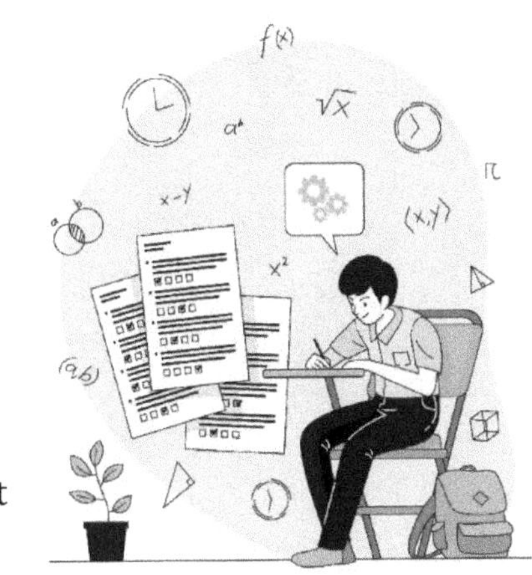

It's almost always better to start the guessing process too early than too late. It only takes a few seconds to remember something and answer the question from knowledge. Carefully eliminating wrong answer choices takes longer. Plus, going through the process of eliminating answer choices can actually help jog your memory.

Summary: Start the guessing process as soon as you decide that you can't answer the question based on your knowledge.

How to Narrow Down the Choices

The next chapter in this book (**Test-Taking Strategies**) includes a wide range of strategies for how to approach questions and how to look for answer choices to eliminate. You will definitely want to read those carefully, practice them, and figure out which ones work best for you. Here though, we're going to address a mindset rather than a particular strategy.

Your odds of guessing an answer correctly depend on how many options you are choosing from.

Number of options left	5	4	3	2	1
Odds of guessing correctly	20%	25%	33%	50%	100%

You can see from this chart just how valuable it is to be able to eliminate incorrect answers and make an educated guess, but there are two things that many test takers do that cause them to miss out on the benefits of guessing:

- Accidentally eliminating the correct answer
- Selecting an answer based on an impression

We'll look at the first one here, and the second one in the next section.

To avoid accidentally eliminating the correct answer, we recommend a thought exercise called **the $5 challenge**. In this challenge, you only eliminate an answer choice from contention if you are willing to bet $5 on it being wrong. Why $5? Five dollars is a small but not insignificant amount of money. It's an amount you could afford to lose but wouldn't want to throw away. And while losing $5 once might not hurt too much, doing it twenty times will set you back $100. In the same way, each small decision you make—eliminating a choice here, guessing on a question there—won't by itself impact your score very much, but when you put them all together, they can make a big difference. By holding each answer choice elimination decision to a higher standard, you can reduce the risk of accidentally eliminating the correct answer.

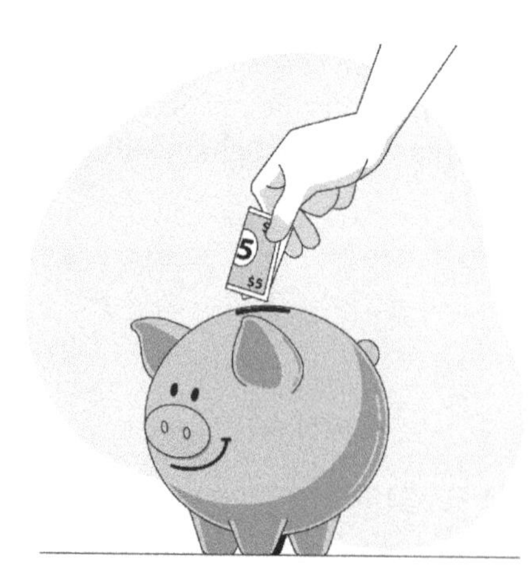

The $5 challenge can also be applied in a positive sense: If you are willing to bet $5 that an answer choice *is* correct, go ahead and mark it as correct.

Summary: Only eliminate an answer choice if you are willing to bet $5 that it is wrong.

Which Answer to Choose

You're taking the test. You've run into a hard question and decided you'll have to guess. You've eliminated all the answer choices you're willing to bet $5 on. Now you have to pick an answer. Why do we even need to talk about this? Why can't you just pick whichever one you feel like when the time comes?

The answer to these questions is that if you don't come into the test with a plan, you'll rely on your impression to select an answer choice, and if you do that, you risk falling into a trap. The test writers know that everyone who takes their test will be guessing on some of the questions, so they intentionally write wrong answer choices to seem plausible. You still have to pick an answer though, and if the wrong answer choices are designed to look right, how can you ever be sure that you're not falling for their trap? The best solution we've found to this dilemma is to take the decision out of your hands entirely. Here is the process we recommend:

Once you've eliminated any choices that you are confident (willing to bet $5) are wrong, select the first remaining choice as your answer.

Whether you choose to select the first remaining choice, the second, or the last, the important thing is that you use some preselected standard. Using this approach guarantees that you will not be enticed into selecting an answer choice that looks right, because you are not basing your decision on how the answer choices look.

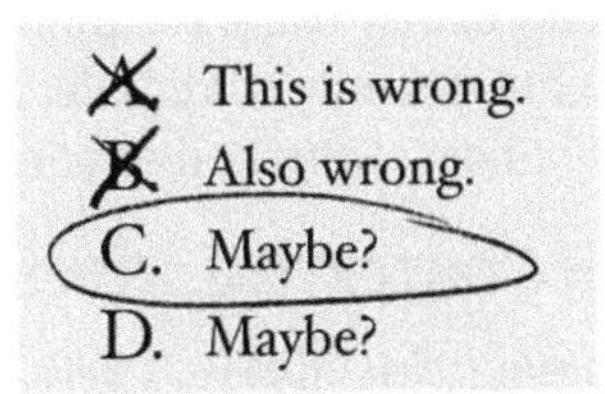

This is not meant to make you question your knowledge. Instead, it is to help you recognize the difference between your knowledge and your impressions. There's a huge difference between thinking an answer is right because of what you know, and thinking an answer is right because it looks or sounds like it should be right.

Summary: To ensure that your selection is appropriately random, make a predetermined selection from among all answer choices you have not eliminated.

every question is different.

Test-Taking Strategies

This section contains a list of test-taking strategies that you may find helpful as you work through the test. By taking what you know and applying logical thought, you can maximize your chances of answering any question correctly!

It is very important to realize that every question is different and every person is different: no single strategy will work on every question, and no single strategy will work for every person. That's why we've included all of them here, so you can try them out and determine which ones work best for different types of questions and which ones work best for you.

Question Strategies

⊘ Read Carefully

Read the question and the answer choices carefully. Don't miss the question because you misread the terms. You have plenty of time to read each question thoroughly and make sure you understand what is being asked. Yet a happy medium must be attained, so don't waste too much time. You must read carefully and efficiently.

⊘ Contextual Clues

Look for contextual clues. If the question includes a word you are not familiar with, look at the immediate context for some indication of what the word might mean. Contextual clues can often give you all the information you need to decipher the meaning of an unfamiliar word. Even if you can't determine the meaning, you may be able to narrow down the possibilities enough to make a solid guess at the answer to the question.

⊘ Prefixes

If you're having trouble with a word in the question or answer choices, try dissecting it. Take advantage of every clue that the word might include. Prefixes and suffixes can be a huge help. Usually, they allow you to determine a basic meaning. *Pre-* means before, *post-* means after, *pro-* is positive, *de-* is negative. From prefixes and suffixes, you can get an idea of the general meaning of the word and try to put it into context.

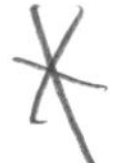

⊘ Hedge Words

Watch out for critical hedge words, such as *likely, may, can, sometimes, often, almost, mostly, usually, generally, rarely*, and *sometimes*. Question writers insert these hedge phrases to cover every possibility. Often an answer choice will be wrong simply because it leaves no room for exception. Be on guard for answer choices that have definitive words such as *exactly* and *always*.

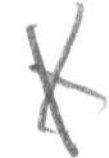

⊘ Switchback Words

Stay alert for *switchbacks*. These are the words and phrases frequently used to alert you to shifts in thought. The most common switchback words are *but, although*, and *however*. Others include *nevertheless, on the other hand, even though, while, in spite of, despite*, and *regardless of*. Switchback words are important to catch because they can change the direction of the question or an answer choice.

common sense

⊘ FACE VALUE

When in doubt, use common sense. Accept the situation in the problem at face value. Don't read too much into it. These problems will not require you to make wild assumptions. If you have to go beyond creativity and warp time or space in order to have an answer choice fit the question, then you should move on and consider the other answer choices. These are normal problems rooted in reality. The applicable relationship or explanation may not be readily apparent, but it is there for you to figure out. Use your common sense to interpret anything that isn't clear.

Answer Choice Strategies

⊘ ANSWER SELECTION

The most thorough way to pick an answer choice is to identify and eliminate wrong answers until only one is left, then confirm it is the correct answer. Sometimes an answer choice may immediately seem right, but be careful. The test writers will usually put more than one reasonable answer choice on each question, so take a second to read all of them and make sure that the other choices are not equally obvious. As long as you have time left, it is better to read every answer choice than to pick the first one that looks right without checking the others.

⊘ ANSWER CHOICE FAMILIES

An answer choice family consists of two (in rare cases, three) answer choices that are very similar in construction and cannot all be true at the same time. If you see two answer choices that are direct opposites or parallels, one of them is usually the correct answer. For instance, if one answer choice says that quantity *x* increases and another either says that quantity *x* decreases (opposite) or says that quantity *y* increases (parallel), then those answer choices would fall into the same family. An answer choice that doesn't match the construction of the answer choice family is more likely to be incorrect. Most questions will not have answer choice families, but when they do appear, you should be prepared to recognize them.

⊘ ELIMINATE ANSWERS

Eliminate answer choices as soon as you realize they are wrong, but make sure you consider all possibilities. If you are eliminating answer choices and realize that the last one you are left with is also wrong, don't panic. Start over and consider each choice again. There may be something you missed the first time that you will realize on the second pass.

⊘ AVOID FACT TRAPS

Don't be distracted by an answer choice that is factually true but doesn't answer the question. You are looking for the choice that answers the question. Stay focused on what the question is asking for so you don't accidentally pick an answer that is true but incorrect. Always go back to the question and make sure the answer choice you've selected actually answers the question and is not merely a true statement.

⊘ EXTREME STATEMENTS

In general, you should avoid answers that put forth extreme actions as standard practice or proclaim controversial ideas as established fact. An answer choice that states the "process should be used in certain situations, if..." is much more likely to be correct than one that states the "process should be discontinued completely." The first is a calm rational statement and doesn't even make a definitive, uncompromising stance, using a hedge word *if* to provide wiggle room, whereas the second choice is far more extreme.

⊘ BENCHMARK

As you read through the answer choices and you come across one that seems to answer the question well, mentally select that answer choice. This is not your final answer, but it's the one that will help you evaluate the other answer choices. The one that you selected is your benchmark or standard for judging each of the other answer choices. Every other answer choice must be compared to your benchmark. That choice is correct until proven otherwise by another answer choice beating it. If you find a better answer, then that one becomes your new benchmark. Once you've decided that no other choice answers the question as well as your benchmark, you have your final answer.

⊘ PREDICT THE ANSWER

Before you even start looking at the answer choices, it is often best to try to predict the answer. When you come up with the answer on your own, it is easier to avoid distractions and traps because you will know exactly what to look for. The right answer choice is unlikely to be word-for-word what you came up with, but it should be a close match. Even if you are confident that you have the right answer, you should still take the time to read each option before moving on.

General Strategies

⊘ TOUGH QUESTIONS

If you are stumped on a problem or it appears too hard or too difficult, don't waste time. Move on! Remember though, if you can quickly check for obviously incorrect answer choices, your chances of guessing correctly are greatly improved. Before you completely give up, at least try to knock out a couple of possible answers. Eliminate what you can and then guess at the remaining answer choices before moving on.

⊘ CHECK YOUR WORK

Since you will probably not know every term listed and the answer to every question, it is important that you get credit for the ones that you do know. Don't miss any questions through careless mistakes. If at all possible, try to take a second to look back over your answer selection and make sure you've selected the correct answer choice and haven't made a costly careless mistake (such as marking an answer choice that you didn't mean to mark). This quick double check should more than pay for itself in caught mistakes for the time it costs.

⊘ PACE YOURSELF

It's easy to be overwhelmed when you're looking at a page full of questions; your mind is confused and full of random thoughts, and the clock is ticking down faster than you would like. Calm down and maintain the pace that you have set for yourself. Especially as you get down to the last few minutes of the test, don't let the small numbers on the clock make you panic. As long as you are on track by monitoring your pace, you are guaranteed to have time for each question.

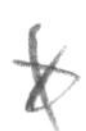

⊘ DON'T RUSH

It is very easy to make errors when you are in a hurry. Maintaining a fast pace in answering questions is pointless if it makes you miss questions that you would have gotten right otherwise. Test writers like to include distracting information and wrong answers that seem right. Taking a little extra time to avoid careless mistakes can make all the difference in your test score. Find a pace that allows you to be confident in the answers that you select.

✓ KEEP MOVING

Panicking will not help you pass the test, so do your best to stay calm and keep moving. Taking deep breaths and going through the answer elimination steps you practiced can help to break through a stress barrier and keep your pace.

Final Notes

The combination of a solid foundation of content knowledge and the confidence that comes from practicing your plan for applying that knowledge is the key to maximizing your performance on test day. As your foundation of content knowledge is built up and strengthened, you'll find that the strategies included in this chapter become more and more effective in helping you quickly sift through the distractions and traps of the test to isolate the correct answer.

Now that you're preparing to move forward into the test content chapters of this book, be sure to keep your goal in mind. As you read, think about how you will be able to apply this information on the test. If you've already seen sample questions for the test and you have an idea of the question format and style, try to come up with questions of your own that you can answer based on what you're reading. This will give you valuable practice applying your knowledge in the same ways you can expect to on test day.

Good luck and good studying!

Clinical Application of Foundational Sciences

Cardiac, Vascular, and Pulmonary Systems

Main Structures of the Heart

Heart chambers, the compartments holding blood during pumping, (in order of blood circulation):

- Right atrium (right upper): receives deoxygenated blood from the venous system via major veins called the superior vena cava (from the head, neck, and upper body) and the inferior vena cava (from the internal organs and lower body).
- Right ventricle (right lower): receives blood from the right atrium, and sends it to the lungs (pulmonary circulation) via the pulmonary artery.
- Left atrium (left upper): receives oxygenated blood from the lungs via the pulmonary veins.
- Left ventricle (left lower): receives blood from the left atrium, and pumps it to the systemic circulation via the ascending and descending portions of the largest artery, the aorta
- Valves between chambers prevent backflow of blood between chambers or chambers and blood vessels:
- Tricuspid valve: located between the right atrium and ventricle
- Pulmonic valve: located between the right ventricle and pulmonary artery.
- Mitral valve: located between the left atrium and ventricle
- Aortic valve: located between the left ventricle and aorta
- Arteries supplying blood to the heart muscles - coronary arteries

Heart Tissues and Functions

The types of heart tissues are:

- Pericardium: the double-walled sac enclosing the heart, with a tough outer surface (fibrous pericardium) and inner serous membrane (serous pericardium); protects against infection and trauma
- Epicardium: the outermost layer of the cardiac wall, the visceral layer of the serous pericardium, protects against infection and trauma
- Myocardium: the central, thick muscular layer of heart tissue, which provides pumping power to ventricles
- Endocardium: the thin tissue layer lining many structures
- Chordae tendineae and associated papillary muscles: tendons and muscles that prevent the eversion (turning inside out) of valves during ventricular systole

The Cardiac Cycle

A cardiac cycle is the time between heart contractions. Each heart chamber has a period of filling or relaxation, called diastole, followed by a period of contraction, called systole. The right side of the heart receives blood from the higher-pressure superior and inferior vena cava veins essentially passively, whereas the left side of the heart requires sufficient high-pressure pumping power to circulate blood.

Each atrium has a phase of atrial diastole followed by atrial systole. During atrial systole, about 70% of the blood empties into the ventricle initially because of the pressure differential; the rest is then expelled through contraction or atrial kick. Ventricular diastole is the ventricular filling, which begins passively, and is followed by stretching of the ventricular walls during the corresponding atrial contraction. Ventricular systole or contraction follows, creating pressure before rapid ejection of the blood. The blood expelled is called the ejection fraction, typically about 60% for the left ventricle.

Cardiac Output

Cardiac output (CO) is the quantity of blood per minute pumped by the heart. At rest, CO is normally between 4 and 8 liters/minute (L/min). During exertion, the maximum possible cardiac output is dependent on two factors: the heart rate (HR) in beats per minute (bpm) and stroke volume (SV), represented as follows:

$$\text{CO (L/min)} = \text{HR(bpm)} \times \text{SV(liters)}$$

Cardiac output is affected by a factor called preload, the amount of tension on the ventricular wall prior to contraction. Preload is defined according to a relationship called the Frank-Starling mechanism, which basically says that a stronger ventricular contraction occurs when there is more stretch on the myocardium and a larger volume of blood (which creates pressure). CO is also affected by afterload, the amount of pressure in the aorta opposing ejection. Afterload is directly related to blood pressure (BP).

Cardiac Conduction System

The heart has three characteristics directly related to electrical impulses: automaticity, the ability to initiate internal electrical impulses; excitability, the capability to respond to electrical stimuli; and conductivity, the transmission of electrical impulses between cells in the heart. The heart also has contractility, the capacity to stretch and recoil as a unit, and rhythmicity, the ability to repeat this sequence with regularity. The cardiac conduction system facilitates contraction and pumping of blood and influences heart rate. It is controlled intrinsically by several areas that transmit electrical impulses.

In order, they are the sinoatrial (SA) node in the right atrium near the entrance of the superior vena cava, the atrioventricular (AV) node in the floor of the right atrium, the bundle of his between the two ventricles, branches from the bundle of his called the right and left bundle branches, and, ultimately, the Purkinje fibers. Successful conduction stimulates the myocardium, initiating ventricular contraction. There are also extrinsic controls, primarily the vagus nerve of the parasympathetic system and the upper thoracic nerves of the sympathetic branches of the autonomic nervous system, which lower or accelerate heart rate respectively.

Hormones Effects on Cardiac Function

A number of bodily hormones affect cardiac function, either by influencing blood volume, causing vasoconstriction, or triggering vasodilation. In the atria of the heart, there are atrial natriuretic peptides that can be stimulated by increased atrial stretch, resulting in lower blood volume. Blood volume can be increased by the hormone aldosterone, which is stimulated when there is hypovolemia or decreased renal perfusion.

Vasoconstriction or the narrowing of blood vessels, which reduces blood flow and increases blood pressure, can be induced by norepinephrine during stress or exercise, or angiotensin or vasopressin in response to decreased arterial pressure. Hormones that can cause vasodilation or widening of blood vessels include epinephrine in response to stress or exercise, and bradykinin and histamine in response to tissue damage.

Systemic Circulation

Systemic circulation is the flow of blood to the body. It is initiated when oxygenated blood is ejected from the left ventricle during systole into the large artery, the aorta. The aorta diverges into smaller arteries, then narrower arterioles, and eventually even narrower capillaries. There is an exchange of gases at the capillary level, in which oxygen (O_2) is distributed to the surrounding tissues and carbon dioxide (CO_2) is taken in. The deoxygenated blood travels from the capillaries into larger venules, then wider veins, and ultimately the vena cava into the heart. The systemic circulation on the venus side is facilitated by muscular contractions and pressures, as well as unidirectional valves that prevent blood backflow.

Pulmonary Circulation

Pulmonary circulation is the flow of blood from the heart to the lungs. It is initiated when deoxygenated blood in the right ventricle is expelled into the pulmonary artery. The pulmonary artery divides into right and left branches, then smaller arteries, narrower arterioles, and eventually even narrower pulmonary capillaries within each lung. These pulmonary capillaries are surrounded by alveoli, which are small air sacs in the lung. The blood becomes oxygenated in the pulmonary capillaries through gas exchange, in which carbon dioxide (CO_2) is expelled and oxygen (O_2) is taken in. The oxygenated blood flows from the capillaries via the pulmonary veins into the left atrium of the heart.

Blood Vessels and Cells

Three Layers of Blood Vessels

All blood vessels have three layers. The innermost layer is called the tunica intima, which is composed of endothelial cells over a basement membrane and provides a smooth surface for laminar blood flow. The middle layer is termed the tunica media, consisting of smooth muscle cells and elastic connective tissue.

The tunica media is also innervated by sympathetic nerves and is the layer responsible for constriction and dilation of the vessel to control blood pressure. The outermost layer is known as the tunica adventitia. This section is made up of collagen fibers (connective tissue), lymph vessels, and other blood vessels that supply it with nutrients.

Three Types of Blood vessels

The three types of blood vessels are arteries, veins, and capillaries. All arteries have a thick middle or tunica media layer that permits them to adjust to pressure changes from the heart. There are large, relatively elastic arteries, such as the aorta, its large branches, and the pulmonary artery; medium-sized ones like the coronary arteries, which are more muscular; and small arteries and arterioles. Most arteries carry oxygenated blood from the heart. Veins come in a range of diameters from small to large. They have a thin tunica media layer but a thick outer tunica adventitia. Veins carry deoxygenated blood to the heart and have valves that thwart backflow of blood and aid in the venous return. Capillaries are the narrowest type of blood vessel, found at the convergence between the arterial and venous systems. Gases, as well as blood cells and fluids, are exchanged at the capillary level. The configuration of each capillary bed or mass is dependent on the circulatory requirements in the area.

Different Types of Blood Cells

Blood cells fall into three categories: erythrocytes, leukocytes, or thrombocytes. Erythrocytes are red blood cells (RBCs) that contain hemoglobin. Hemoglobin consists of four protein chains attached to pigment complexes containing iron. It transports oxygen to tissues through the attachment of oxygen to the iron, forming oxyhemoglobin. Leukocytes are white blood cells

(WBCs). There are five varieties of leukocytes, all of which play some role in immune defense and fighting off infection. WBCs include neutrophils, basophils, eosinophils, lymphocytes, and monocytes. The third type of blood cell is a platelet (Plt) or thrombocyte, which is involved in clot formation.

Functions of Blood

Blood is involved in oxygen and carbon dioxide transport through hemoglobin binds. Nutrients and metabolites are transported by binding to plasma proteins. The plasma portion of blood carries hormones throughout the body, waste products to the liver and kidneys, and cells and other molecules involved in the immune response to infection sites. Many of the blood's functions are related to regulation of bodily functions. These include maintenance of fluid balance through adjustment of blood volume, optimal body temperature via vasoconstriction or dilation, and acid-base balance. Blood also preserves hemostasis by clotting and halting bleeding and hemorrhaging.

Lymphatic System Structure

The lymphatic system is responsible for immune defenses and movement of fluid between the bloodstream and interstitial fluid. It consists of lymph vessels, lymph fluid, and specific lymph tissues and organs. Lymph is a fluid that contains white blood cells, primarily lymphocytes, drained from tissue spaces by the lymph vessels. Lymph is produced from excess interstitial fluid and other large molecules, which enter lymphatic capillaries, as well as lipids taken on in the small intestine. Lymph nodes are specialized organs in various regions of the body that filter the lymph prior to its inclusion in the circulation. The system has assorted ducts, which feed into the largest lymphatic ducts, the thoracic and right lymphatic ducts. These ducts drain into the veins in the cervical area. Several lymphatic organs have specific roles, including the thymus at the base of the neck, where thymosin is secreted and T lymphocytes (T cells) associated with cellular immunity mature; the spleen in the abdominal area, which filters bacteria and other matter from the blood and destroys old red blood cells; and the tonsils, located in the back of the oral cavity and which defend us against bacteria.

Respiratory System

Anatomy

The upper respiratory or pulmonary system consists of the nose, pharynx, and larynx. The nose is comprised of two nasal cavities lined with mucous membranes and supported by bone and cartilage. It is the channel through which air enters and where that air is filtered, warmed, and humidified. At the back of the nasal cavity is the pharynx, which connects the nasal and oral cavities to the larynx and the oral cavity to the esophagus. It serves as a conduit for both air and food. At the bottom of the upper respiratory tract is the larynx, or passageway between the pharynx and trachea; it is responsible for voice production and stops food from entering the lower respiratory tract.

The lower respiratory system consists of the trachea and various parts of the bronchial tree. The trachea is a flexible tube made of cartilage where inspired air is cleaned, warmed, and moistened. The trachea divides into the left and right main stem bronchi of the bronchial tree within the two lungs. The bronchial tree branches into smaller secondary and tertiary bronchi and, ultimately, the bronchioles, which terminate in alveoli, tiny sacs were gas exchange occurs. Both lungs are covered with serous membranes called pleurae.

Review Video: Respiratory System
Visit mometrix.com/academy and enter code: 783075

Inspiration and Expiration Processes

The primary inspiratory muscles are the diaphragm, the external intercostals, and the internal intercostals. There are also a number of accessory muscles that become involved in inspiration during exercise or if a person has cardiopulmonary disease. These accessory muscles include the trapezius, sternocleidomastoid, scalenes, the pectorals, and others. Inspiration, or the drawing in of air to the lungs, is an active process involving contraction of the diaphragm to increase lung volume (controlled by the phrenic nerve), rotation of the ribs by the external intercostals to increase thoracic volume, and elevation of the ribs by the internal intercostals.

Expiration, or the process of breathing out, primarily occurs passively as inspiratory muscles relax. Forcible expiration is facilitated by the rectus abdominis and the external and internal oblique muscles. All of the inspiratory and expiratory muscles are innervated by specific nerves.

The Appearance of and Landmarks Associated with the Positioning of the Lungs in the Thorax

The thorax is the upper part of the torso. It contains the lungs and heart, is divided vertically by the sternum or breastbone, and is enclosed by 12 pairs of ribs. The top seven ribs are true ribs that are connected to the sternum by costal cartilage and articulate with thoracic vertebrae. The remaining five so-called ribs are actually false, as ribs 8 to 10 are just attached via cartilage to rib 7 and ribs 11 and 12 are merely floating. The two lungs are different in appearance from the front. The right lung has three lobes or divisions, the right upper lobe extending from the collarbone down, the right middle lobe essentially below it, and a low, outer portion called the right lower lobe. The left lung has only two lobes, the left upper lobe, approximately equivalent to the combined upper and middle portions of the right lung, and the left lower lobe. For both lungs, the posterior view only shows upper and lower lobes for each.

Neural Control of Respiratory Functions

Involuntary, rhythmic breathing is regulated by the medullary respiratory center in the brain stem. Respiratory rate and depth is controlled by the pneumotaxic center in the pons area of the brain. Voluntary breathing is directed by the cerebral cortex, which sends messages via motor neurons to respiratory muscles. Respiration is also under chemical control, principally the arterial levels (pressures) of oxygen (P_{O2}) and carbon dioxide (P_{CO2}) and the concentration of hydrogen ions (H^+). Respiratory rate will increase or decrease as carbon dioxide or oxygen levels respectively increase. Respiratory rate and depth can change in response to irritants or stressors.

Pulmonary Physiology Processes

Pulmonary physiology involves ventilation, respiration, diffusion, and perfusion. Ventilation is the flow of air into and out of the lungs. It is controlled as discussed on another card both involuntarily and voluntarily. Respiration is the act of breathing, which is basically related to pressure changes in the thorax and the difference between atmospheric and alveolar pressure. Inspiration occurs when the alveolar pressure is less than the atmospheric pressure, and expiration occurs when the alveolar pressure is greater than the atmospheric. The process of diffusion takes place at the alveolar-capillary membrane, where inspired oxygen (O_2) can diffuse into the bloodstream and, conversely, carbon dioxide (CO_2) can be taken in due to a concentration gradient. Perfusion is the transfer of dissolved gases between the lungs and blood cells via the cardiovascular system. Gas exchange is optimal when the ventilation/perfusion ratio (V/Q) is close to 1:1. Oxygen is ultimately transferred from the lungs to bodily tissue, about 97% through chemical combination with hemoglobin and about 3% dissolved in plasma.

Activity and Exercise Effects

Indications of Cardiac Patient Instability That Impact Performance of Physical Therapy

If a cardiac patient is unstable, he should receive medical attention before any physical therapy is performed. Unqualified indications that a patient is unstable and physical therapy should be withheld include the presence of decompensated congestive heart failure, heart blocks that are either third-degree or second-degree with premature ventricular contractions (PVCs), excessive or multifocal PVCs, a dissecting aortic aneurysm, recent onset atrial fibrillation, or chest pain with new ST segment changes.

There are other situations that suggest instability and modification or withholding of physical therapy. These include a resting heart rate of more than 100 bpm, a myocardial infarction or its extension within the last two days, ventricular ectopy or atrial fibrillation while resting, the presence of uncontrollable metabolic diseases, patient psychosis, or indications of resting hypertension or hypotension. These are defined as blood pressure readings of greater than 160 mm Hg systolic/90 mm Hg diastolic for hypertension and less than 80 mm Hg systolic BP for hypotension.

Heart Rate Monitoring and Blood Pressure to Indicate Patient Tolerance for Activity Level

There are eight parameters that can be used to gauge a patient's tolerance for a particular activity level. Heart rate (HR) monitoring is one of the best indications as heart rate and work are linearly related. HR is used in a number of ways, such as choosing activities that result in a HR 20 to 30 beats above resting or within a safe range (typically 60 to 80% of the maximum). Heart rate recovery (HRR), which is the difference in heart rate at its peak during activity and 60 seconds later, should normally be more than 18 bpm or 12 bpm depending on whether or not there has been a cool-down period. Blood pressure (BP) is also monitored to make sure it does not indicate extreme hypertension (> 180 mm Hg systolic, > 110 mg Hg diastolic) or that the systolic component does not go down more than 10 mm Hg below resting. BP can also be used to determine intensity in patients with non-rate-modulated pacemakers.

The Borg Scales

There are three Borg Scales: the Borg RPE Scale, the Borg CR10 Scale, and the Borg CR100 Scale. All are utilized to rate how the patient perceives exertion during physical activity. The Borg RPE (rating of perceived exertion) Scale is the gold standard for subjective rating by the patient of exercise intensity, breathlessness, or muscle fatigue; it uses a scale from 6 to 20. The Borg CR10 and Borg CR100 (centiMax) Scales also measure RPE, just using different scales indicated by their names. Borg CR10 uses a scale of 1 to 10; Borg C100 uses 1 to 100. These subjective measurements are useful because in general it is recommended that individuals only exercise to point 13 on the Borg RPE or point 5 on the Borg CR10 Scales. They are also very useful for patients taking beta-blockers because these individuals cannot be monitored via heart rate as these drugs regulate heart activity.

Parameters Other Than HR, BP, and RPE Used to Evaluate Patient's Tolerance Activity Level

The rate pressure product (RPP) can be calculated as (HR x systolic BP) to provide an indication of myocardial oxygen demand. Auscultation can be used to listen for normal and abnormal heart sounds and breath sounds. Continuous monitoring with an electrocardiogram (ECG) is generally done during conditioning exercises like treadmill use for cardiac patients. The main reason an ECG is performed is to identify divergences from a patient's normal heart rhythm and potential decline in cardiac status. ECG indications of declining status include ST changes, increased occurrence or areas of premature ventricular contractions (PVCs), progression of heart blockage, and development of atrial fibrillation.

Indications That a Patient's Response to Activity or Exercise Is Unstable

Regardless of whether an individual's underlying cardiac issue is related to ischemia, pump failure, or congestive heart failure, patients present with similar symptoms during activity or exercise if they are unstable. Unstable congestive heart or pump failure can present as a greater than 10 mm Hg increase in pulmonary artery pressure and/or a deviation in central venous pressure of more than 6 mm Hg. Otherwise, unstable patients can be observed to have cyanosis, sweating, nasal flaring, increased use of accessory muscles for respiration, a subjective increase in RPE (rate of perceived exertion), pallor, confusion, and symptoms of ischemia, notably angina (chest pain). Patients usually have symptoms of congestive heart failure whether or not that is the underlying problem. Certain ECG changes occur with instability, including ST segment changes, development of multifocal PVCs, and increased occurrence of ventricular ectopy. Instability is also indicated by a systolic BP drop of more than 10 mm Hg, a diastolic BP change in either direction of more than 10 mm Hg, and a heart rate drop of more than 10 bpm.

Musculoskeletal System

Musculoskeletal System Components

The musculoskeletal system is comprised of the bony skeleton and soft tissues. The soft tissues include contractile muscles, tough fibrous tendons and ligaments, joint capsules, and relatively elastic cartilage. The musculoskeletal system enables movement and performance of fine-motor tasks, absorbs shock, converts and generates energy, and protects vital organs and the central nervous system. The musculoskeletal system is intimately related to the nervous system as nerves stimulate the muscles. Functional deficits are often related to impairment of the musculoskeletal system through traumatic injuries or degenerative alterations.

Patient History in Musculoskeletal Evaluation

In addition to general medical questions, there are specific areas related to possible musculoskeletal problems that should be addressed in the patient history. The examiner should ask about the individual's chief complaint or history of the present illness, the mechanism of injury, the rapidity of onset of symptoms, areas that bother the patient, types of sensations and their locations, and particularly the history and characterization of the involved pain (discussed further elsewhere). Mechanism of injury refers to whether there was a provoking trauma (macrotrauma) or a repetitive activity (microtrauma) involved. Previous history of musculoskeletal, rheumatologic, or neurologic diseases should be noted along with prior injuries and surgeries, use of assistive devices or adaptive equipment, and history of falls. The history should also include potentially relevant information, such as the use of analgesics, steroids, or other medications; physician precautions regarding weight bearing, activity level, or positioning; lab and imaging information; and familial or developmental history of diseases, such as cancer or arthritis and other serious systemic illnesses.

Pain Related to Musculoskeletal Problems

There can be many causes of pain in addition to musculoskeletal, for example, a number of system diseases ranging from cancer to infection, psychological, etc. The patient should be asked whether the pain is acute, meaning generally new and severe, or chronic, persistent but generally less intense. The patient should identify the area of pain, which is generally peripheralized (large in area and more distal to the lesion) when the lesion is worse, or centralized (smaller and more localized) during improvement. Generalized pain in any area may be referred pain sensed at a location other than the injury due to common innervation. The pain should be described in terms of the movements or activities causing it and the length of the problem (acute: 7 to 10 days; sub-acute: 10 days to 7 weeks; chronic: more than 7 weeks). The constancy of the pain should be noted as constant, periodic (or occasional), or episodic due to specific activities; musculoskeletal pain is usually periodic or episodic. The intensity, duration, frequency, and changes in each should be noted. The pain should be described in terms of its daily timing and its type or quality (sharp, deep, aching, etc.).

Principles of Arthrokinematics

Arthrokinematics describes joint motion in terms of joint shapes, types of joint motion, and other accessory motions. A joint is the connection between two bony partners. The joint shape is either ovoid, where one surface is convex and the other concave, or sellar, in which both surfaces have convex and concave components. Movement of the body lever around the joint is its swing, generally described as flexion, extension, abduction, adduction, or rotation. There are also three potential types of motion between the bony surfaces: rolling of the surface in the same direction as the bony lever movement; sliding (translating) of one surface over the other to a new position, often combined with rolling; or spinning, rotation of one segment about a stationary axis. Other accessory motions include compression, reduction of the space between bony partners; traction, a longitudinal pull; and distraction, separation of bony partners.

Muscle Performance

Muscle performance is the facility of a muscle to perform work, the amount of energy generated by a force moving through a distance. Muscle performance is related to muscle strength, the force output of a contracting muscle as a function of the amount of tension it can produce; muscle power, the amount of work produced by the muscle per unit of time (force x distance/time); and muscle endurance, the capacity of a muscle to contract repetitively over a long period of time against a load or resistance, while reducing and maintaining tension and resisting fatigue.

Muscle Performance Training

Two types of training are associated with muscle performance. The first is strength training to develop muscle strength by systematically doing low-repetition or short-duration exercises involving lifting, lowering, or controlling heavy loads. The other is endurance training to improve aerobic power and length of muscle use by doing high-repetition, low-intensity muscle contractions over a prolonged time period. Both are considered resistance exercise or training. Resistance exercise is based on the principle of overload, meaning muscle performance can only improve when the load is above its metabolic capacity.

Effective Resistance Training Terms

Alignment: proper positioning of patient or body segments

Duration: total number of weeks or months in the exercise program

Effective resistance training programs incorporate use of appropriate terminology:

Exercise order: the sequence of utilization of muscle groups

Frequency: the number of training periods per day or week

Integration of function: use of exercises approximating

Intensity: the amount of load applied

Mode of exercise: definitions provided in terms of type of contraction, weight- or nonweight-bearing position, form of resistance (manual, mechanical, etc.), short- or full-arc range of movement, or energy system involved (anaerobic, aerobic)

Periodization: the amount of variation

Rest interval: the rest time between exercise sets or sessions

Stabilization: the steadying of proximal or distal joints (on a surface or through body weight) to prevent substitution

Velocity: speed of exercise

Volume: the product of the total number of repetitions and sets done in a session multiplied by the resistance utilized

Neuromuscular and Nervous Systems

Nervous System and Nerve Cells Types

Structurally, the nervous system consists of the central nervous system (CNS), which includes the brain, cerebellum, brain stem, and spinal cord; and the peripheral nervous system (PNS), which encompasses all parts of the nervous system outside the CNS. The PNS is split into two portions in terms of physiological function: the somatic nervous system, involving sensory organs and responsible for voluntary muscle activity; and the autonomic nervous system (ANS), which controls involuntary bodily processes, such as breathing. Nerve cell types comprising the CNS are neurons and neuroglia. Neurons transmit electrochemical impulses. Functionally, they may be afferent, or sensory, neurons, which carry sensory input from peripheral sources through tracts to the CNS; efferent, or motor neurons, that convey messages from the CNS ultimately to peripheral muscles; or interneurons, which link two other neurons. Neuroglia does not transmit nerve responses, but they perform important associated functions. Neuroglia include astrocytes, which are mainly responsible for vascular connections to neurons; oligodendrocytes, which primarily insulate axons (message sending portion of the neuron); and microglia that assist with nervous system repair.

Neuron

A neuron, or nerve cell, is made up of dendrites, extensions that collect information from other neurons; the cell body, comprised of a nucleus and other organelles, where this data is processed; and the axon, a longer extension that transmits impulses to target cells like muscle cells. Most axons are covered with sections of white insulating material made of protein and fats (called myelin sheath) interrupted by unsheathed areas called the nodes of Ranvier. Myelinated axons transmit messages more quickly than unmyelinated ones. Regions of the nervous system, such as the brain and spinal cord, are primarily myelinated and are referred to as white matter. Gray matter, as seen in the part of the brain called the cerebrum, is a highly concentrated area of nerve cell bodies and dendrites. The gap between the axon of one neuron and the dendrite of another is the synapse. Transmission of information across a synapse is facilitated by chemicals called neurotransmitters, some of the most important being acetylcholine, glutamate, dopamine, and norepinephrine.

The Brain

The Cerebrum

The cerebrum is the major portion of the brain. It is highly convoluted and covered by gray matter, with white matter internal to that. It consists of four lobes:

- The frontal lobe in the front, which controls complex, voluntary motor activities and much of cognitive function
- The parietal lobe behind the frontal lobe, where sensory information is processed and short-term memory resides
- The temporal lobe, centrally located below the frontal and parietal lobes, which performs functions, such as the interpretation of sounds and music and long-term memory
- The occipital lobe in the back of the head, which is the major visual cortex

There are association areas, or cortex, between the parietal, temporal, and occipital lobes. The brain, including the cerebrum, has several protective layers, starting with the outer bony skull or cranium. Below that are three membranous layers, or meninges, with spaces between each: the dura mater; the arachnoid; and the pia mater, which is attached to the brain. The cerebrum is divided into right and left hemispheres, which are responsible for different functions (discussed on another card); neuronal connections between them are called the corpus callosum. There are also deeper brain structures and other brain portions called the cerebellum and brain stem (discussed elsewhere).

Cerebral Hemispheres and the Effects of Brain Damage

The side of the brain's cerebrum that controls someone's language is deemed the dominant cerebral hemisphere. Ninety-five of the populace is left hemisphere dominant, encompassing all right-handed people and about half of left-handed individuals. There are behaviors that have been associated with the left or right hemisphere.

The left hemisphere is the verbal or analytic aspect of the brain. It is associated with behaviors, such as sequential, linear cognitive processing; processing and production of language; reading skills; mathematical computation; sequencing and performance of movements and gestures; and articulation of positive emotions. Damage to the left hemisphere can result in deficits like apraxia (inability to perform complex movements) or lowered speech comprehension.

The right hemisphere is linked to nonverbal and artistic abilities. Behaviors associated with the right hemisphere are information processing in a more holistic manner, overall comprehension of concepts, ability to process nonverbal stimuli, visual-spatial perception, mathematical reasoning (as opposed to calculation), posture, sustaining movement, and expression of negative emotions. Right hemisphere damage can lead to poor judgment, irritability, etc.

Subcortical Structures and Their Roles in Motor Function

Deep, subcortical structures in the brain include the internal capsule, the diencephalon, the basal ganglia, and the limbic system:

- The internal capsule is the area through which descending fibers from motor areas of the frontal area pass; damage to it can result in contralateral deficits of voluntary movement and ability to perceive touch and positioning.

- The diencephalon is quite deep and consists of the thalamus and hypothalamus. It is the zone where the sensory tracts and visual and auditory pathways synapse. The thalamus portion accepts all sensory input (excluding sense of smell) and directs it to the correct cortical area. The hypothalamus lies beneath the thalamus at the base of the brain, and its primary purpose is regulation of homeostasis and autonomic functions.
- The basal ganglia, at the base of the cerebrum, regulate motor functions like posture and muscle tone, as well as cognitive functions. Damage to basal ganglia can result in neurological diseases, such as Parkinson's disease and postural instability.
- The limbic system runs through various areas of the diencephalon and cortex; its functions are memory-related and include regulation of certain behaviors (sexual interest, pleasure, etc.).

Cerebellum and Brain Stem

The cerebellum is comprised of two symmetric hemispheres situated below the occipital lobe of the cerebrum of the brain and behind the brain stem. It plays a role in balance and posture maintenance. It also regulates complex muscular movements in a number of ways, including coordinating multi-joint movements, controlling a number of parameters related to muscle contraction, and sequencing of muscle firing during certain movements.

The brain stem is situated between the base of the cerebrum and the spinal cord. It is comprised of three sections with different functions:

1. The midbrain: at the upper portion; acts as a conduit between the diencephalon and pons; has reflex centers for sight, sound, and touch
2. The pons: below the midbrain; houses axon bundles that connect the cerebellum to other parts of the central nervous system; has functions such as regulation of breathing, orientation of the head, and transmission of facial motor and sensory information (via cranial nerves V to VIII)
3. The medulla: below the pons; contains fiber tracts into the spinal cord, which control neck and mouth motor and sensory functions, the heart, and respiratory rate

The brain stem also contains the reticular activating system, which controls things like the sleep-wake cycle.

Spinal Cord Anatomy

The spinal cord extends from the medulla in the brain stem, through the vertebral column that protects it, down the level of the initial lumbar vertebra. Starting at the top is the cervical segment, followed by the thoracic segment, the lumbar segment, the sacral segment, and, finally, the dural sac, including the cauda equina (an area of nerve roots for spinal nerves L2 to S5) and the filum terminale connecting to the coccyx. There are eight cervical nerves, 12 thoracic nerves, five lumbar nerves, five sacral nerves, and one coccygeal nerve. The center of the spinal cord consists of gray matter in a sort of butterfly pattern. The upper dorsal, or posterior horn, of this region transmits sensory stimuli, while the lower ventral, or anterior horn, conveys primarily motor impulses. The outer portion of the spinal cord is white matter, containing tracts of groups of nerve fibers. There are two main afferent (ascending) sensory tracts: the dorsal column, which transmits information about position, vibration, deep touch, and two-point discrimination; and the anterolateral spinothalamic tract, conveying data about light, touch, and pressure. There is one major efferent (descending) motor tract, called the corticospinal tract, which directs skilled movements in extremities, as well as other descending tracts with specific motor functions.

Anterior Horn Cells, Motor Units, and Muscle Spindles

An anterior horn cell is a larger neuron in the central gray matter of the spinal cord. Its axons ultimately connect to peripheral nerves that innervate muscle fibers. One type of anterior horn cell, called an alpha motor neuron, innervates skeletal. A motor unit is therefore defined as one alpha motor neuron and the muscle fibers it innervates. There are also gamma motor neurons that convey messages to the muscle spindle, which is a sensory organ in skeletal muscle primarily involved with the stretch response and deep tendon reflexes. The muscle spindle is important because it directly transmits sensory input to the spinal cord without the need for higher cortical interpretation.

Somatic Nervous System

The somatic (body) nervous system is the portion of the peripheral nervous system (PNS) that is involved with voluntary reactions to stimuli. It is composed of 12 pairs of cranial nerves, 31 pairs of spinal nerves, and related ganglia and cell bodies. The 12 cranial nerves are situated in the brain stem, and they have various names related to their primary sensory or motor function in the head region (for example, cranial nerve I is olfactory, involved with the sense of smell). Each spinal nerve has a sensory and motor component that comes through an intervertebral foramen between vertebra, where they divide into rami or divisions, beginning the PNS. The uppermost spinal nerves are eight cervical nerves, of which C1 to C4 form the cervical plexus innervating muscles in the neck and shoulder region. The C5 to C8 cervical and T1 thoracic nerve roots comprise the brachial plexus, whose five main nerves innervate most upper-extremity musculature. There are actually 12 thoracic nerves, the rest of which are primarily involved with trunk functions. Lower-extremity muscles are innervated by the nerves forming the lumbosacral plexus, the five lumbar (L1 to L5) and first three (S1 to S3) of five sacral nerves. Peripheral nerves connect to the system efferently, eventually innervating motor end plates in muscles; or afferently, originating in the skin, muscle tendon, or Golgi tendon organ.

Autonomous Nervous System

The autonomous nervous system (ANS) is the portion of the peripheral nervous system involved with regulation of involuntary functions, such as respiration and metabolism. Control centers for the ANS are situated in the hypothalamus and brain stem, and regulation within the system is achieved through a two-way pathway between the central nervous system and organs. The ANS is comprised of two types of nerve fibers: sympathetic nerve fibers that originate in the thoracic and upper lumbar parts of the spinal cord and regulate functions in the abdominal region affected by stress, such as heart rate, blood pressure, and temperature; and parasympathetic fibers responsible for homeostasis or maintenance of fundamental bodily functions. Parasympathetic responses are derived from cranial nerves III, VII, IX, and X in the brain stem (X being the important vagus nerve, which innervates the myocardium and lung and digestive tract smooth muscles) and sacral nerves S2 to S5, which regulate bowel, bladder, and external genitalia functions. The primary neurotransmitters involved are norepinephrine and acetylcholine for sympathetic and parasympathetic divisions, respectively.

Blood Circulation in Nervous System Functionality

Neurons within the brain must receive an adequate blood supply constantly as they are incapable of performing glycolysis (the breakdown of carbohydrates to produce energy) or storing glycogen. Most of the cerebrum is supplied with blood through the carotid and cerebral arteries, which ascend originally from the aortic arch anteriorly. The brain stem and part of the occipital and temporal lobes are supplied blood via the basilar artery and its branches, which are other cerebral arteries. A protective mechanism that alleviates the potential danger of blood vessel occlusion in the brain is the circle of Willis at its base, where the basilar artery and several carotid and cerebral arteries are interconnected.

Events Subsequent to Nerve Cell Damage

Neurons in any portion of the nervous system that are denied oxygen cannot regenerate and, thus, die. They also release excess glutamate, which can damage neighboring nerve cells. Nerve cell death usually occurs in the central nervous system within minutes of artery obstruction. Typically, within a day or so, the necrotic tissue liquefies and forms a cyst and then a glial scar. Within four or five days, adjoining healthy axons move in to form compensating networks. Peripheral nerve injuries are not usually due to obstruction but rather situations like stretching, compression, or disease. Therefore, the compensatory mechanism is typically different. Here, basically, there is axonal necrosis distal to the site, separation from the myelin sheath, phagocytosis by Schwann cells, and wallerian degeneration of postsynaptic cells. If the peripheral nerve injury is minimal involving only the axon, regeneration may occur through sprouting at the proximal end and the corresponding muscle may eventually be re-innervated.

Motor Control

Motor Control

Motor control is the capacity to sustain and change posture and movement. It involves both the neurologic and muscular systems. It is an interaction between the individual, the task at hand, and the surrounding environment. Motor control utilized for specific tasks is a function of the person's cognitive and perceptual status, which can change over time. Motor control must be utilized within milliseconds to be functional, making deficits potentially dangerous. Sensory stimuli can elicit reflexive motor responses, and there are higher levels of motor control, the utmost being voluntary movement.

Hierarchic Theory of Motor Control

The hierarchic theory of motor control states that the cortex of the brain exerts ultimate control over motor functions, the development of certain motor behaviors in childhood is related to maturation of the brain, the highest stage of motor control is the ability to perform voluntary movement, and reflexes are the basic motor control units. It defines a reflex as the coupling of a sensory stimulus and motor response, which for simple reflexes requires only three neurons: the sensory neuron and the associated interneuron and motor neuron derived from the spinal cord. There are also higher-level tonic reflexes, affecting muscle tone and posture and involving the brain stem, and complex postural responses, associated with the midbrain and cortex, such as righting reactions, equilibrium reactions, and protective reactions in extremities.

Stages of Motor and Postural Control According to the Hierarchal Theory

According to hierarchal theory, infants go through four stages of motor control: mobility, random movement during approximately the first three months of life; stability or static postural, the capacity to maintain a stable, weight-bearing, antigravity posture; controlled mobility (also known as dynamic postural control), mobility combined with postural stability; and skilled movement patterns, such as reaching or walking.

There are two types of stability: tonic holding, which is mainly isometric (for example, prone extension); and co-contraction, which involves static contraction of antagonistic muscles at a joint for stability. Co-contraction is the mechanism invoked for various prone positions, a semi-squat, and standing. Combined with weight shifting or movement to another position, co-contraction becomes controlled mobility. Postural control, the capacity to maintain body alignment and balance, develops sequentially, as well, in the following order: righting reactions, head and trunk movements facilitating orientation or alignment; protective reactions, extremity movements in response to displacement, such as moving a limb to prepare for falling; and equilibrium reactions, counteracting responses that maintain the center of gravity within a base of support.

Systems Models of Motor Control

There are various systems models of motor control. Some of the basic tenets of each are that:

- Motor control is a complex interaction between a number of bodily systems, including the nervous, musculoskeletal, and cardiopulmonary systems, and posture.
- Posture and movement occur in a logical fashion.
- Movement control is either dependent on past success through feedback (a closed-loop model) or a cued, preprogrammed response (open-loop model).

Postural control, the correlation between posture and movement, is essential to motor control in these models. Further, there are seven components to postural control: staying within the limits of stability, which means having the center of gravity within one's base of support; adaptation of posture to the current environment; functioning musculoskeletal and neurologic systems; a predictive central set (anticipatory postural readiness); muscular coordination or timely sequencing; stabilization of the eyes and head; and sensory organization. Sensory organization, in terms of posture and balance, means use of functioning visual, vestibular (balance-related functions initiated in the ear), and somatosensory (touch, proprioception) systems.

Nashner's Model of Postural Control

Nashner's model of postural control is a paradigm for control of standing balance. It posits that there are three sway strategies that allow balanced standing. In adults, the first is the ankle strategy, in which the person sways from the ankles, always coming back to midline through use of the anterior tibialis and gastrocnemius muscles. Another is the hip strategy, where the individual sways from the hips, activating in sequence proximal to distal muscles. This strategy is useful on narrow bases of support, such as balance beams. The last is the stepping strategy, where the person steps while swaying. Some children employ the ankle sway strategy as early as 18 months and occasionally the hip strategy, but the expected use of sway strategies as quickly as adults occurs at 7 to 10 years of age.

Motor Learning Stages

Motor learning is the process by which a lasting change in motor performance occurs through practice or experience. For infants, motor learning involves the perfection of certain tasks, such as learning to walk. For any given individual, the time it takes to learn a specific motor task is contingent on the task's difficulty, the person's motivation to learn it, the amount of practice completed, and the amount of feedback received. People go through three phases of motor learning before perfecting a new task. The first is the cognitive phase, where the individual uses sensory input, such as verbal directions and vision, to figure out what the task involves. This stage requires a high degree of attention to the task at hand and is difficult for patients who have undergone brain injuries or cerebrovascular accidents. The second period is a longer associative phase, in which the individual makes a number of trials and uses sensory feedback to get better with time by detecting errors and correcting them. The last stage is the autonomous phase, where the task has been mastered and can be completed with little attention to it and minimal sensory input.

THEORIES OF MOTOR LEARNING

Prevalent theories of motor learning include:

- Adams' closed-loop theory: This theorizes that intrinsic (internally derived) feedback and extrinsic feedback (knowledge of results) are used to develop the correct feel of new movements. It explains how slow movements might be learned but not faster ones.
- Schmidt's schema theory: This theory says that once a motor program, or a learned motor task, is developed, it can be recalled with minimal cognitive or cortical input because muscle commands are preprogrammed unless parameters change. Further, it expounds that feedback during movement can be derived from the muscles as they contract during the movement, the portions of the body that are moving, and/or the surrounding environment.

Thus, learned actions are under both open-loop and closed-loop control. These assumptions explain learning of both slow and fast movements.

LIFE-SPAN APPROACH TO DEVELOPMENT

Developmental change throughout life can be viewed in a number of ways. These views include a triangular view, with development peaking during maturity and declining with age; a plateau view, which is similar, except maturity is more prolonged; a continuous circle or life-cycle view, where the beginning and end are similar; or as multidimensional and intertwined. The latter view is consistent with the life-span approach to development as espoused by Bates, which says that development has five characteristics; it is life-long; multidimensional; plastic and flexible; contextual; and entrenched in history. Thus, a life-span view of motor development regards change as a continual process from conception to death.

DEVELOPMENTAL TIME PERIODS

The developmental time periods follow:

- The first developmental time period is infancy, defined as from birth to two years of age, when sensory data is used to cue movement and explore the environment.
- Childhood spans from age two years to the time of adolescence, which differs for girls (age 10) and boys (age 12). Childhood is the time period when an individual learns movement strategies and solutions for daily problems, primarily centered around themselves with parental help during early childhood and more interactive and concrete later.
- Adolescence is defined as the time directly proceeding and continuing into and after puberty, which is roughly 10 to 18 years of age for females and 12 to 20 years of age for males. It is a period of intense physical and emotional changes, including establishment of individual identity, formation of values, development of vocational aspirations, and development of the ability to solve abstract problems.
- Adolescents slowly transition into early adulthood, which starts approximately at age 18 for females and 20 for males and extends to age 40.
- Middle and older adulthood have been defined as from 40 to 65 years and from 65 years to death, respectively. Older adulthood has been further divided into the young-old (65 to 74 years), middle-old (75 to 84 years), and old-old (85 years or older).

THEORIES OF DEVELOPMENT

PIAGET'S THEORY OF INTELLIGENCE AND STAGES OF COGNITIVE DEVELOPMENT

Piaget's theory of intelligence divides life-span periods up to pubescence into stages in which characteristic cognitive developments occur. According to Piaget, these ages encompass four stages:

1. During infancy, there is a sensorimotor stage, in which the infant learns to associate sensory input and motor reflexes, eventually leading to purposeful activity.
2. This is followed during the preschool period by a preoperational stage of intelligence, in which the child develops a one-dimensional awareness of the environment and starts to use spoken language as symbols.
3. School age (about age 7 to 11 in Piaget's view) is the concrete operational stage of cognitive development, in which the child learns to solve real problems and classify things (for example, math skills).
4. Pubescence period starts at age 12, according to Piaget, and is the formal operational stage, in which the individual learns to solve abstract problems through induction and deduction.

MASLOW'S HIERARCHY AND ERIKSON'S STAGES OF DEVELOPMENT

Maslow's hierarchy and Erikson's stages of development are ways of looking at the gamut of development throughout life, as opposed to Piaget's theory (discussed elsewhere) that covers only to pubescence. Maslow's hierarchy does not isolate specific life periods, but rather says that development is hierarchical. At the base of the hierarchy is satisfaction of basic physiological and survival needs, such as eating, drinking, and elimination. Next are skills that provide safety, followed by those that satisfy the needs for love and belonging, then those providing self-esteem, and, lastly, those allowing the person to be self-actualized (self-assured and independent, able to solve problems, etc.) Each stage is retained and builds upon the previous one.

Erikson's scheme defines eight stages in terms of life span and the characteristics that are struggled with during each. These stages are:

1. Trust versus mistrust during infancy
2. Autonomy versus shame or doubt during late infancy
3. Initiative versus guilt during the preschool childhood period
4. Industry versus inferiority during school age
5. Identity versus role confusion in adolescence
6. Intimacy or isolation during early adulthood
7. Generativity versus stagnation during middle adulthood
8. Integrity of one's ego versus despair in late adulthood

COMMON DEVELOPMENTAL CONCEPTS

All developmental concepts embrace the notion that motor development is epigenetic, meaning it develops through successive gradual changes, and that there is a series of gross-motor milestones children pass. There are two types of concepts regarding development: directional and kinesiologic.

Directional concepts include: cephalocaudal development, the idea that head movements are mastered before trunk ones; proximal to distal, meaning that an infant works to establish midline control in the head and neck before shoulders, pelvis, and extremities; mass to specific movements, in other words mastering whole body movements before isolated or dissociated ones; and gross to fine, proceeding from large muscle to more discreet movements.

Kinesiologic concepts are based upon the observation that shortly after birth, infants are in physiologic flexion, meaning their limbs and trunk are naturally in a flexed position. Only over time do they move toward antigravity extension and later antigravity flexion, then lateral flexion, and, ultimately, rotation.

Developmental Processes

The three processes involved in development are growth, maturation, and adaptation:

1. Growth is defined as any expansion in dimension or proportion, usually quantified in terms of parameters like height, weight, and head circumference.
2. Maturation is the full development of certain internal body processes as genetically programmed, such as internal organs becoming more complex or the emergence of secondary sexual characteristics.
3. Adaptation is the course by which physical changes occur in response to environmental stimuli, such as the way in which musculoskeletal strength is developed through performance of functional activities.

Gross- and Fine-Motor Milestones in Infants

Gross- and fine-motor milestones refer to expected developmental milestones involving large movements and small muscle movements, respectively. The expected gross-motor milestones are head control by 4 months; log rolling followed by segmental rolling, achieved by 6 to 8 months; independent sitting by 8 months; cruising (walking sideways using hands or tummy) by 9 months; reciprocal creeping by 10 months; and walking by age 12 months (range 7 to 18 months).

The expected fine-motor milestones of development include a palmar grasp reflex present at birth; hand awareness or regard at 2 months; raking at 5 months; and development of a voluntary palmar grasp by age 6 months. This voluntary grasp should develop further over the next few months to become radial palmar (adduction of thumb) at 7 months; radial digital (use of fingers as well) by 9 months; use of thumb with index finger in various arrangements (inferior and superior pincher) by 12 months; and a three-jaw chuck grasp in the same time period. Infants should be able to release a grasped object voluntarily at about 7 to 9 months, with further control developed within the next few months.

Infant Development Up to 10 Months

During the first two months of life, the infants' internal body processes stabilize, essential biologic rhythms are developed, and they can spontaneously grasp and release and do unilateral head lifting on all fours. At ages 3 to 4 months, infants have developed forearm support, head control, and midline orientation. This enables them to do things such as support themselves while prone on their elbows, perform primitive rolling without rotation, and hold their head upright while being held vertical or tilted. At 4 to 5 months, they start to gain antigravity control of the extensors and flexors, and they can do bottom lifting and dissociate head and limb movements. They often assume a posture that looks like swimming. By 6 months, the infant has strong extension-abduction of the extremities and complete extension of the trunk. They pivot in a circle on their tummy and right themselves using the Landau reflex, can do segmental rolling (essential for transitions), can sit up if placed and supported, can be pulled up to sitting or standing, and can do some reaching. By 7 to 8 months, their trunk control has developed to the point that they can do balanced sitting, have some spontaneous trunk rotation, and can ambulate via pre-walking mechanisms like belly crawling. By ages 9 to 10 months, movement progresses to crawling, creeping, pulling themselves up to stand, and cruising.

Infant Development During Toddler Phase

A toddler is a young child learning to walk, the phase generally defined as starting at age 1 year and extending through age 2. By 12 months of age, the infants typically try slow independent walking using their hands for guarding. Their skill at walking usually progresses by age 16 to 17 months to the point where they can carry or pull objects at the same time, walk sideways and backwards, and navigate stairs one step at a time. They have learned to rise from supine to standing through rolling, four-point prone, plant grade, squat, and semi-squat positions. Most toddlers demonstrate adult gait characteristics, such as reciprocal arm swing and heel strike by 18 months. They should be able to squat easily and pick up toys by age 20 to 22 months and ambulate quickly with arm swing closely approximating an adult by age 24 months. Older toddlers can do easy types of jumps, typically done from one-foot landing on the other at 18 months, jumping up from and landing with two feet at 24 months, and progressing to increasingly more difficult types.

Movement Developed During Childhood

The majority of experts concur that most children achieve a mature gait pattern by age 3 years and almost all do by age 4. Three-year-olds can also accomplish other reciprocal activities, such as climbing a ladder and more difficult jumps than before. Children acquire good enough static and dynamic balance by age 4 to do things like prolonged one-foot standing, sequential hopping, galloping, and catching a ball. These skills are developed further by age 5, when they also encompass things such as skipping on alternating feet and kicking. Hand dominance, the regular use of one hand over the other for tasks like throwing or eating, is established by this time period. Balance and coordination are further developed by age 6, and the child can master other forms of locomotion like bike riding. Adult approximations of activities, such as running, are possible in the 6-to-10-year age range. Movement patterns, while generally established by age 10, can be changed at later ages into adulthood. In older individuals, these pattern changes are often related to pathological changes, such as stiffening of joints; these persons often revert to a more asymmetrical pattern as seen in young children, rather than the symmetrical patterns typical from adolescence through adulthood.

Postural Changes Associated with Aging

When babies are born, they have a forward flexed curve in the thoracic region and another in the sacral region. As they proceed through infancy and learn movements, convex forward cervical and lumbar curves also develop. When viewed laterally, a young person in standing posture has a vertical gravity line that goes linearly at a right angle to the ground through the middle of the earlobe, the middle of the acromion process of the shoulder, the greater trochanter of the hip, the knee behind the patella but in front of the joint, and a point slightly in front of the lateral malleolus of the ankle. Essentially posture is quite straight.

However, as we age, the secondary spinal curves tend to decrease, intervertebral discs often stiffen and flatten, and other changes may occur as a result of a sedentary lifestyle or prolonged sitting. The typical standing posture of an older person is more forward and less straight than that of a younger person. This may be accompanied by demineralization of bone, decreased flexibility at the joints, loss of strength, and changes in gait and balance.

Balance and Gait Changes Associated with Aging

Older adults may have significant problems related to balance and falling. Many of these problems are associated with neurologic changes. Sensory receptors involved with positioning, head movement, awareness of vibration, or vision are often changed structurally by this point, thus reducing the quality of information received. In addition, musculoskeletal changes, such as loss of some joint range of motion and muscular strength, make it more difficult to respond quickly and establish balance. Gait changes associated with aging include decreased cadence and stride length and use of a wider base of support for increased balance.

Nerve Root Types and Their Effects on Musculoskeletal Pain

A dermatome is a section of skin supplied by a single nerve root of the spine. Peripheral nerves are generally supplied by more than one nerve root and do not necessarily correspond to a single nerve root. A nerve root is the section of the spine from which innervation originates. Beginning at the skull going down, there are eight cervical (C1 to C8), 12 thoracic (T1 to T12), five lumbar (L1 to L5), and four sacral (S1 to S4) nerve roots. A myotome is a group of muscles whose initial innervation is a single nerve root. Injury to a single nerve root causes only incomplete paralysis of the muscles in the myotome, whereas a lesion in a peripheral nerve causes complete paralysis of the associated muscles. A sclerotome is a bone or connective tissue region supplied by a single nerve root. The significance of dermatomes, myotomes, and sclerotomes is the differentiation between referred and localized pain. This is important in terms of musculoskeletal pain because it is often referred pain.

Integumentary System

Overall Structure

The skin and associated appendages make up the integumentary system. The skin has two overall layers: the relatively thin, avascular, external epidermis and the thicker, extremely vascularized dermis below. Each consists of several strata, or layers (discussed further on another card). The associated appendages of the integumentary system are the hair and hair shafts, nails, and the sebaceous and sweat glands, most of which originate in the dermis. Skin thickness ranges from 0.5 mm to 4.0 mm, depending on the gender and body region; the thickest skin is found in adult (not elderly) males. Below the dermis lies subcutaneous tissue and fat linking to muscle and bone, as well as larger blood vessels that feed into the smaller ones in the skin.

Strata of the Epidermis and Dermis

Starting externally, the epidermis is made up of the tough outer stratum corneum, containing dead keratinocytes; the pigment layer, containing melanocytes; the stratum granulose, made up of mature keratinocytes and Langerhans' cells; the stratum spinosum, containing keratinocytes; and the stratum basale, which is comprised of new keratinocytes and Merkel's cells. Mature keratinocytes make keratin for waterproofing of the skin; melanocytes manufacture a pigment called melanin, which prevents ultraviolet absorption; Langerhans' cells have immune functions; and Merkel's cells are associated with touch.

The outer layer of the dermis is the papillary layer, consisting of areolar connective tissue for adhesion, blood and lymph vessels for circulation and drainage, Meissner's corpuscles for sensation of light touch, and free nerve endings that detect pain and heat. Below this level is the reticular layer, made up of collagen, elastin, and fibers for strength and pliability; followed by the hypodermis, which consists of subcutaneous fat for insulation and shock absorption; and free nerve endings and Pacinian cells, which sense cold and pressure respectively.

Main Functions

The seven main functions of the integumentary system are:

1. Body temperature regulation: a system that works via adjustment of sweat production and/or superficial blood flow
2. Protection: a protective barrier against microbes, ultraviolet radiation, dehydration, abrasions, and chemicals

3. Sensation: the detection of pain, temperature, and touch
4. Excretion: the extrusion of sweat, water, and heat
5. Immunity: both elimination of surface microorganisms through periodic loss of epidermal cells and transportation of external antigens for the production of protective antibodies
6. Blood reservoir: a conduit for blood that can be moved to organs or muscles as required
7. Vitamin D synthesis: production of Vitamin D from cholesterol derivatives with ultraviolet radiation exposure

Other Systems

Metabolic and Endocrine Systems

Primary Endocrine Glands

Starting at the head and working downward:

- There are two endocrine centers in the head. First are the hypothalamic nuclei in the hypothalamus, the portion of the brain responsible for controlling involuntary functions, such as hormone release and body temperature. At the base of the brain is the pituitary gland, which produces hormones that control other glands and affect growth.
- Located in the neck region are the thyroid and parathyroid glands. The thyroid gland secretes several hormones that control metabolism and growth. The parathyroid gland, which is smaller than and near the thyroid gland, controls the deposition of calcium and phosphorus in bones.
- The adrenal glands are situated above each kidney and secrete epinephrine and steroids.
- Slightly lower near the stomach, the pancreas releases juices into the small intestine and insulin, glucagon, and somatostatin into the bloodstream.
- The reproductive organs are considered endocrine glands; the female ovaries releasing estrogen and progesterone and the male testes producing sexual hormones and sperm. Both located in the pelvic region.

Thyroid Gland

Three hormones are secreted by the thyroid gland. Thyroxine (T_4) and triiodothyronine (T_3) are dependent on the presence of iodine and have systemic targets. Adequate levels of T_4 and T_3 stimulate growth and development of many cells, especially nerve cells; increase metabolism; and promote the effects of the neurotransmitter catecholamine. The third hormone, calcitonin or thyrocalcitonin, targets the bones, inhibiting their resorption and depressing blood levels of calcium.

Thyroid gland functions are regulated by another hormone called thyroid-stimulating hormone (TSH, also known as thyrotropin), produced by the pituitary gland, which is in turn controlled by the hypothalamic hormone called thyrotropin-releasing hormone (TRH). TSH and T_4 have an effect on each other via a negative feedback loop.

Pituitary Hormones

The anterior lobe of the pituitary gland secretes:

Growth hormone: is released systemically to promote growth of bones, muscles, and other organs; also targets the liver for creation of somatomedin, another hormone stimulating bone and muscle growth; Thyrotropin: influences the production and secretion of thyroid hormones to stimulate growth; Adrenocorticotropin: produces the same types of effects targeting the cortex of the adrenal gland; Follicle-stimulating hormone (FSH) and luteinizing or interstitial cell-stimulating hormone

(LH): both target reproductive organs (ovaries or testes); in women, FSH stimulates development of follicles and secretion of estrogen, while in men, it encourages development of somniferous tubules and spermatogenesis; LH influences ovulation, development of the corpus luteum, and release of progesterone in females, while in men, it prompts secretion of testosterone; Prolactin or lactogenic hormone: is sent to mammary glands for milk secretion; Melanocyte-stimulating hormone: targets skin for production of pigmentation

The posterior lobe secretes:

- Antidiuretic hormone (vasopressin): targets the kidneys for reabsorption of water and fluid and electrolyte balance
- Oxytocin (stored in the pituitary but produced in the hypothalamus): is sent to the arterioles, uterus, and breast for blood pressure control, contraction, and milk expression respectively

Adrenal Gland Hormones

The adrenal glands above the kidneys each have an outer cortex and an inner medulla. The outer cortex secretes mineralocorticoids, the primary one being aldosterone, that target the kidney and aid in the reabsorption of sodium and water and the elimination of potassium. It also releases glucocorticoids, such as cortisol, into the bloodstream, where they contribute to the metabolism of carbohydrates, proteins, and lipids; depress immune responses; suppress inflammation; and are involved in the stress response. also, in addition, the outer cortex secretes several systemic sex hormones, including androgens, progesterone, and estrogen, which are involved with childhood growth and development of secondary sexual characteristics.

The inner medulla secretes the catecholamines epinephrine and norepinephrine. Epinephrine, also known as adrenaline, affects cardiac and smooth muscles and is responsible for speeding up and increasing the force of heart pumping during emergencies by stimulating the sympathetic nervous system as a stress response. Norepinephrine acts as a sympathetic neurotransmitter in major organs and the skin and also increases peripheral resistance.

Gastrointestinal System

Primary Organs Associated with Digestion

The primary organs associated with digestion are the oral cavity, pharynx, esophagus, stomach, small intestine, and large intestine. The oral cavity is the gastrointestinal system's entrance, where mechanical and chemical digestion is initiated. Behind the oral cavity is the pharynx, or throat, which mechanically aids in swallowing and food movement. Below the pharynx is a long tube called the esophagus, which conveys food to the stomach. The stomach is a large sac that processes food in several ways. Mechanically, it stores, mixes, and pulverizes food and controls its passage into the small intestine. Physiologically, the stomach has exocrine functions, such as secretion of hydrochloric acid and other digestive substances, as well as endocrine functions, secreting hormones that promote the release of digestive enzymes in other organs. The subsequent small intestine consists of three segments: the duodenum, which neutralizes acids and introduces pancreatic and bile secretions; the jejunum, which takes in nutrients, water, and electrolytes; and the ileum, which absorbs bile acids and other components. Lastly, the large intestine serves to absorb water and electrolytes and eliminate feces. It consists of the cecum, appendix, colon (ascending, transverse, descending, and sigmoid), rectum and anus.

Review Video: Gastrointestinal System
Visit mometrix.com/academy and enter code: 378740

Accessory Organs Associated with Digestion

The accessory organs associated with digestion are the teeth, tongue, salivary glands, liver, gallbladder, and pancreas. The teeth break up food for combination with saliva. The tongue is a sensory (taste) organ, but it also directs the food. The salivary glands secrete saliva, which moistens and dissolves food. Saliva is composed of water, mucin, enzymes, and other proteins. The other accessory organs are located near the stomach. The liver has several functions. It produces digestive fluid bile; regulates serum levels of fats, carbohydrates, and proteins; and aids drug metabolism and the production of red blood cells and vitamin K. The gallbladder is a small sac on the underside of the liver, where bile is stored and concentrated before release into the duodenum. The pancreas serves two types of functions: an exocrine one, in which bicarbonate and digestive enzymes are conveyed to the duodenum; and an endocrine, in which various hormones are released into the bloodstream for regulation of blood glucose. Nearby is the spleen, which is not technically a digestive organ but does filter out foreign substances.

Genitourinary System

Structure of the Genitourinary System

The genitourinary system consists of structures related to urinary and reproductive functions. The urinary structures, starting at the top (in an upright position), are:

- Two kidneys in the abdomen, where waste is filtered
- Two ureters, or urinary ducts, that carry urine to the bladder
- The bladder, which stores urine
- The urethra, where urine is discharged

The system also consists of reproductive structures. In men, these structures are the prostate gland, near the urethra; the testicles, where sperm is produced; and the attached tube, called the epididymis. Female reproductive organs include the uterus, or womb, for fetal development; fallopian tubes; ovaries, where eggs and hormones are produced; the muscular tube, called the vagina; the external genitalia; and the perineum.

Main Functions of the Genitourinary System

The genitourinary system is responsible for excretion of cellular waste products through the creation of urine and the process of micturition, or voiding. Urine is formed in each kidney by filtration of blood, reabsorption, and secretion in the nephrons, small tubes in the renal cortex and medulla regions. Regulation of several other parameters is related to the amount of excretion or composition of the excreted urine, including blood volume, electrolyte concentrations, acid-base balance, and arterial blood pressure. If the system is working properly, a state of homeostasis, or equilibrium, is maintained. The genitourinary system is also involved in erythropoietin secretion for red blood cell manufacture, gluconeogenesis to form glucose, and reproductive functions.

Multi-System

Pregnancy

Organ Systems Affected During Pregnancy

During pregnancy, the uterus expands exponentially in terms of size, weight, and particularly capacity. This is facilitated by the surrounding connective tissues, primarily ligaments. Urinary system changes include an approximate 1 cm increase in kidney length and development of a perpendicular relationship between the ureters and bladder due to uterine enlargement, which encourages urinary infections. The depth of pulmonary respiration increases, creating a natural condition of hyperventilation with its attendant difficulties during later pregnancy. The pulmonary system is also affected by the hormonal changes, resulting in early edema and congestion in the tract, changes in rib position even before uterine enlargement, and elevation of the diaphragm. Blood volume increases at a greater rate than RBCs do, creating a so-called "physiologic anemia." Blood pressure, particularly the diastolic component, decreases, and other venous pressures change as well. Heart changes include increased size, elevation, heart rate, cardiac output, and, sometimes, rhythm disturbances. The contractile ability of the abdominal muscles is diminished, the pelvic floor muscles drop, and ligaments lose their tensile strength. Basal metabolic rate and heat production are both higher.

Postural, Balance, and Weight Changes During Pregnancy

During pregnancy, the average women gains 25 to 27 pounds, with the greatest amount attributed to the fetus, closely followed by blood and other fluids, then the uterus and breasts. The latter causes the women's center of gravity to shift upward and forward, necessitating postural changes. Compensatory mechanisms include increased curvature in the lower back, hyperextension of the knees, rounding of the shoulder girdle and upper back, changes in the eye's suboccipital muscles to maintain eye level, and shifting of weight back toward the heels. In order to maintain balance, a pregnant woman usually ambulates with a wider base of support and more external hip rotation. She increasingly has difficulty with activities of daily living and behaviors that require fine balance or directional changes.

Pelvic Floor Musculature

The basic functions of pelvic floor musculature are support of the pelvic organs, preservation of continence, sexual response, reproduction, and resistance to intra-abdominal pressure. Viewed from below the deep pelvic diaphragm, which provides the main muscular support, the system consists of the coccygeus and the levator ani, which have functions that include moving the pelvic floor and closing the rectum. Above that are several parts of the urogenital diaphragm, or perineal membrane, involved with compression of the urethra and vaginal wall; even higher are the superficial or outlet structures involved with functions like clitoral erection and compression of the anal canal. In women, the pelvic floor must provide room for the urethra, vagina, and rectum. Pelvic floor muscles are controlled by nerves originating from the S2 to S4 portions of the sacral plexus.

Aerobic Exercise

Physiological Effects of Aerobic Exercise During Pregnancy on the Mother

Aerobic exercise diverts some blood flow away from the mother's organs and fetus to the muscles in use, which can reduce the nutrients and oxygen available to the fetus (possibly stimulating early labor). A pregnant woman can only do mild exercise because her respiratory rate cannot accommodate greater workloads; she has less cardiac reserve during exercise. Starting at the fourth month of pregnancy, she also has less cardiac output and can have orthostatic hypotension due to compression of the inferior vena cava by the uterus; thus, protracted lying down or static standing is inadvisable. Pregnant women are prone to hypoglycemia and need additional caloric consumption of about 500 calories daily, if exercising. Exercise can increase core temperature, but if the pregnant woman is fit, she can control this. The force and frequency of uterine contractions can increase during exercise because levels of the neurotransmitter norepinephrine are elevated.

Physiological Effects of Maternal Aerobic Exercise on the Fetus

Most studies indicate that maternal aerobic exercise during pregnancy has no harmful effects on the fetus. For example, uterine blood flow would have to be diminished by at least 50% to have a detrimental effect on the fetus, which never occurs. Maternal exercise can increase the fetal heart rate (FHR) for up to a half-hour, causing temporary fetal bradycardia and asphyxia, but a vigorous fetus is able to endure this. Women who exercise into late pregnancy statistically have somewhat lower birth weight newborns, but their head circumference and heel-crown length fall within normal range and neurodevelopment during early childhood is actually improved.

Examination/ Foundations for Evaluation, Differential Diagnosis, & Prognosis

Cardiac, Vascular, and Pulmonary Systems

Patient History for Cardiac Evaluation

In terms of cardiac evaluation, the patient history should address whether the patient has chest pain, cardiac risk factors, palpitations (fast or irregular heartbeats), prior myocardial infarction (MI) or cardiac-related tests, a family history of cardiac disease, or a history of dizziness or fainting. The history should also include the related medical treatment administered and its effect. Chest pain or angina should be described in terms of its location and radiation, its frequency, the quality of the pain (for example crushing, numbing, or burning), what the patient is describing as chest pain (for example, shortness of breath, dizziness, jaw pain, etc.), and the factors that precipitate, aggravate, and alleviate the pain. Chest pain generally indicates lack of blood to the heart.

Cardiac Risk Factors

Cardiac risk factors should be addressed in the patient's history. The main independent risk factors for cardiac problems are smoking, hypertension, diabetes mellitus, aging, and a poor cholesterol profile (high total and high LDL and/or low HDL). Other factors that can predispose individuals to cardiac issues should also be included in the history and include physical inactivity; a body mass index of > 30 kg/m^2; obesity, particularly abdominal (high waist-hip ratio, waist > 40 in for men and > 35 in for women); family history of early heart disease; psychosocial issues; and ethnic background. There are a number of substances in the blood which, when elevated, may also be indicative of cardiac risk. These include triglycerides, homocysteine, lipoprotein (a), or inflammatory markers. The presence of small LDL particles, C-reactive protein (CRP), or fibrinogen can also indicate cardiac risk.

Physical Examination

Cardiac Issues

There are four components of a physical examination related to cardiac issues: observation, palpation, blood pressure measurement, and auscultation. The patient should be observed for facial and skin color and tone, the presence of diaphoresis (sweating), respiratory rate, edema or swelling in the extremities, trauma possibly caused by cardiac procedures, and the existence of jugular venous distention. The latter is indicative of fluid backup related to congestive heart failure (CHF). A semirecumbent patient with his head turned to the side should have pulsations just above the sternum in the internal jugular neck area; if these are absent or in a higher spot, there is jugular venous distention.

Pulse Palpation

Palpation is a method of clinical evaluation that uses gentle pressure with the fingers. In terms of cardiac evaluation, it is used to measure the person's pulse or to check extremities for pitting edema. Some of the more common spots for checking the pulse are the radial artery in the wrist, the carotid artery in the neck, or the brachial artery at the bend of the arm. Pulses give an indication of circulation quality, heart rate (HR), and rhythm. Pulse amplitude is classified on a scale from 0 to 4+. A "0" indicates no pulse or circulation, a "1+" designates a diminished pulse (from factors like increased vascular resistance and lowered stroke volume and ejection fraction),

"2+" is a normal resting pulse, "3+" indicates a moderately increased pulse, and "4+" means a markedly increased or bounding pulse. The latter two are associated with varying degrees of increased stroke volume and ejection fraction. Possible pulse abnormalities include pulsus alternans (alternating strong and weak pulses indicative of left ventricular failure), pulsus paradoxus (weak pulse and low blood pressure during inspiration associated with a number of cardiopulmonary problems), and bigeminal pulses (every other pulse weak and premature due to preventricular contractions).

Pitting Edema Palpation

Palpation is used during a physical examination as part of a cardiac evaluation to measure the patient's pulse (discussed elsewhere) or to check the extremities bilaterally for pitting edema. Edema is swelling due to a buildup of excess fluid which, among other things, could be due to circulation problems. The pitting edema scale ranges from 1+ to 4+ as follows:

1+: trace; scarcely perceptible depression observed with palpation

2+: mild; up to a 0.6 cm easily identified depression (EID), meaning the skin rebounds in less than 15 seconds

3+: moderate; between a 0.6 and 1.3 cm EID, which rebounds within 15 to 30 seconds

4+: severe; a 1.3 to 2.5 cm EID, with a rebound that takes more than 30 seconds

Blood Pressure

How Blood Pressure Is Taken and What It Indicates

Blood pressure (BP), a vital sign, should be taken as part of a physical examination. BP measurement indirectly quantifies the force against arterial walls during the phases of ventricular systole (pumping) and diastole (filling). A cuff with an inflatable bladder and pressure gauge, called a sphygmomanometer, is used. The patient should be seated with his arm resting at heart level. At the outset, readings should be taken on both arms and the arm with higher readings should be used. At least two readings separated by as much time as possible should be taken. The appropriate size cuff is wrapped around the arm approximately 1 inch above the antecubital crease. The bladder is inflated with the attached bulb to a pressure 20 to 40 mm Hg above the systolic pressure, which is indicated when a radial pulse (palpated simultaneously) disappears. The bladder is then deflated at a rate of 3 mm Hg/second while the clinician uses a stethoscope to listen for characteristic Korotkoff sounds indicating first systolic (initial faint tapping) and then diastolic pressure (muffled or absent). These sounds are discussed further on another card. BP can also be taken on the thigh with auscultation at the popliteal artery at the knee.

Characterize the Korotkoff Sounds Heard During Blood Pressure Measurement

Korotkoff sounds are characteristic sounds heard with a stethoscope while deflating the sphygmomanometer around 2 to 3 mm Hg/second. A phase one Korotkoff sound, which is a faint tapping noise that gets louder, should be heard first. This indicates the systolic pressure or point at which the blood starts to flow through the compressed artery. As the bladder is deflated more, a phase two swishing sound is heard, followed by phase three louder tapping. As deflation continues, at some point, the sounds become more muffled (phase four). In children younger than 13 years of age or adults who are exercising, pregnant, or hyperthyroid, this muffling indicates the diastolic pressure. However, for normal resting adults, the diastolic pressure is not reached until the Korotkoff sounds disappear (phase five), which is generally 5 to 10 mm Hg lower than phase four.

Auscultation for Heart Sounds

Auscultation is the use of a stethoscope to listen to the sounds of an individual's organs. Auscultation is most often used to listen to heart sounds; a stethoscope with a bell and diaphragm is used to hear low- and high-pitched sounds, respectively. Four areas should be examined: the pulmonic area, the aortic area, the region near the tricuspid valve, and that near the mitral valve area and apex. All of these areas should normally have two sounds (S1 and S2) that indicate closure of the atrioventricular and semilunar valves and correspond to the initiation of ventricular systole and diastole, respectively. Additional sounds are generally abnormal. These include an S3 sound right after S2 or an S4 sound right before a subsequent S1. A soft fluttering sound or murmur heard in a valve region indicates regurgitation of blood at that valve. Another abnormal sound is a creaking or rubbing noise called a pericardial friction rub found at the third or fourth intercostal space. This is a sign of pericarditis, inflammation of the pericardium.

Normal Blood Pressure Ranges

Blood pressure (BP) is always expressed as two numbers, the first of which is the systolic pressure and the second being the diastolic pressure. Normal values depend on age.

Normal blood pressure values are:

- At age 8: systolic 85 to 114 mm Hg,diastolic 5 to 85 mm Hg
- At age 12: systolic 95 to 135 mm Hg,diastolic 58 to 88 mm Hg
- Adults: systolic < 120 mm Hg,diastolic < 80 mm Hg

For adults, prehypertension and hypertension (high blood pressure indicative of arterial disease) are defined as:

- Prehypertension: systolic 120 to 139 mm Hg; diastolic 80 to 89 mm Hg
- Hypertension:
  - Stage 1: systolic 140 to 159 mm Hg; diastolic 90 to 99 mm Hg
  - Stage 2: systolic ≥ 160 mm Hg; diastolic ≥ 100 mm Hg

Individuals who are exercising are expected to have increased systolic pressure of 5 to 12 mm Hg per MET (metabolic equivalent) in workload while their diastolic readings should remain within 10 mm Hg of their normal value.

Electrocardiogram

An electrocardiogram (ECG) is a diagnostic tool for detecting a number of heart defects. It graphically illustrates electrical activity in the heart. In a hospital, a patient may be hooked up to three to five leads and continuously monitored using an ECG technique called Holter monitoring. Data is recorded on tape or by telemetric ECG monitoring, which sends signals in real-time to a monitor for observation. There are also diagnostic ECG methods using 12 leads. Holter monitoring can determine heart rate variability (HRV), which if low suggests cardiac issues, such as new hypertension or risk of cardiac mortality. ECGs are interpreted by looking at the duration and amplitude of different waves or segments. These segments are the P wave, indicative of atrial depolarization; the PR interval, or time between atrial and ventricular depolarization; the QRS complex, where there is ventricular depolarization and atrial depolarization; the ST segment or time between the finish of ventricular depolarization and the start of repolarization; the QT interval or duration between the beginning and end of repolarization; and the T wave, where ventricular repolarization occurs.

Review Video: 12 Lead ECG
Visit mometrix.com/academy and enter code: 962539

BLOOD CELL COUNTS

COMPLETE BLOOD CELL COUNTS

A complete blood cell count (CBC) is an important evaluation tool for an individual's cardiac and vascular systems. It consists of several results, including a red cell count (RBC), white cell count (WBC), a WBC differential, the hematocrit (Hct), hemoglobin (Hgb) measurement, and platelet (Plt) count. The RBC count indicates the number of red blood cells per microliter (μl) of blood drawn. It is mainly used to see whether the patient has lost blood or has anemia. The WBC indicates the number of white blood cells in 1 μl of blood; its primary purpose is to assess whether there is infection or inflammation. The WBC differential lists the percentages of the five types of white blood cells present, providing a better picture of possible infection. The hematocrit indicates the percentage of RBCs that are in the patient's whole blood; it can point to blood loss or fluid imbalance. Hemoglobin values represent the amount of hemoglobin in 100 ml of blood (the percentage); they also are diagnostic for anemia, blood loss, and associated imbalances. Platelet counts signify the number of platelets per μl of blood; they are mainly used to gauge thrombocytopenia, low platelet counts associated with hemorrhaging.

THE NORMAL VALUES FOR A COMPLETE BLOOD CELL COUNT, AND WHAT ABNORMAL VALUES CAN INDICATE

CBC Test: Red blood cell count (RBC) Normal Value: Female: 4.2 to 5.4 x 10^6/μml; Male: 4.7 to 6.1 x 10^6/μml Possible Indications of Abnormal Results: Elevated: augment-ed risk for blood flow stoppage; can indicate COPD, dehydration, or poisoning; Reduced: possible anemia, leukemia, fluid overload, or new hemorrhage

CBC Test: White blood cell count (WBC) Normal Value: 5 to 10 x 10^3/μml

Possible Indications of Abnormal Results: Elevated: infection; leukemia; tissue death, Reduced: bone marrow suppression (for example, during radiation or chemotherapy)

CBC Test: WBC differential Normal Value: Neutrophils: 55- 70% Lymphocytes:20-40% Monocytes: 2 to 8% Eosinophils: 1-4% Basophils: 0.5-1%

Possible Indications of Abnormal Results: Different combinations used to establish various infectious states and leukemia

CBC Test: Hematocrit (Hct) Dehydration Normal Value: Female: 37 to 47% Male: 42 to 52%

Possible Indications of Abnormal Results: Elevated: polycythemia; Reduced: anemia; severe blood loss; hemodilution

CBC Test: Hemoglobin (Hgb) Normal Value: Female: 12 to 16 g/100 ml Male: 14 to 18 g/100 ml

Possible Indications of Abnormal Results: Elevated: dehydration; polycythemia Reduced: anemia; new hemorrhage; fluid overload

CBC Test: Platelets (Plt) Normal Value: 150,000 to 450,000/μml

Possible Indications of Abnormal Results: Elevated: malignancy; splenectomy; Polycythemia; Reduced: anemia; coagulation disorders; hemolysis; AIDS and other viral infections; splenomegaly

Three Erythrocyte Indices

The three erythrocyte indices are generally calculated from CBCs. They are:

- Mean corpuscular volume (MCV) = Hematocrit (Hct) x 10/red blood cell count (RBC) This is a measure of the mean size of a single red blood cell in a microliter of blood, normally 80 to 100 ug^3. MCV outside the normal range is often associated with anemias. Increased volume indicating macrocytic, folic, or vitamin B deficiency types, and decreased volume is suggestive of microcytic, iron-deficiency, or hypochromic types. Low volumes may also suggest liver disease or recent alcohol consumption, while high ones are associated with thalassemia and lead poisoning.
- Mean corpuscular hemoglobin (MCH) = Hemoglobin (Hgb) x 10/RBC This index reports the amount of hemoglobin in one RBC, the normal value being 26 to 34 pg (picogram)/cell. MCH is increased in macrocytic anemia and decreased with microcytic anemia. Hgb deficiency is associated with a low MCH.
- Mean corpuscular hemoglobin concentration (MCHC) = Hgb/Hct x 100 MCHC represents the proportion of each RBC that contains hemoglobin, normally 31 to 37 g/dl (deciliter).

Erythrocyte Sedimentation Rate

An erythrocyte sedimentation rate (ESR, also called sed rate) determines the rate of fall of red blood cells in anticoagulated blood. The erythrocyte sedimentation rate is a non-specific test related to the presence or extent of inflammation, which can be associated with a variety of disease states ranging from systemic infections to collagen vascular diseases. There are several ways of doing an ESR, yielding different normal values. The greatest utility of the test is that it is generally directly related to the course of disease if taken sequentially. Patients with certain conditions tend to have a low ESR, for example, those with liver disease or sickle-cell disease.

Coagulation Profile

A coagulation profile provides information about blood clotting times. Partial thromboplastin time (PTT) and prothrombin time (PT) are measured. PTT can be measured directly or rapidly in activated form (APTT). It is used to assess heparin therapy or to screen for bleeding problems. Depending on the method, normal values are 60 to 70 seconds (PTT) or 30 to 40 seconds (APTT). This time is increased with heparin or warfarin therapy, liver disease, DIC, and clotting deficiencies, while it is low in widespread malignancy or early DIC. PTT looks at common intrinsic clotting factors (I, II, V, VIII, IX, X, and XI), while PT looks at common extrinsic clotting factors (I, II, V, VII, and X). The prothrombin time is generally compared to the International Normalized Ratio (INR), which is the ratio between the patient's PTT and a laboratory standard. PT, normally between 11 and 12.5 seconds, is mainly used to gauge the effectiveness of warfarin therapy (which increases it) or to screen for bleeding disorders. Increased PT can indicate bile duct obstruction, salicylate intoxication, disseminated intravascular coagulation (DIC), etc., while decreased levels suggest concerns, such as a high-fat diet.

Review Video: The Coagulation Profile
Visit mometrix.com/academy and enter code: 423595

Blood Lipid Tests and Normal Values

Blood lipid tests generally measure total cholesterol, low-density lipoproteins (LDLs), high-density lipoproteins (HDLs), and often triglycerides. All are some form of lipid, a fat constituent insoluble in water. High total cholesterol puts an individual at risk for atherosclerosis (blood flow obstruction due to plaques) and ischemic heart disease. LDLs comprise the portion that sticks to the inner walls of blood vessels; therefore, a high LDL level is also associated with a propensity toward coronary artery disease (CAD). The larger HDLs do not adhere to internal walls but flow freely and actually lower risk of CAD. High triglyceride levels have also been associated with CAD.

Current normal values are:

Total cholesterol =< 200 mg/dl (> 240 mg/dl considered high)
LDLs =< 100 mg/dl
HDLs => 33 mg/dl for males; > 43 mg/dl for females

The ratio of total cholesterol to HDL should be between three and five.

C-Reactive Protein

C-reactive protein (CRP) is a blood indicator of inflammation. Its measurement is important in terms of cardiovascular disease because it has been found that high levels are predictive for coronary event recurrence and increased mortality in patients with unstable angina and acute myocardial infarction. A special CRP assay, called the high-sensitivity C-reactive protein (hs-CRP) test, is performed to determine its concentration. The hs-CRP test places people into one of three groups: those at lower, average, or high risk for development of cardiovascular disease generally have an hs-CRP value of less than 1.0 mg/L, from 1.0 to 3.0 mg/L, or greater than 30 mg/L, respectively.

Creatine Kinase, Tropinin T, and Tropinin I

The biochemical markers creatine kinase, tropinin T, and tropinin I are used to confirm the diagnosis of a myocardial infarction (MI), or heart attack. Creatine kinase (CK) is an enzyme that is liberated after cell death or injury, such as that which occurs in a segment of the heart muscle during a MI. CK comes in three forms, or isoenzymes, with the CK-MB isoenzyme associated with cardiac muscle injury or death. Serum CK and its CK-MB form rise several hours after an MI, generally peaking within 24 hours. Reperfusion is related to clearance or a return to normal CK levels; CK-MB should subside within 72 hours for reversible damage. Tropinins are contractile proteins found in cardiac as well as skeletal muscle. The tropinin I isotype (cTnI) is cardiac specific and rises only after a MI, whereas the tropinin T isotype (cTnT) rises after cardiac damage, muscle injury, and liver failure. Both tropinin isotypes typically rise within 2 to 4 hours after an MI, peak at 24 to 36 hours, but do not return to normal levels until 10 to 14 days later. Normal values for these markers are 55 to 71 IU CK (with ≤ 3% being CK-MB), < 0.2 pg/liter troponin T, and < 3.1 pg/liter troponin I.

Natriuretic Peptides

The term natriuretic refers to the excretion of sodium. There are three natriuretic peptides termed atrial natriuretic peptide (ANP), brain natriuretic peptide (BNP), and C-natriuretic peptide (CNP). ANP and BNP have additional diuretic and vasodilation properties and are involved in homeostasis and blood pressure control; plasma levels of these two peptides are known to be elevated in individuals with heart failure. ANP and BNP are accrued in the right atrium and ventricles, respectively, and released when there is increased pressure in those areas. CNP is predominantly detected in the vasculature, but its role is somewhat unclear.

Arterial Blood Gas Analysis

Arterial blood gas analysis looks at the acid-base balance, ventilation, and oxygenation levels of a patient. Typically, arterial blood is sampled via an indwelling arterial line, although other sites are sometimes tested. Acid-base balance is necessary for optimal cellular metabolism and is indicated by the pH value (the degree of acidity or alkalinity in the blood). Ventilation is measured by Pa_{CO2} or P_{CO2}, the partial pressure of dissolved carbon dioxide (CO_2) in the plasma. Oxygenation is indicated by the Pa_{O2} or P_{O2}, the partial pressure of dissolved oxygen (O_2) in the plasma. The percentage of hemoglobin sites filled with O_2, the O_2 saturation (Sa_{O2}), may also be expressed. In addition, the concentration of bicarbonate (HCO_3) is determined.

Normal values for each component of blood gas analysis are:

$$pH = 7.35 \text{ to } 7.45$$
$$Pa_{CO2} = 35 \text{ mm Hg to } 45 \text{ mm Hg } (> 50 \text{ mm Hg considered hypercarbia, excessively high levels})$$
$$Pa_{O2} = > 80 \text{ mm Hg}$$
$$HCO_3 = 22 \text{ to } 26 \text{ mEq/liter}$$

Interpretation of Arterial Blood Gas Analysis

A patient is in acidemia caused by acidosis when his arterial blood gas pH is less than 7.4; the patient is considered acidotic. Conversely, the patient is in alkalemia caused by alkalosis when the pH is higher than 7.4; this patient is considered alkalotic. Both conditions indicate an acid-base imbalance and potential underlying respiratory or metabolic disorders that must be addressed to normalize the pH. In other words, a low pH in combination with a high P_{CO2} suggests uncompensated respiratory acidosis, while a high pH along with a low P_{CO2} indicates uncompensated respiratory alkalosis. The HCO_3 levels will be outside the normal range if the primary disorder is metabolic in origin. Both pH and HCO_3 are low in uncompensated metabolic acidosis, while both are high for an uncompensated metabolic alkalosis. Metabolic and respiratory processes sometimes compensate for one another, in which case the HCO_3 or P_{CO2} may shift toward correcting the other. The oxygen pressure or levels measured by the P_{O2} are used to determine hypoxia, referring to inadequate oxygen levels of less than 80 mm Hg.

Conditions That Cause Acid-Base Imbalances

Acid-base imbalances, as measured by arterial blood gas analysis, are a result of an underlying respiratory or metabolic dysfunction. Patients with acidosis have a pH of less than 7.4, while those with alkalosis have a pH higher than approximately 7.4. Respiratory acidosis can be caused by chronic obstructive pulmonary disease (COPD), pneumothorax (air in the pleural cavity), pulmonary edema, or trauma to the chest wall. It can also result from less obvious sources, such as sedation, drug overdose, head trauma, sleep apnea, or central nervous system disorders. Metabolic acidosis manifests from lactic acidosis or ketoacidosis. The latter may be attributed to diabetes, diarrhea, starvation, alcohol abuse, or use of parenteral nutrition. Respiratory alkalosis can be due to a pulmonary embolism, hypoxia, pulmonary edema, asthma, or acute respiratory distress syndrome, as well as less obvious issues like anxiety, pregnancy, sepsis, and fever. The condition is also indicative of congestive heart failure (CHF). Metabolic sources of alkalosis include vomiting, the use of diuretics or steroids, nasogastric suction, low blood potassium, ingestion of excessive amounts of antacids, administration of bicarbonate, Cushing's syndrome, or transfusions.

Echocardiography

Echocardiography is an ultrasound technique that evaluates heart function. There are two types performed: transthoracic echocardiography (TTE) and transesophageal echocardiography (TEE).

TTE can measure things such as ventricular volume and valve integrity. The procedure is often done in conjunction with stress exercise testing on a bicycle or treadmill to look at wall-motion abnormalities due to blockage. It may also be done in conjunction with an exercise stress test induced by the agent dobutamine. Dobutamine is both an alpha-1 and beta-receptor agonist, and it increases contractility. It is infused in increasing amounts up to 0.04 kg/kg body weight. Patients that have increased contractility with dobutamine tend to respond better to an exercise program.

With TEE, patients fast before the procedure; during the procedure, they are somewhat sedated and their oropharynx is anesthetized in order to insert a catheter with an attached piezoelectric crystal into the esophagus. TEE is appropriate when conditions, such as regurgitation around a valve, bacterial endocarditis, septal defects, or emboli in the heart, are suspected. Echocardiography is often enhanced with the use of an intravenously injected contrast agent.

Exercise Testing in Cardiac Patients

The Indications and Contraindications for the Use of Exercise Testing in Cardiac Patients

Exercise, or stress testing, is the methodical and progressive use of some form of activity accompanied by concurrent ECG readings, blood pressure measurements, patient observation, and possibly pulmonary function analysis. It is most often used to diagnose the presence of coronary artery disease (CAD) and is also useful for predicting disease prognosis or severity, evaluating other cardiac problems like congestive heart failure or arrhythmias, and looking at functional capacity. Exercise testing can also be used to determine the person's safe heart rate range for activity. Exercise testing is contraindicated during acute illness and for cardiac patients who have had a myocardial infarction within the last 48 hours or who have unstable angina, acute pericarditis, ventricular or fast arrhythmias, untreated advanced heart block, or decompensated congestive heart failure.

How Exercise Testing Is Performed

The patient is subjected to increasingly intense activity while being monitored. The typical types of exercise include treadmill walking, stationary biking with an ergometer, stair climbing, or arm ergometry. The patient is typically monitored by ECG analysis, blood pressure readings, subjective analysis like the Borg's Rate of Perceived Exertion (RPE), and perhaps expired gas analysis. Exercise testing can be maximal, in which the patient is pressed to his maximum predicted heart rate (HR), or submaximal, where the test stops earlier, for example at 75% of maximal HR.

Common Pharmacologic Variants of Stress Testing

Exercise testing introduces stressors during which cardiac parameters are measured. Pharmacologic agents or radioactive materials are often injected intravenously in addition to or instead of the exercise component. Thallium stress testing is a quite sensitive variation in which radioactive thallium is injected intravenously during peak exercise or symptoms.

Afterward, the patient is subjected to a nuclear scanner for distribution of thallium uptake and myocardial perfusion. Another pharmacologic variation is Persantine thallium stress testing. The supine patient is given dipyridamole (Persantine) intravenously to dilate coronary arteries for four minutes followed by thallium and is then put under a nuclear scanner to examine myocardial perfusion. Areas with coronary atherosclerosis will not dilate from the Persantine, and blood will be shifted elsewhere, which can be observed by a lack of thallium uptake.

Metabolic Equivalents

Metabolic equivalents (METs) represent the ratio between an individual's metabolic rate while performing a particular activity compared to the metabolic rate while seated and resting (1 MET). Most fit people can perform maximally around 8 METs. Some typical exercise test protocols push people to higher limits, around 13 METS, such as the Bruce Protocol for the treadmill and some bike ergometer protocols. METs are actually a measurement of oxygen consumption. The formula for calculation of METs is:

$$\text{METs} = \text{oxygen requirements in ml } O_2\text{/kg/minute } (V_{O2})/3.5$$

Walking pace (feet/minute) on a level surface is related to oxygen consumption. If a patient cannot sustain a particular walking pace for one minute, that pace is near their optimal METs or oxygen consumption. If they cannot maintain a particular walking pace for 10 minutes, then that rate is higher than their anaerobic threshold. A pace that can be sustained for 1 to 10 minutes should be used interspersed with rest for exercise testing.

Atrial Rhythm Disturbances

Atrial rhythm disturbances include supraventricular tachycardia, atrial flutter, atrial fibrillation, and premature atrial contractions:

Supraventricular tachycardia is characterized on an ECG by a regular rhythm and a high heart rate of 160 to 250 bpm. It is often due to rheumatoid heart disease (RHD), mitral valve prolapse, cor pulmonale, or digitalis toxicity. A physical therapist should not treat such a patient until the supraventricular tachycardia subsides.

Atrial flutter is distinguished by a high atrial rate of 250 to 350 bpm, with or without a regular rhythm. It is generally due to coronary artery disease, mitral stenosis, or hypertension. The physical therapist should evaluate how well the patient tolerates atrial flutter before treating.

Atrial fibrillation (AF) is an irregular rhythm with an absent atrial component (just quivering). It can occur in association with many types of cardiac disease, including CHF, CAD, RHD, cor pulmonale, and hypertension. Chronic cases can be treated carefully, but new ones should be attended to medically first.

Premature atrial contractions are seen as a normal heart rate (60 to 100 bpm) that displays irregular rhythm, sometimes sporadic. They can be attributed simply to lifestyle issues, like caffeine ingestion, but may also indicate CAD, CHF, or electrolyte imbalance—the patient may be asymptomatic. These contractions can precede development of AF.

Ventricular Rhythm Disturbances

Ventricular rhythm disturbances include ventricular tachycardia, multifocal VT, premature ventricular contractions, ventricular fibrillation, and idioventricular rhythm: Agonal rhythm is an irregular rhythm with an extremely low rate of < 20 bpm and no P wave, indicating the patient is close to death and should not be treated. Ventricular tachycardia (VT) is generally a regular rhythm with a rate of > 100 bpm and absent P wave or retrograde conduction. The usual cause is coronary artery disease subsequent to acute MI. Patients require immediate medical attention, not physical therapy. Multifocal VT, or torsades de pointes, is similar on an ECG except that the rate is higher, > 150 bpm. It is usually induced by the use of antiarrhythmic drugs, MI, low electrolyte levels of potassium or magnesium, or hypothermia. Again, medical attention, not physical therapy, is indicated. Premature ventricular contractions (PVCs) are described in terms of the number of ectopic foci occurring and are characterized on ECG by an irregular rhythm, such as a beat skipped at certain intervals, and generally normal rate. They can occur in normal individuals subsequent to things like caffeine use but are also associated with CAD, MI, and other cardiac diseases. Treatment depends on the rate of occurrence. Ventricular fibrillation shows a messy ECG pattern indicative of severe heart disease. Medical attention, not physical therapy, is indicated. Idioventricular rhythm is regular but in the range of 20 to 40 bpm, indicating advanced cardiac disease that generally should be left untreated.

Junctional Rhythm Disturbances

Junctional rhythm disturbances include junctional escape rhythm and junctional tachycardia:

- Junctional escape rhythm is characterized on an ECG by a regular rhythm and a low rate of 20 to 40 bpm. The ECG also shows an inverted P wave on either side of the QRS complex and ectopic foci in the atrioventricular junction tissue. Junctional escape rhythm usually occurs as a physiological response to AV blockage, sinus bradycardia, atrial fibrillation, sinoatrial block, or drug intoxication. Most of the time, the physical therapist can treat these patients.
- Junctional tachycardia is similar to junctional escape rhythm on ECG except that the rate is higher, in the range of 100 to 180 bpm. It is generally seen in patients with chronic atrial fibrillation and sometimes other cardiac diseases. Physical therapy should only be provided if the patient can endure it, otherwise medical attention should be given first.

Atrioventricular Blocks

Atrioventricular (AV) blocks include first-degree AV block, second-degree AV block type 1, second-degree AV block type II, and third-degree AV block (a complete heart attack): First-degree atrioventricular (AV) blocks are characterized on an ECG by a normal rhythm and rate but a prolonged PR interval greater than 0.2. They are usually seen in elderly patients with heart disease, acute myocarditis, or during acute myocardial infarction. The underlying heart disease really determines how to treat these patients, and new blockage should be monitored for progression.

Second-degree AV blocks are characterized on the ECG by an irregular rhythm and an atrial rate higher than the ventricular one. There are two types. Patients with type I, generally due to acute infection or MI, have a long PR interval and no QRS complex on the ECG and are usually asymptomatic. Patients with type II, the cause of which is anteroseptal myocardial infarction, show a constant PR interval and QRS complex on the ECG. They often need physical therapy as they may have congestive heart failure or other symptoms. Third-degree AV block is a complete heart block characterized on an ECG as a regular rhythm and an atrial rate higher than the ventricular one. This can occur subsequent to many types of cardiac disease, including anteroseptal MI and coronary artery disease, as well as other issues like conduction problems or electrolyte imbalance. These patients have severe CHF and need medical attention.

Valvular Heart Disease

There are three basic types of valvular heart disease: stenosis, the narrowing of a valve; regurgitation, reverse blood flow through a valve due to incomplete closure; or prolapse, the displacement of a valve due to enlarged cusps. The end result of valvular heart disease can be pumping problems or heart failure. Valvular heart disease usually occurs at the aortic valve or mitral valve. Aortic stenosis, chronic aortic regurgitation, and acute aortic regurgitation are common manifestations involving the aortic valve, all of which can be reasons for left ventricular failure and all of which can be indicated by murmurs. Stenosis, chronic regurgitation, acute regurgitation, and prolapse all often occur at the mitral valve. An enlarged left atrium suggests possible mitral stenosis or chronic regurgitation with pulmonary vascular congestion as a major symptom. Mitral valve prolapse usually presents as a systolic click, but symptoms may be absent or present simply as fatigue or palpitation.

Types of Myocardial Heart Disease

Myocardial heart diseases, also known as cardiomyopathies, are disorders in which the heart muscle, or myocardium, is affected in some way. Functionally, there are three types of cardiomyopathies: dilated, hypertrophic, and restrictive.

- The dilated type, in which the ventricle is dilated and contractility is diminished, results in systolic dysfunction.
- The hypertrophic type, in which the ventricular myocardium is thickened resulting in less compliance and filling, adversely affects diastolic function.
- The restrictive type, in which there is endocrinal scarring of the ventricles, decreases both compliance during diastole and contractile force during systole.

Cardiomyopathies are also often classified in terms of their etiology, for example, as inflammatory (infarctions due to viruses or bacteria), metabolic (often due to diabetes), genetic (such as Duchene's muscular dystrophy), infiltrative (due to malignancies or sarcoidosis), physical agents (such as radiation or hypothermia), and others.

Types of Pericardial Heart Disease

Pericardial heart diseases are the result of some sort of issue with the pericardium, the fibrous sac enclosing the heart. The four basic types are acute pericarditis (inflammation of the pericardium), constrictive pericarditis, chronic pericardial effusion, and pericardial tamponade.

- Patients with acute pericarditis have pericardial friction rub, retrosternal chest pain, difficulty breathing, a cough, difficulty swallowing, fever, and chills.
- Constrictive pericarditis is suggested by jugular vein distention. Symptoms include abdominal swelling, peripheral edema, vague retrosternal chest pain, shortness of breath, dizziness, and pulmonary venous congestion.
- People with chronic pericardial effusion (fluid) have muffled heart sounds and possibly pericardial friction rub. They tend to have a vague fullness in their anterior chest, a cough, hoarseness, and difficulty swallowing.
- Pericardial tamponade occurs when the fluid buildup is enough to increase and equalize pressures to parts of the heart thus reducing cardiac output. Signs include jugular vein distention and cardiomegaly (heart enlargement). Patients present symptoms associated with low cardiac output, such as dyspnea, dizziness, and possibly retrosternal chest pain.

On an ECG, all of these diseases show a decreased QRS voltage.

General Signs and Symptoms of Heart Failure

Heart failure is a decrease in cardiac output. The heart cannot pump enough blood to meet bodily needs so that if left untreated, death can result. Heart failure is usually called congestive heart failure (CHF), which is descriptive of the buildup of blood in the heart that often enlarges it.

CHF can be classified as a left-sided heart failure, where the left ventricle is affected and there is back flow to the lungs, or right-sided, in which the right-side failure causes back flow to the systemic venous system. It can also be described as a high- or low-output failure, meaning that it is either secondary to renal system failure (i.e. fluid is not filtered off) or that the output is so low that circulation cannot be sustained. Heart failure can also be a systolic or diastolic dysfunction.

Many signs suggest CHF, including cold, pallid, possibly cyanotic extremities, peripheral edema, distention of the jugular vein, chest rales, an enlarged liver, and sinus tachycardia. The patient may have gained weight and have a diminished capacity for exercise and physical work. Many symptoms are breathing-related, including shortness of breath, spastic nighttime breathing, rapid breathing, orthopnea, and cough. The heart during inadequate circulation is said to be "decompensated" as opposed to "compensated" when medically stabilized.

Congestive Heart Failure

Recently, staging for congestive heart failure was described by J. Dekerlegand as follows:

- Stage A: Patient is at risk for development of left ventricular dysfunction; treatment is directed toward modifying risk factors.
- Stage B: Patient has asymptomatic left ventricular dysfunction; management is focused on risk factor modification to avoid symptoms.
- Stage C: Patient presents with symptomatic left ventricular dysfunction; treatment is focused on mitigation of symptoms and thwarting disease progression.
- Stage D: Patient is diagnosed with advanced refractory disease; the condition is managed aggressively with drugs, surgical devices, and/or transplantation.

Review Video: Congestive Heart Failure
Visit mometrix.com/academy and enter code: 924118

Classifications of Heart Disease

The American Heart Association (AHA) places patients with diseases of the heart into one of four classes based on objective assessment and functional capacity. They are as follows:

- Class I: no objective evidence of cardiovascular disease; functionally, no limitations with respect to physical activity; no symptoms while performing activity
- Class II: tangible evidence of minimal cardiovascular disease; physical activity only slightly limited; activity results in symptoms of anginal pain, dyspnea, palpitations, or fatigue
- Class III: objective signs of moderately severe cardiovascular disease; noticeable limitations in regard to physical activity; exhibits symptoms (as mentioned for class II) with low level activities
- Class IV: objective evidence of severe cardiovascular disease; all physical activities and possibly even rest are uncomfortable; symptoms (as listed for class II) increase upon exertion

Respiratory Evaluation

Patient History Relative to a Respiratory Evaluation

A respiratory evaluation should consist of patient history, physical examination, and analysis of certain specific diagnostic tests. The patient history should contain information relevant to respiratory evaluation, namely smoking history, use of oxygen therapy at rest and/or during activity, history of dyspnea (shortness of breath) at rest and/or during activity, any use-assisted or mechanical ventilation, documentation of episodes of pneumonia, and notation of thoracic procedures and other surgeries. The patient history should also document factors, such as environmental and occupational exposure to asbestos or other toxins, notation of activity level prior to admission, history of baseline sputum production, and the patient's sleeping position and number of pillows.

Inspection Portion of a Respiratory Evaluation

The physical examination of a patient undergoing evaluation for respiratory issues should include five parts: inspection, auscultation, palpation, mediate percussion, and cough examination. A meticulous inspection of the patient should examine factors, such as appearance, alertness, phonation, carriage and chest shape, skin color, notation of use of supplemental O_2 or other medical interventions, and the presence of digital clubbing or surgical incisions. In addition, a large element of the inspection should be observation of the patient's respiratory pattern for rate, depth, inspiration/expiration ratio, the succession of chest wall movements, the way different muscles appear to be used, and the general ease of breathing. A normal respiratory rate is 12 to 20 breaths per minute, and the customary inspiration/expiration ratio is one or two. Specific breathing abnormalities are described on another card.

Auscultation for Breath Sounds During Respiratory Evaluation

For respiratory evaluation, the clinician uses auscultation (the use of a stethoscope) to listen for normal, abnormal, and adventitious breath sounds, as well as extrapulmonary sounds and voice sounds. He uses the flat diaphragm of the stethoscope to hear sounds on the anterior, lateral, and posterior portions of both lungs. The patient, who is seated or prone, breathes through the mouth. Normal breath sounds should include loud tubular tracheal and main stem bronchial sounds with a pause between inspiration and expiration, similar sounds without a pause in bronchovesicular areas, and softer vesicular sounds in more distal areas. Breath sounds that are heard in uncharacteristic areas are considered abnormal and probably due to the fluid consolidation associated with pneumonia. Diminished sounds result from hypoventilation, congestion, or emphysema, and missing sounds suggest pneumothorax or lung collapse. Adventitious sounds are due to airflow alteration. Continuous adventitious sounds are due to some type of airway obstruction and include continuous wheeze, lower-pitched rhonchi, or very high-pitched stridor, the latter being a medical emergency. Discontinuous crackles indicate the presence of fluid or abrupt airway opening.

Auscultation for Voice Sounds During Respiratory Examination

Voice sounds, or phonation, can be heard with an intensity related to the area of the bronchial tree, just as with breath sounds. Voice sound tests with auscultation corroborate breath sound findings. Three kinds of voice sound tests are suggested. The first is whispered pectoriloquy, in which the individual whispers "one, two, three." If these sounds can be heard in distal lung areas, there is consolidation present, and if they are barely audible in distal portions, then hyperinflation is indicated. A similar test is bronchophony, in which the patient repeatedly says the phrase "ninety-nine"; indications are the same as for pectoriloquy. The third suggested voice sound test is egophony, in which the person repeats the letter "e" during auscultation; if it sounds like "a" in the distal areas, then the presence of fluid in the lung parenchyma or air spaces is implied.

Palpation During Respiratory Evaluation

During respiratory evaluation, palpation, or medical examination using finger pressure, should be performed on the upper, middle, and lower lung fields. The clinician faces the patient and uses the thumb and fingers on both hands to palpate near the collarbone, in the middle of the chest, and slightly lower, respectively. He should note whether there is fremitus or vibrations during respiration; these occur during voice production but also indicate the presence of secretions. Palpation should also be used to elucidate areas and reproducibility of pain or tenderness, skin temperature, pattern of chest expansion, existence of rib fractures and/or bony anomalies, and the presence of subcutaneous emphysema. The latter results from air in subcutaneous tissues due to pneumothorax, poor central line placement, or thoracic surgery, and manifests during palpation as bubbles that pop.

Mediate Percussion During Respiratory Evaluation

Mediate percussion is a technique in which a clinician places the palm side of his index and/or middle finger along an intercostal space in the chest wall and then uses the tips of the index and/or middle finger of the other hand to thump against the tip of the finger resting on the chest wall. The front and back areas of the chest are thus evaluated. The sounds heard during mediate percussion are characteristic; normal lung tissue should sound resonant. Possible abnormalities include sounds that are hyper resonant, indicating emphysema or pneumothorax; tympanic or vibrating, if there is abdominal gas; dull when there is decreased air in the lungs or dense tissues; and flat or very dull in areas of extremely dense tissue. Mediate percussion is also used to determine the position of the diaphragm during regular and deep breathing and the relative shift, or diaphragmatic excursion, on each side of the posterior chest wall.

Cough Examination During Respiratory Evaluation

Cough examination involves either instructing the patient to cough or observing as he naturally coughs. Coughing should consist of four stages, each of which must be seen. Normally, the first phase is full inspiration, followed by the second, closure of the glottis accompanied by augmented intrathoracic pressure. The third phase is the abdominal contraction, and the final is the quick expulsion of air. If any step is not done properly, pulmonary secretion clearance is impacted. During cough examination, the clinician should observe the patient for the effectiveness of secretion clearance, capacity to control coughing, the quality of clearance (wet, dry, or spastic), the rate of occurrence, and characteristics of the sputum, including presence of hemoptysis (the expectoration of blood).

Specific Breathing Abnormalities

Specific breathing abnormalities and the associated defects include:

- Apnea: no airflow to the lungs for longer than 15 seconds; due to airway obstruction, cardiopulmonary arrest, or narcotic overdose
- Respiratory rate abnormalities: Bradypnea: less than 12 bpm; due to sedative or alcohol use, fatigue, or certain neurologic or metabolic disorders Tachypnea: more than 20 bpm; results from acute respiratory distress, anemia, etc. Respiratory depth abnormalities:
    - Hyperpnea: increased depth; associated with congestive heart failure (CHF), pulmonary infections, or activity Cheyne-Stokes respirations: increasing depth trailed by a phase of apnea; due to CHF, narcotic overdose, or elevated intracranial pressure

Combined or paradoxical abnormalities:

- Hyperventilation: rate and depth increased with depressed P_{CO2}; due to anxiety or metabolic acidosis
- Hypoventilation: rate and depth decreased with increased P_{CO2}; due to metabolic alkalosis or anything that depresses respiration, such as sedation or overmedication
- Biot's respirations: rate and depth increased trailed by a phase of apnea; due to high intracranial pressure or meningitis
- Kussmaul's respirations: higher but regular rate and depth; due to diabetic ketoacidosis or renal failure
- Orthopnea: dyspnea while lying down; causes generally chronic lung disease or CHF
- Paradoxical respirations: abdominal or chest wall moves in upon inspiration and out upon expiration; due to paralysis or trauma
- Sighing respirations: sighing more than two to three times a minute; associated with dyspnea, angina, or fear

Respiratory Status

Pulse Oximetry as a Diagnostic Tool for Respiratory Status

Pulse oximetry is a technique in which finger or ear sensors detect arterial oxyhemoglobin saturation (Sa_{O2}). The oxyhemoglobin saturation is related to the partial pressure of oxygen (PaO_2) fairly linearly until high saturation is achieved. Thus, pulmonary reserve and the possibility of hypoxia, or oxygen deprivation, can be indirectly determined using pulse oximetry. High oxyhemoglobin saturation of 97 to 99% generally precludes hypoxia and corresponds to 90 to 100 mm Hg oxygen partial pressure. An Sa_{O2} of 95% corresponds to 80 mm Hg PaO_2 and generally presents symptomatically as tachypnea and/or tachycardia. Patients with 90% oxyhemoglobin saturation have only an oxygen partial pressure of 60 mm Hg and main signs of hypoxia, including the aforementioned as well as things like impaired judgment, vertigo, and/or nausea. Once the saturation levels are at 85% or lower, the patient will have other critical symptoms of hypoxia, such as labored respiration, cardiac dysrhythmias, and disorientation.

Diagnostic Use of Chest X-Rays for Respiration Status

Chest x-rays or radiographs (CXR) are used for differential diagnosis of pulmonary states. They are useful for diagnosing and monitoring conditions such as airspace consolidation (present in a number of cardiopulmonary diseases), identifying airspaces, diagnosing lobar atelectasis or collapse, pinpointing nodules or abscesses, evaluating certain structural features, or figuring out where to place tubes or lines. CXRs are generally described in terms of where the x-ray beam enters and exits, with the three most prevalent types being posterior-anterior (P-A), anterior-posterior (A-P), and lateral. The preferred position for all types is upright sitting or standing. The A-P type may be taken semi-reclined or lying down, while the lateral type might be shot as the patient lies on his side. Denser structures, such as bone, appear whiter or radiopaque on a CXR; intermediate ones, like the heart and pulmonary vessels, are shades of gray; and airspaces should be relatively dark or radiolucent.

Flexible Bronchoscopy

Flexible bronchoscopy is a technique in which a bendable, fiberoptic tube, or bronchoscope, is inserted into the bronchial tree for visualization and aspiration. The bronchoscope is placed through an endotracheal or tracheal tube if the patient is being mechanically ventilated or through one of the nostrils if not. Flexible bronchoscopy is used diagnostically, as well as therapeutically. Some of the diagnostic purposes include the evaluation of neoplasms in the area, assistance with endotracheal intubation, following anastomosis procedures involving the bronchial tree, and the examination of a number of unexplained or suspected pulmonary issues. Therapeutic indications include the removal of secretions, foreign material, or obstructive tissue; lavage, intubation, or stent placement; and maintenance of the airway.

Ventilation/Perfusion Scans

Ventilation/perfusion or V/Q lung scans are done in tandem. The ventilation portion involves the inhalation of inert radioactive gases by the patient, projections are then taken after the first breath, at equilibrium, and during washout. The perfusion scan involves intravenous injection of a radioisotope, after which six projections are obtained. The perfusion portion, which distinguishes deficient blood flow, is useful for detecting a variety of pulmonary diseases or lesions, as well as hypoventilation. Comparison between ventilation and perfusion scans is done to evaluate the V/Q matching, which should be about 0.8.

Computerized Tomographic Pulmonary Angiography

Computerized tomographic pulmonary angiography (CT-PA) is a technique primarily used to visualize the pulmonary artery and find pulmonary embolisms or thrombi.

Pulmonary Function Tests

Pulmonary function tests (PFTs) are a series of measurements of an individual's lung volumes during various phases of breathing, a number of associated capacities, and inspiratory and expiratory flow rates. PFTs are performed for reasons such as the detection and quantification of pulmonary diseases, differentiation between obstructive and restrictive lung diseases, determination of the extent of pulmonary contribution to systemic diseases, appraisal of disease progression, assessment of the viability of and response to certain respiratory therapies, and determination of the extent of impairment. Pulmonary function tests are performed using instruments that the patient breathes into, called spirometers (volume, flow, or gas dilution), or utilizing enclosed body plethysmography. Normal values are dependent on a number of factors, such as age and height, and are predicted from available nomograms (scaled graphs), or regression equations. There are quite a few PFTs, which are discussed in detail on other cards, but the most important ones are those that indicate airway patency during expiration. These are forced expiratory volume in 1 second (FEV_1), forced vital capacity (FVC), and their ratio (FEV_1/FVC).

Tests that Measure Lung Volumes

Pulmonary function tests measuring lung volume include:

- Inspiratory reserve volume (IRV): the maximum volume of air normally inspired; a decreased value suggests obstructive pulmonary disease
- Expiratory reserve volume (ERV): the maximum volume of air normally expired; a decreased value suggests ascites, pleural effusions, or pneumothorax
- Tidal volume (TV): the volume of air taken in or breathed out during one breath while resting; a decreased value suggests restrictive lung diseases, malignancy
- Residual volume (RV): the volume of air still present in lungs at the end of maximum expiration; distinguishes between obstructive (increased RV) and restrictive (decreased RV) lung disease
- Total lung capacity (TLC): the total lung volume at the conclusion of maximal inspiration; calculated as the sum of all above volumes (IRV+ ERV + TV + RV); also distinguishes between obstructive (increased) and restrictive (decreased) lung diseases
- Vital capacity (VC): the maximum air volume that can be expired slowly; expressed as the sum of VT + IRC + ERV
- Functional residual capacity (FRC): the air volume still in the lungs at the conclusion of normal expiration; equal to the sum of ERV + RV; indicative of obstructive (increased) versus restrictive (decreased) disease
- Inspiratory capacity (IC): the largest possible inspiratory volume after resting expiration; the sum of VT + IRV; a decreased value suggests restriction
- RV:TLC x 100: the relative percentage of unexpired residual volume to total lung capacity; suggests obstructive disorders if greater than 35%

Pulmonary Spirometry Tests

Pulmonary spirometry tests performed include:

- Forced vital capacity (FVC): air volume is forcefully and quickly expired subsequent to maximum inspiration; usually equal to vital capacity (VC), except in obstructive diseases (decreased)
- Forced expiratory volume timed (FEV_t): the air volume forcefully expired during a specific time interval, generally 1 second (FEV_1), which is decreased in both obstructive and restrictive lung disorders
- FEV%: the percentage of FVC expired during a specific time interval, generally 1 second, thus calculated usually as $FEV_1/FVC \times 100$; used to distinguish between obstructive (decreased) and restrictive (increased) disorders
- Forced expiratory flow 25 to 75% ($FEF_{25-75\%}$): the average airflow in the middle of measuring FEV; indicative of peripheral airway resistance; if decreased, medium-sized airways are obstructed
- Peak expiratory flow rate (PEFR): maximal achievable airflow rate during FEV testing
- Maximum voluntary ventilation (MVV): the maximal achievable air volume breathed in 1 minute voluntarily; generally calculated by measuring for 10 to 15 seconds and multiplying accordingly; indicative of the status of respiratory muscles, airway and tissue resistance, and lung and thorax compliance
- Flow-volume loop (F-V) loop: graphic representation of maximal FEV and maximum inspiratory flow volume

Ventilation and Gas Exchange Tests

There are three types of ventilation tests:

1. Minute volume (VE), or minute ventilation, is the entire volume of air inspired or expired in one minute. It is calculated as: VE = VT(tidal volume) x respiratory rate. VE is often measured during exercise or stress testing as it increases when the patient is hypoxic, has too much carbon dioxide in the blood, or has acidosis.
2. The respiratory dead space (VD) is the air volume ventilated but not perfused. VD is important because it is indicative of the surface area accessible for gas exchange. More dead space means decreased gas exchange.
3. Alveolar ventilation (VA) indicates the air volume participating in gas exchange, estimable as (VT - VD). VA estimations of oxygen availability are generally backed up with arterial blood gas measurements.

The gas exchange test performed is the diffusing capacity of carbon monoxide (DLCO), in which the patient inhales a mixture of carbon monoxide and helium. After exhaling for 10 seconds, the gases are quantified. DLCO is indicative of the gas exchange area, the extent of contact between a functioning pulmonary capillary bed and functioning alveoli.

Obstructive vs. Restrictive Lung Disease

Obstructive lung diseases or conditions are states where there is diminished airflow out of the lungs due to narrowing of the airway lumen. The general result is more dead space and decreased surface area available for gas exchange. Obstructive pulmonary conditions include asthma, chronic bronchitis, emphysema, cystic fibrosis, and bronchiectasis. Obstructive situations in which there are airflow limitations that cannot be completely reversed are collectively referred to as COPD, chronic obstructive pulmonary disease.

With restrictive lung disease, there is decreased lung compliance, making expansion and breathing difficult. Often the underlying issue is tissue scarring. Restrictive lung disorders include atelectasis, pneumonia, pulmonary edema, adult respiratory distress syndrome (ARDS), pulmonary embolisms (PE), and lung contusions.

Asthma

Asthma is an obstructive lung disorder exacerbated by an immunologic reaction to allergens, exercise, stress, cold, bacterial infections, or gastroesophageal reflux. During an asthma attack, bronchial smooth muscles constrict, leukocytes increase with a subsequent increase in mucus production, and bronchial mucosa become inflamed and thicken. Symptoms of an asthma attack include rapid and pursed lip breathing, use of accessory muscles, fatigue, active expiration, and, in critical cases, cyanosis. Palpation reveals a rapid heart rate with weak pulse, and the chest diameter is enlarged. The individual will wheeze upon expiration and have diminished breath sounds by auscultation; they generally have a very stiff, nonproductive cough. Asthmatics will produce a normal chest x-ray between exacerbations, but during them, the CXR will show translucent lung fields, a flat diaphragm, a larger chest diameter, and horizontal ribs. Asthma is managed with the use of bronchodilators, corticosteroids, and, if necessary, supplemental oxygen or IV fluid administration. The simplest management is avoidance of the precipitating agent.

Chronic Bronchitis

Chronic bronchitis is an obstructive lung disorder defined as chronic coughing and pulmonary secretion expectoration; chronic is characterized as a minimum three months/year for two successive years. Cigarette smoking, air pollution, and infections have been implicated as causative agents. The bronchial mucosa become inflamed, resulting in narrowing of the large and, later, small airways. The bronchial smooth muscle cells and mucous glands become enlarged, air is trapped, and the alveoli become hyperinflated. The results are bronchospasm and increased secretion retention. People with chronic bronchitis have rapid and pursed lip breathing, use of accessory muscles, and fatigue. They tend to have a characteristic stocky, edematous build with elevated shoulders and a barrel chest. Palpation reveals rapid heart rate, hypertension, and increased chest diameter. One can hear low-pitched rhonchi, crackles, and diminished breath sounds upon auscultation. The cough is intermittent and more likely to be productive in the morning. Chest x-rays show translucent lung fields, compressed diaphragms, and possibly an enlarged heart. Chronic bronchitis is managed with bronchodilators, steroids, expectorants, and. if necessary, antibiotics, diuretics, oxygen, or assisted ventilation. Smoking cessation is a primary tool.

Emphysema

Emphysema is an obstructive lung disorder in which alveolar walls and surrounding capillaries are gradually destroyed by diminished pulmonary elasticity, airway collapse, and the formation of air pockets called bullae. This produces decreased lung elasticity, trapping of air, and hyperinflation. Emphysema may be related to the same types of irritants as chronic bronchitis: cigarette smoking, infections, or pollutants. Some cases are hereditary in which there is a deficiency of alpha-1-antitypic, allowing unchecked alveolar destruction. Symptoms of emphysema are similar to chronic bronchitis and include rapid, difficult breathing and use of accessory muscles; emphysema patients usually have cachexia, generalized weakness, and debilitation. Palpation reveals tachycardia, hypertension, and increased chest diameter, and auscultation generally shows extremely diminished breath sounds, wheezing, and crackles. Cough is generally absent. A chest x-ray should show translucent lung fields, compressed diaphragms, bullae (air pockets), and possibly a small heart. Emphysema is managed with bronchodilators, supplemental oxygen, and nutritional support.

Cystic Fibrosis

Cystic fibrosis (CF) is a hereditary disorder affecting the exocrine glands. The result is fibrosis of the pancreas and buildup of secretions in many bodily systems, including the lungs, where it is a relatively fatal obstructive lung disease. After babies with CF experience an infection, their bronchial and bronchiolar walls get inflamed; the bronchial glands and goblet cells enlarge, producing persistent secretions; and clearance of the secretions is diminished. Pulmonary abnormalities associated with CF include bronchospasm, augmented airway resistance, V/Q mismatch, and increased susceptibility to respiratory infections. CF patients display rapid breathing, accessory muscle use, generalized weakness, and a barrel chest. Palpation reveals tachycardia, hypertension, and increased chest diameter, and auscultation should show diminished breath sounds, rhonchi, and crackles. Patients have a controlled or intermittent cough with very thick, greenish, possibly bloody sputum. Their chest x-rays show fibrosis, atelectasis, an enlarged right ventricle, streaks, translucent lung fields, and flattened diaphragms. CF patients are managed with antibiotics, bronchodilators, mucolytics, supplemental oxygen, often lung transplantation, and other support.

Bronchiectasis

Bronchiectasis is a lung disorder in which there is both obstruction and restriction. It is technically defined as the permanent expansion of larger airways, i.e. typically, those with a diameter > 2 mm. The causative agents include bacterial respiratory infections, cystic fibrosis, tuberculosis, and ciliary defects. Bronchiectasis is characterized by the destruction of bronchiole walls and the mucociliary escalator; dilation, fibrosis, and ulceration of the bronchioles; and enlargement of the bronchial artery. Signs are similar to cystic fibrosis, namely rapid breathing, accessory muscle use, generalized weakness, and a barrel chest. Physical examination findings are comparable to CF as well, including a rapid heart rate, hypertension, expanded chest diameter, diminished breath sounds, crackles, and rhonchi. The sputum from a bronchiectasis patient's cough is purulent, smells foul, and may contain blood. Chest x-rays reveal patchy infiltrates, often atelectasis, increased markings on blood vessels and bronchi, and, if severe, a honeycombing appearance. Treatments include antibiotics, bronchodilators, corticosteroids, supplemental oxygen, dispensation of IV fluids, bronchopulmonary hygiene, nutritional sustenance, lung transplantation, and sometimes pain medication.

Atelectasis

Atelectasis is a restrictive lung condition in which alveoli, one or more lung segments, or one or more lobes have collapsed partially or totally. It is usually a result of hypoventilation or unsuccessful pulmonary secretion clearance, but it can also occur for other reasons, such as after a bout of pneumonia, situations that restrict the diaphragm (e.g., paralysis), and/or the compression of lung tissue. A ventilation/perfusion mismatch, shunting, and vasoconstriction result ultimately in hypoxemia. The patient may or may not present with rapid breathing, shallow respirations, and/or fever. The main observations on palpation are a decreased tactile fremitus, vocal resonance, and sometimes a rapid heartbeat. Auscultation reveals crackles, where the atelectasis has occurred, and reduced breath sounds. If a lobe has collapsed, breath sounds are missing or bronchial. The sputum characteristics depend on the underlying cause; characteristic chest x-ray findings feature linear opaque areas at the site, fissures, displacement of the diaphragm, and, in cases of lobar collapse, a dense, white triangular area. Atelectasis is managed by using incentive spirometry, supplemental oxygen, bronchopulmonary hygiene, and mobilization.

Pneumonia

Pneumonia is a restrictive pulmonary disease characterized by inflammation of the smaller airways, resulting in ventilation/perfusion mismatch and hypoxemia. It can be caused by the inhalation of a number of bacteria and viruses, as well as foreign substances, chemicals, dusts, gastric matter, and post-radiation therapy. As the disease progresses, the alveoli first become edematous and exudative up to day three, then are infiltrated with bacteria and various blood cells (days two to four). Consolidation occurs there typically days four through eight. Sometime after day eight, resolution with expectoration or enzymatic destruction of the infiltrates occurs; complete clearance may not occur until six weeks. Signs include tachypnea, shallow respirations, and/or fever. Physical examination shows decreased local chest wall expansion, dull percussion, occasionally rapid heart rate, crackles, rhonchi, and bronchial breath sounds in consolidation regions. Patients initially have a dry cough, which becomes more productive; the sputum is colored. The characteristic chest radiograph finding is a well-delineated density at the involved lobe, possibly accompanied by an air bronchogram or pleural effusion. Patients are treated with antibiotics, oxygen, IV fluids, mobilization, and bronchopulmonary hygiene.

Pulmonary Edema

Pulmonary edema, the buildup of excess fluid, is a restrictive pulmonary condition divided into two categories depending on origin: cardiogenic pulmonary edema and noncardiogenic pulmonary edema. Cardiogenic pulmonary edema is characterized by the backflow of blood from the heart (due to left ventricular hypertrophy, etc.), which encourages fluid movement from the pulmonary capillaries into the alveolar spaces. This ultimately results in fluid buildup in many areas of the bronchial tree. Capillary permeability changes can also occur subtly subsequent to other conditions, such as pneumonia or adult respiratory distress syndrome, resulting in noncardiogenic pulmonary edema. In either case, patients develop atelectasis, V/Q mismatch, and hypoxemia. Signs present as rapid breathing, anxiety, accessory muscle use, and orthopnea, which is significant because the physical therapist should avoid treating these patients while supine. Physical findings include increased tactile and vocal fremitus on palpation, symmetric wet crackles, possible wheezing on auscultation, and relatively clear sputum. Chest radiographs show increased hilar vascular markings, short horizontal lines, left ventricular hypertrophy, fluffy opaque heart areas, and sometimes pleural effusion. Treatment includes diuretics, oxygen, hemodynamic monitoring, and possibly other drugs.

ARDS

ARDS, or adult respiratory distress syndrome, is the acute, critical inflammation of the lung due to aspiration or some other type of trauma. In ARDS, an exudative stage occurs within hours or days and is characterized by augmented capillary permeability, edema, hemorrhage, and consolidation. This is followed by a proliferative phase characterized by fibrosis, atelectasis, V/Q disparities, critically low blood oxygen, and pulmonary hypertension. Patients with ARDS present with labored and rapid breathing and increased pulmonary artery pressure. Physical examination shows hypotension, decreased bilateral chest wall expansion, dull percussion, rapid or slow heart rate, diminished breath sounds, crackles, wheezing, and rhonchi. Patients usually do not cough up sputum unless there is also an infection. The characteristic chest x-ray finding is pulmonary edema with scattered, patchy opaque areas. Management strategies include mechanical ventilation, IV fluids, homodynamic monitoring, and nitrous oxide therapy. Prone positioning can be used by experienced professionals as it allows greater aeration to dorsal segments, better V/Q matching, and improved drainage of secretions.

PULMONARY EMBOLISM

Pulmonary embolism (PE) is the occlusion of pulmonary blood vessels. The vast majority of cases are due to thromboembolism, a blockage from a blood clot. Other sources of blockage include air introduced through catheterization, fat droplets, or tumor pieces. The consequences include decreased pulmonary blood flow distal to the obstruction, atelectasis, local edema, bronchospasm, and occasionally tissue death. PE is an acute, potentially critical state. Patients undergoing a pulmonary embolism experience rapid onset tachypnea, dysrhythmia, dizziness, and often chest pain. Physical examination shows hypotension, rapid heart rate, locally decreased chest wall expansion, wheezing, crackles, and diminished or missing breath sounds distal to the embolism. A chest radiograph should display decreased lung volume, a dilated pulmonary artery with markings, and possibly atelectasis and/or density at the infarct location with distal radiolucency. Therapies include anticoagulation measures, hemodynamic stabilization, oxygen, mechanical ventilation, thrombolysis, embolectomy, and filters inserted into the inferior vena cava. Physical therapy should not be performed during a PE.

INTERSTITIAL LUNG DISEASE AND LUNG CONTUSION

These are two types of restrictive lung disease: interstitial lung disease and lung contusion. Interstitial lung disease (ILD) is the universal name for any condition in which respiratory membranes in many areas of the lung are destroyed through inflammation and fibrosis. There are many potential causes of ILD, and the main observed symptom is dyspnea upon exertion.

Lung contusion is a situation in which some type of trauma initially causes lung tissue to compress against the chest wall producing a rupture at the alveolar-capillary membrane with subsequent hemorrhaging. Decompression then follows, stretching the tissues. Blood and fluid buildup in the alveoli and interstitial areas, causing shunting and other problems, with an end result of hypoxemia. Patients present with tachypnea, bleeding along the chest wall, and cyanosis, if advanced. Physical examination reveals hypotension, tachycardia, crackling noises due to broken ribs, diminished or missing breath sounds at the site, wet crackles, and sometimes a weak cough with relatively clear sputum. CXR shows patchy but localized opacities and consolidation, if present. Lung contusions are treated with pain management, oxygen, mechanical ventilation, and IV fluids.

PLEURAL EFFUSION

Pleural effusions are extrapulmonary, meaning they are external to the visceral pleura, but if present they impact pulmonary function. A pleural effusion occurs when there is fluid in the pleural space, enclosed by the thin membrane surrounding the lung called the pleura. The effusion can be transudative or exudative, primarily cardiac or lymphatic in origin respectively. Patients with pleural effusions will have a rapid breathing, decreased chest expansion on the side with the effusion, and often discomfort. Physical examination findings on palpation generally include decreased tactile fremitus, dull percussion, possibly tachycardia. Breath sounds on auscultation vary from normal to diminished to bronchial at the area of effusion. The fluid present will obscure the diaphragm and move with position changes on chest radiographs, the dependent lung will appear homogeneously dense, and in severe cases the mediastinum will shift. Management strategies include supplemental oxygen, diuretics, chest tube placement, pleurodesis (artificial obliteration of the pleural space through use of chemicals or surgery), pain management, and thoracocentesis (introduction of a cannula to remove fluid or air).

PNEUMOTHORAX

Pneumothorax (PTX) is a restrictive extrapulmonary condition in which there is air in the pleural space. The three common causes are puncturing of the visceral pleura (spontaneous PTX), perforation of the chest wall and parietal pleura (traumatic or iatrogenic PTX), or gas from bacteria associated with empyema (discussed elsewhere). In terms of air movement, the pneumothorax can be described as:

- Closed: independent of breathing, meaning the chest wall is intact
- Open: related to breathing movements, meaning the pleural space is in contact with the atmosphere
- Tension: where air movement occurs only during inspiration

Signs and physical findings are very similar to pleural effusion, for example, decreased chest expansion on the involved side along with rapid breathing and heart rate. However, breath sounds upon auscultation will be diminished at the site or absent in the case of tension PTX. Characteristics on chest radiographs are a translucent area usually at the apex of the lung, a narrow white line representing the visceral pleura, and, if severe, things like a depressed diaphragm, atelectasis, lung collapse, and/or shifting of the mediastinum. Moderate- to large-sized PTX should be treated with chest tube placement, supplemental oxygen, and pain management, if needed.

Review Video: Pneumothorax
Visit mometrix.com/academy and enter code: 186841

Hemothorax, Empyema, and Flail Chest

Hemothorax is the existence of blood in the pleural space due to some type of injury to the pleura. It presents symptomatically, through physical findings, and on chest radiographs very similarly to pneumothorax, air in the pleural space. If there is associated lung contusion, hemoptysis (the coughing up of blood) can distinguish it from pneumothorax. Management strategies include supplemental oxygen, chest tube placement, pain control if needed, and blood transfusions. Patients with hemothorax should be monitored for shock and treated, if necessary. Hemopneumothorax means there is both blood and air in the pleural space.

In empyema, pus from anaerobic bacteria invades the pleural space due to some type of trauma. There is pleural swelling, exudate formation, fibrin accretion on the pleura, and fibroblast formation.

A flail chest is a situation in which three or more contiguous ribs are broken due to some type of chest injury or forceful cardiopulmonary resuscitation. Changes in pressure gradients cause paradoxical breathing where the ribs move in opposition to normal patterns, there is contused lung tissue underneath, and mediastinal shifting may occur.

Adrenocortical Steroids for Respiratory Abnormalities

Adrenocortical steroids, also known as glucocorticoids, primarily affect the immune response by preventing the accumulation of inflammatory cells at an infection site and impeding the release of lysosomal enzymes and chemical mediators. They also reduce dilation and permeability of capillaries. There are systemic, inhaled, and intranasal forms available. Well-known glucocorticoids include dexamethasone, beclomethasone, and prednisone. Glucocorticoids are known to have many adverse side effects, such as vomiting, thromboembolism, hypertension, adrenal insufficiency, oral thrush with inhaled varieties, and a risk of osteoporosis. Patients receiving systemic steroids should be monitored for blood pressure and blood glucose.

Bronchodilators

Bronchodilators alleviate ongoing bronchospasm in one of three ways:

1. Anticholinergic bronchodilators, like ipratropium bromide, block acetylcholine in bronchial smooth muscle and decrease mucus secretions. Possible adverse effects include palpitations, dry mouth, dizziness, and bronchitis.
2. Another category of bronchodilators includes beta2agonists, which affect beta2receptors and relax bronchial smooth muscle. Unfortunately, they often also cause palpitations and tachycardia. There are short- and long-acting types, such as albuterol and salmeterol, respectively.
3. The third type of bronchodilator is theophylline, which acts through a number of other mechanisms. If theophylline is administered, the patient should be closely monitored and a therapeutic concentration of 5 to 20 mcg/ml maintained because there are many potential adverse effects. At high concentrations, patients can develop ventricular tachycardia, premature ventricular contractions, and seizure.

Antihistamines, Leukotriene Modifiers, and Mast Cell Stabilizers

Respiratory abnormalities are generally treated with drugs from one or more of five classes: adrenocortical steroids, antihistamines, bronchodilators, leukotriene modifiers, and mast cell stabilizers.

- Antihistamines work by competing for histamine binding sites, thus diminishing inflammation and bronchoconstriction. Some common antihistamines are chlorpheniramine maleate, diphenhydramine, and cetirizine.
- Leukotriene modifiers are used primarily for asthma control and act as selective antagonists for leukotriene receptors. Montelukast and zafirlukast are examples.
- Mast cell stabilizers are used for more long-term control of asthma and other allergic diseases. Their mechanism of action is blocking histamine release from mast cells. Cromolyn is the most well-known example.

Common Types of Respiratory Dysfunction

Types of respiratory dysfunction include:

- Hypoxemia and hypoxia: low levels of oxygen in the blood and tissues, respectively
- Air trapping: retention of gas in the lung due to airway obstruction
- Bronchospasm: the contraction of smooth muscle in the walls of bronchi and bronchioles, causing constriction
- Consolidation: replacement of alveolar air with transudate, exudate, or tissue fragments
- Hyperinflation: overexpansion of the lungs at rest due to air trapping
- Respiratory distress: a condition in which inadequate gas exchange causes a combination of shortness of breath, respiratory muscle fatigue, aberrant respiratory pattern and rate, nervousness, and cyanosis; usually leads to respiratory failure if untreated
- Respiratory failure: incapacity of respiratory system to maintain adequate oxygen-carbon dioxide gas exchange

Acute Coronary Syndrome

Acute coronary syndrome occurs with an inadequate myocardial oxygen supply relative to demand that results in myocardial ischemia or lack of blood. The ischemia may be attributed to a coronary arterial spasm that impairs blood flow, known as variant or Prinzmetal's angina. More often, it is due to coronary atherosclerotic disease (CAD), in which the coronary walls are narrowed by thrombus formation that occurs subsequent to the deposition of fatty plaques on arterial walls. Clinically, CAD can manifest as stable, exertional angina (chest pain) responsive to nitroglycerin, unstable angina (USA) that is more severe, or myocardial infarction (MI), in which myocardial cells have died due to a severe occlusion in some part of a coronary artery.

Myocardial Infarctions

Myocardial infarctions (MIs) are defined in terms of the wall affected and potential occlusion. These include:

- Anterior MI: in anterior left ventricle due to left coronary artery occlusion
- Inferior MI: in inferior left ventricle due to right coronary artery occlusion
- Anterolateral MI: in anterolateral left ventricle with occlusion in left anterior descending region
- Anteroseptal MI: in the septal region between the left and right ventricles due to left anterior descending area occlusion
- Posterior MI: in the posterior of the heart due to right coronary area region blockage
- Right ventricular MI: blockage in the right coronary artery
- Transmural or subendocardial MI: full- or partial-thickness MI occurring in any artery, also described as Q-wave MI or non-Q-wave MI, respectively
- Anterior and inferior MIs often result in complications like atrioventricular (AV) blocks or congestive heart failure (CHF). Anterolateral and anteroseptal MIs often precipitate brady- or tachyarrhythmias. Posterior MI is associated with bradycardia and heart blocks, and right ventricular MI can lead to right ventricular failure and subsequent cardiogenic shock.

Cardiac Rhythm and Conduction Disturbances

There are four general categories of cardiac rhythm or conduction disturbances, and each has characteristic electrocardiographic (ECG) patterns. The four categories are:

- Atrial rhythm disturbances includes supraventricular tachycardia, atrial flutter, atrial fibrillation (AF), and premature atrial contractions
- Ventricular rhythm disturbances: includes ventricular tachycardia (VT), multifocal VT (also called torsades de pointes), premature ventricular contractions, ventricular fibrillation, and idioventricular rhythm
- Junctional rhythm disturbances: includes junctional escape rhythm and junctional tachycardia
- Atrioventricular (AV) blocks: includes first-degree AV block, second-degree AV block type 1, second-degree AV block type II, and third-degree AV block (a complete heart attack)

Dean's Hierarchy

Components of Dean's Hierarchy

Dean's hierarchy for treatment of patients with impaired oxygen transport addresses bronchopulmonary hygiene. It is based on the assertion that individuals have optimal physiologic function when they are upright and moving.

The nine components and their goals are:

1. Mobilization and exercise: to reach an exercise level that impacts the oxygen transport pathway
2. Body positioning: to position the patient as close to upright and moving as possible, whether active, assisted, or passive

3. Breathing control maneuvers: to promote alveolar ventilation, mucociliary transport, and coughing
4. Coughing maneuvers: to encourage mucociliary clearance with few cardiopulmonary side effects
5. Relaxation and energy-conservation intercessions: to lessen the work of breathing, reduce unnecessary oxygen demand, and minimize heart rate
6. Range-of-motion (ROM) exercises: to stimulate alveolar ventilation and change its distribution
7. Postural drainage positioning: to assist airway clearance using gravity
8. Manual techniques: to facilitate airway clearance in combination with specific body positioning
9. Suctioning: to remove of airway secretions

Physical Therapy Interventions for Dean's Hierarchy

The nine components of Dean's hierarchy and suitable physical therapy interventions or desired effects are:

1. Mobilization and exercise: techniques ideally should result in acute, long-term, and preventive effects
2. Body positioning: specific positioning should impact hemodynamics due to fluid shifts and improve many cardiopulmonary functions, such as ventilation, perfusion, matching, and gas exchange
3. Breathing control maneuvers: specific maneuvers of value include coordination of breathing during activity, incentive spirometry, pursed-lip breathing, eucapnic breathing, sustained maximal inspiration, and maximal tidal breaths
4. Coughing maneuvers: maneuvers of value include active and spontaneous coughing with closed glottis; modified techniques with open glottis, such as a forced expiration or huffing; and active-assisted coughing
5. Relaxation and energy-conservation intercessions: use of relaxation procedures while resting and active may produce energy conservation and pain control
6. Range-of-motion (ROM) exercises: work may be active, assisted-active, or passive
7. Postural drainage positioning: the use of bronchopulmonary segmental drainage positions
8. Manual techniques: procedures of value include autogenic drainage, manual percussion, vibration, use of deep breathing, and coughing
9. Suctioning: systems include open suction, closed suction, tracheal tickle, instillation with saline, and bagging

Bronchopulmonary Hygiene

To institute a bronchopulmonary hygiene program for patients with respiratory issues, physical therapists need a basic understanding of the underlying pathophysiology. They must understand concepts, such as reversibility versus irreversibility and obstructive versus restrictive lung disorders. They must also be familiar with a wide range of modalities for bronchopulmonary hygiene and know which ones require prior physician approval, such as bronchodilators, other drugs, and supplemental oxygen. Physical therapists must be flexible in planning as physical therapy and other interventions can affect patient status. To maximize continuity, they should familiarize themselves with each patient's normal bronchopulmonary hygiene pattern. Some baseline and/or monitoring measurements are generally recommended, including baseline sputum production and pulse oximetry monitoring. Physical therapists should be familiar with procedures to increase a patient's cough effectiveness, such as splinting, positioning, and nasotracheal suctioning of secretions.

Activity Progression with Respiratory Impairments

Patients with respiratory impairments should be monitored with measurements related to respiratory function, such as the Dyspnea scale, the rating of perceived exertion, and O_2 saturation rather than heart rate. Activity progression programs should concentrate on short, frequent sessions at times when the patient will not be fatigued. Bronchopulmonary hygiene prior to the session often increases activity tolerance. The patient may need supplemental oxygen during exercise, even if not required at rest. Progression or regression should be documented, including items like type, frequency, and duration of rest periods.

American Thoracic Society (ATS) Dyspnea Scale

Dyspnea refers to difficulty breathing and is usually pulmonary or cardiac in origin. The degree of dyspnea observed is useful not only diagnostically but also as a tool to evaluate the response to activity progression. The ATS Dyspnea Scale grades dyspnea from 0 to 4, ranging from none to severe as described below:

- Grade 0: no dyspnea; patient is not troubled with breathlessness except during strenuous exercise
- Grade 1: slight dyspnea; patient is breathless only when hurrying on a level plane or walking on slight incline
- Grade 2: moderate dyspnea; patient is a slow walker for age group due to breathlessness or must stop to catch breath when walking on the level
- Grade 3: severe dyspnea; patient has to stop to catch breath while walking on the level approximately every 100 yards or several minutes
- Grade 4: very severe dyspnea; patient is so breathless that activities of daily life are impacted

Patient Information in a Vascular Evaluation

A physical examination that includes information relevant to the vascular system should incorporate specific components of history, inspection, palpation, auscultation, vascular tests, and diagnostic studies. The history should reveal pertinent medical history (for example, history of diabetes, hypertension, high lipid levels, etc.), exercise habits, use of tobacco or alcohol, and periods of lengthy bed rest or vascular surgery. A large part should be devoted to the documentation of pain because it can be indicative of vascular occlusion and claudication (reduced blood supply to the leg muscles). Therefore, pain in the extremities, nocturnal pain, pain at rest (suggesting advanced occlusion), intermittent claudication, and claudication in the buttock, hip, or thigh (a sign of obstruction in the aorta and iliac arteries) should all be detailed. The patient's history or current presence of edema, which also suggests vascular problems, should be documented.

Evaluation of Vascular Function

Physical Inspection

During a vascular evaluation, the clinician should inspect certain features to determine the location and magnitude of vascular disease and whether it is localized in the arteries or veins. He should observe the patient's extremities (particularly the legs) for discolorations in skin color at the distal extremities and nail beds, dilated or purplish veins, digital clubbing, patchy hair distribution, and the presence of cellulitis, petechiae spots, and/or skin lesions. Clinicians should also observe the patient for gait abnormalities, and edema or atrophy in extremities, in particular, should be carefully observed and documented. Bilateral peripheral edema suggests right-sided congestive heart failure; unilateral peripheral edema suggests chronic venous insufficiency, obstruction of lymphatics, or trauma. The physical therapist should use a tape measure to quantify the circumference of the person's forefoot, the smallest part above the ankle, the biggest part of the calf, and the mid-thigh with knee extended. Edema is implied if the metric differs more than 1 cm from a normal value or the measurement from the other side above the ankle or 2 cm at the calf.

Palpation and Auscultation in a Physical Examination to Evaluate Vascular Function

The most important part of palpation for vascular function is measuring the peripheral pulses in terms of strength and rate. The typical peripheral pulses to evaluate are the carotid, brachial, radial, temporal, ulnar, femoral, popliteal, posterior tibial, and dorsalis pedis. Note that carotid arteries should not be palpated at the same time as that can reduce blood flow to the brain. Each pulse should be graded from 0 to +4 as follows: 0, absent on palpation; 1, diminished or hardly palpable; 2, brisk as expected; 3, full or increased; and 4, bounding. Weak peripheral pulses suggest decreased fluid volumes and possible corresponding upticks in heart and respiratory rates. However, some adults have normally absent peripheral pulses. Patients with diabetes, hypertension, or peripheral vascular disease should have their pulses tested before, during, and after activity to look at changes. Palpation can also inform the physical therapist about pain at a particular site, the presence/absence of edema, the temperature of the skin, etc.

Auscultation for vascular function should include an assessment of systemic blood pressure and listening for bruits, whooshing sounds associated with turbulent blood flow due to obstruction.

Vascular Tests Used to Evaluate Perfusion

Perfusion can be evaluated with three tests:

- Capillary refill time: Used for the assessment of vascular perfusion and circuitously cardiac output, the test involves squeezing the nail beds of fingers or toes until blanched and then releasing. Blanching should go away in less than 2 seconds.
- Elevation pallor: To assess arterial perfusion, this exam involves elevating the limb 30 to 40 degrees for 15 to 60 seconds and monitoring whether color changes are observed. Pallor or gray color changes indicate occlusive disease. The condition is considered severe if color changes at 25 seconds, moderate if it occurs at 25 to 40 seconds, and mild at 40 at 60 seconds.
- Ankle-Brachial Index (ABI): Calculation of the ratio between perfusion pressures in the lower leg and upper extremity helps check for evidence of arterial insufficiency. The patient lays down while blood pressure readings are taken in two spots for brachial readings (one on each arm) and two on the lower leg (dorsalis pedis and posterior tibial). The larger readings for each are used to calculate ABI as:
  - ABI = highest ankle pressure/highest brachial pressure.
  - ABI ranges and their indications are: ABI ≥ 1.0 to 1.3, normal; ≥ 0.6 to 0.8, borderline; ≤ 0.5, severe ischemia; and ≤ 0.4, critical ischemia in the limb.

Trendelenburg's Test for Vascular Function

The Trendelenburg's test for vascular function, also known as the retrograde filling test, is used to look at whether varicosities are due to superficial or deep veins and their valves. The distended veins in question are marked while the patient is standing. The person then lies down and raises the leg for approximately a minute to drain the veins. The patient stands up again, and the physical therapist observes the time it takes to fill up the veins. Veins should normally take a minimum of 30 seconds to refill. If they fill more quickly, the patient should lie down again, elevating the leg for a minute. A tourniquet is put on the upper thigh, the patient stands, the tourniquet is taken off, and vein filling is observed again. Rapid filling at less than 30 seconds suggests the perforating vein and deep vein valves are incompetent. In order to locate the site of the incompetent valve, the procedure involving the tourniquet is repeated below the knee and around the upper calf. If rapid filling (< 30 seconds) persists, superficial vein valves allowing backflow should be presumed.

Other Vascular Tests

Additional vascular tests include:

- Manual compression test: Used to distinguish whether a valve in a vein is competent or not, this test involves palpation of the dilated vein and compression and palpation with the other hand about 8 inches higher. The absence of impulse is normal, while the presence of impulse at the higher spot indicates incompetent valves in the segment.
- Allen's test: To evaluate the patency of arteries (radial and ulnar) and circulation in the hand, the patient is asked to bend his arm, holding the hand above the elbow. The clinician compresses the radial and ulnar arteries at the wrist, while the patient clenches the fist then opens it, and one of the arteries is released (repeated later with the other artery). The released artery area should change from blanched to flushed in a matter of seconds if circulation is normal (positive); if abnormal, local circulation is deficient (negative).
- Homan's sign: For the detection of deep vein thrombosis, the calf muscle is squeezed or the foot is rapidly bent back. If the patient experiences pain, deep vein thrombosis is suggested. There are a high degree of false positives.

Noninvasive Vascular Diagnostic Studies

There are both noninvasive and invasive studies that can be performed to diagnose vascular abnormalities. The noninvasive vascular diagnostic studies for the evaluation of vascular flow include:

- Exercise testing: measurement of ankle pressure and peripheral vascular resistance after exercise; lowered ankle pressure suggestive of arterial disease
- Doppler ultrasound: local skin application with a probe of high-frequency, low-intensity sound waves; used to detect, determine the direction of, and characterize blood flow
- Color duplex scanning or imaging: use of ultrasound with a pulsed Doppler detector; visualizes vessels and possible plaques; generates distinctive color changes in regions
- Plethysmography: measures volumetric changes, in this case, the volume of blood distal to a particular area to indicate occlusion
- Computed tomography (CT): x-ray imaging technique used, in this case, to visualize the arterial wall
- Magnetic resonance imaging (MRI): imaging technique using electromagnetic radiation to visualize soft tissues, in this instance, the arterial system
- Magnetic resonance angiography (MRA): utilization of blood as a contrast medium, along with magnetic resonance imaging, to look at the structure of and blood flow through major blood vessels

Invasive Vascular Diagnostic Studies

Contrast angiography or arteriography is the only frequently used type of vascular diagnostic study. It involves injection of a radiopaque dye into the brachial, axillary, femoral, or lumbar arteries; the acquisition of a radiograph; and then, often, use of digital subtraction angiography to remove bony structures from the image. Contrast angiography is useful for the visualization of blood flow dynamics, vascular anatomy, and tumors. It is usually done prior to or during interventions like angioplasty, surgical bypasses, or thrombolytic therapy.

Possible complications may be associated with the injected contrast agent (such as anaphylactic sensitivity reactions), the puncture site (for example, local thrombosis), or the catheter used (these must be checked). Patients who have undergone this procedure should rest for four to eight hours. During this time, they should be given IV fluids to get rid of the contrast dye and monitored for BUN, creatinine, and vital signs. Pressure dressings should be applied at the injection site (observing for hematomas). Patients previously on heparin should not be restarted on the medication until a minimum of four hours after the procedure.

Hematologic Evaluation

A hematologic evaluation should include appropriate history, inspection, and palpation, as well as a number of laboratory studies. The history portion should address patient or familial history of anemia and other blood disorders, malignancies, hemorrhage, and infections. It should document presenting symptoms and their onset and should include questions regarding prior blood transfusions, chemotherapy, radiation therapy, drug therapy, environmental contact with toxins, ease of bruising and wound healing, presence of night sweats or fever, and excessive bleeding or menstrual periods. The patient should be observed for general indications of malaise, presence of petechiae spots or ecchymosis (bruising), respiratory rate, and the color (pale or flushed) of the skin, mucous membranes, nail beds, and palm creases. The doctor usually does the palpation portion of the examination, but the physical therapist might use palpation to evaluate bone and joint pain, range of motion, paresthesia, blood pressure, and heart rate, all of which could have some relevance to hematologic or vascular function. Laboratory studies, such as complete cell counts and coagulation profiles, are discussed elsewhere.

Peripheral Blood Smears and D-Dimer Assay

Peripheral blood smears are taken, and the three types of blood cells—red blood cells (RBCs), white blood cells (WBCs), and platelets—are observed microscopically. The parameters of interest are the size, shape, and hemoglobin distribution of RBCs, the percentage of immature cells among WBCs, and the number and shape of platelets.

The D-dimer assay is used to confirm disseminated intravascular coagulation (DIC) and deep vein thrombosis (DVT) as it is elevated in these conditions, as well as other conditions associated with thrombosis. The assay quantifies D-dimer, a fibrin degradation product that is correlated to blood clot formation.

Arterial vs. Venous Vascular Disorders

Various physical findings either differ in arterial and venous vascular disorders or they may be present in one and not the other. Edema, for example, may be present in arterial disorders but is more characteristic of venous disorders. Only arterial problems, not venous, are associated with loss of muscle mass; diminished or absent pulse is also characteristic of arterial disorders. Pain patterns differ as well. People with arterial conditions tend to have intermittent claudicating, cramping, and more pain with elevation, whereas those with venous conditions tend to have pain that is more aching and is improved with elevation and exercise. Individuals with arterial disorders may have painful ulcers at pressure points, patchy hair areas, thick toenails, and tight skin on their legs, whereas those with venous issues tend to have painless ankle or leg ulcers. Cyanosis, bluish skin due to low blood oxygen levels, is seen in both types of disorders, but people with arterial disorders are pallid while those with vein problems have brown discoloration. The temperature of the skin may also differ, feeling cool in arterial disorders and occasionally warm with venous disorders.

Atherosclerosis

Atherosclerosis is an arterial disorder in which blood flow is impeded by the progressive narrowing of blood vessels due to hemorrhaging, cellular proliferation, and the deposition of lipid-containing plaques. There are a number of risk factors predisposing individuals to atherosclerosis, including hypertension, diabetes, high cholesterol, obesity, cigarette use, family history, and even male gender. Predictors include C-reactive protein (CRP), waist circumference, and weight gain. The vessel stenosis causes blood flow turbulence and diminished perfusion distal to it. The major symptom, pain, is generally not observed until the blood flow is reduced by at least 50%. Other signs include reduced or missing peripheral pulses, existence of bruits upon auscultation of larger arteries, cool and pale skin, high blood pressure, and pain in the toes at rest and in the calf or leg when walking (known as intermittent claudicating). Treatment modalities may incorporate risk factor changes, use of anticoagulant and thrombolytic drugs, surgical resection, and grafting. Atherosclerosis in the extremities may be referred to as peripheral vascular or arterial disease (PVD, PAD).

Intermittent Claudication and Pseudoclaudication

Intermittent claudication refers to tight, cramping pain in the extremities, generally the calves, due to an inadequate blood supply to the muscles. The condition is caused by atherosclerosis or narrowing of the blood vessels. It is induced by exercise and alleviated by rest, standing still, or stopping the activity. The location of the pain experienced is found on one side only, in the buttock, hip, thigh, calf, and/or foot. Intermittent claudicating almost always occurs at a predictable interval when walking on the level, which may or may not decrease when walking uphill or increase when walking downhill.

Pseudoclaudication is pain that is neurologic in derivation, such as stenosis of the lumbar canal or disk disease. Associated leg pain is bilateral, and there is often back pain. People with pseudoclaudication feel pain when standing, which is alleviated by sitting and may or may not be induced by activity. It is often mistaken for intermittent claudication as the pain may be similar in nature; or, instead, the pain may be characterized by tingling, weakness, and clumsiness. The onset of pseudoclaudication is unpredictable and, contrary to the intermittent type, occurs later when walking uphill and earlier when walking downhill.

Aneurysms

An aneurysm is an arterial disorder in which the arterial wall becomes weakened due to a fluid-filled sac or bulge in it. Technically, an aneurysm is defined as at least a 50% increase in vessel diameter with deterioration in all three layers. Aneurysms are believed to be due to things like hereditary collagen abnormalities, degeneration of elastin, atherosclerotic destruction of both of these proteins, and augmented proteolytic enzyme action. Aneurysms can impede blood flow or rupture if they become very large or if there is too much internal pressure. They occur in many areas of the body, potentially producing symptoms such as increased intracranial pressure (cerebral aneurysm), brain hemorrhage, lower back pain (referred pain due to aortic aneurysm), abdominal pain, dyspnea or dysphasia due to compression, and signs associated with local lack of blood supply. Aneurysms are currently managed via surgical resection, graft replacement, or endovascular repair.

Arterial Thrombosis and Arterial Emboli

Arterial thrombosis is the adhesion and aggregation of platelets resulting in clotting in arterial regions of low or stagnant blood flow. An embolus is a mass, generally a blood clot, which blocks a blood vessel. When there is stagnant or erratic blood flow in the heart or aorta, the occlusion is referred to as arterial emboli. About 80% of emboli are cardiac in origin, due mostly to atrial fibrillation or myocardial infarction. Some combination of thrombi and/or emboli is the result. Treatment regimens include anticoagulation measures, with or without partial surgical removal of the atherosclerotic regions, or use of antithrombotic agents (such as tissue factors), possibly in conjunction with aspirin, thienopyridine, and/or warfarin. Patients experiencing an acute arterial embolus must be treated immediately.

Aortic Dissection

Aortic dissection is the internal tearing of the aorta resulting in a false lumen between the middle and outer layers. Aortic dissections are classified as ascending (type A or DeBakey I or II) or descending (type B or DeBakey III). Patients with aortic dissection can present with acute, excruciating pain in the chest or upper back, which moves toward the path of dissection; fainting, diminished, or absent pulses; a murmur associated with aortic regurgitation; and neurological issues. Diagnosis is made by transesophageal echocardiography (TEE) or CT scanning as electrocardiograms readings are very vague.

Hypertension

Hypertension is the elevation of both components of arterial blood pressure while resting. Hypertension can be essential or idiotypic, unrelated to an explicit medical cause. Some predisposing factors are genetics, smoking, obesity, diabetes, atherosclerosis, a high-fat or high-sodium diet, and vasomediator imbalance. There is also secondary hypertension, which is related to known medical sources like hereditary coarctation (constriction) of the aorta, the pituitary disorder Cushing's disease, renovascular diseases, and adrenal tumors. Essential and secondary hypertension can be distinguished by having the patient stand up after sitting; the diastolic BP should rise with essential type, and BP should fall with secondary type. Hypertension can affect the brain, causing cerebrovascular accidents or encephalopathy; the eyes, manifesting as blurred or impaired vision or encephalopathy; the kidneys, in the form of renal insufficiency, possibly progressing to renal failure; and the heart, as myocardial infarction, congestive heart failure, myocardial hypertrophy, or dysrhythmias. Management tools include behavioral modification, exercise, and drugs, such as diuretics, beta and calcium-channel blockers, vasodilators, and angiogenesis-converting enzyme inhibitors.

Review Video: Hypertension
Visit mometrix.com/academy and enter code: 999599

Systemic Vasculitis

Systemic vasculitis refers to tissue damage and the eventual narrowing of blood vessels due to inflammation. The underlying causes of systemic vasculitis are often related to the immune system, as well as infectious agents, tumors, drugs, or unknown causes. Vasculitis can secondarily result in thrombosis, aneurysm development, hemorrhage, occlusion, weight loss, and/or generalized malaise.

Raynaud's Disease and Phenomenon

Raynaud's disease and phenomenon both occur in a cold environment, the former with idiopathic or unknown origin and the latter due to autoimmune, myeloproliferative, or arterial occlusive disorders. The characteristic sign of both is a color change in the digits or tip of the nose from white to blue to red (corresponding to vasoconstriction, cyanosis, and vasodilation). These changes occur symmetrically in Raynaud's disease and erratically in Raynaud's phenomenon. Raynaud's disease is not serious and is often controllable, but Raynaud's phenomenon can lead to atrophy of fat pads and, eventually, gangrene. Management includes a conservative means of warming and shielding affected areas, exercise, administration of calcium-channel blockers and sympatholytics, alternative medical procedures, and diets plentiful in antioxidants and fish oils.

Types of Systemic Vasculitis

The known types of systemic vasculitis are:

- Polyarteritis nodosa: acute necrotizing vasculitis of small or medium arteries; possibly due to hepatitis B virus infection; characteristic manifestations include skin lesions, vasculitic neuropathy, and aneurysm development; managed with corticosteroids, cytotoxic, and antiviral drugs.
- Warner's granulomatosis: granulomatous destruction of small and medium blood vessels, particularly in the respiratory tract and kidneys; symptoms similar to pneumonia; treated with immunosuppressive drugs, corticosteroids, and, if needed, anti-infective agents.
- Giant cell arteritis (GCA): granulomatous destruction of internal elastic lamina of larger arteries; cause unknown; common presentation as temporal arthritis characterized by headache, visual disturbances, jaw and tongue soreness, and possibly polymyalgia rheumatica; can also manifest as Takayasu's arteritis, mainly in upper extremities.
- Thromboangiitis obliterans (Buerger's disease): thrombotic, abscessed occlusions of small and medium arteries of distal extremities; probably collagen or autoimmune disorder; associated with heavy cigarette use; symptoms include rest pain and intermittent claudication in feet; treated with smoking cessation, corticosteroids, vasodilators, anticoagulants, etc.
- Raynaud's disease and phenomenon: discussed elsewhere.

Complex Regional Pain Syndrome

Complex regional pain syndrome (CRPS) is an uncommon disorder of the extremities that can occur after healing post-trauma or surgery. Undiminished sensory nerve signals to the spinal cord cause augmented sympathetic signals to the extremities. CRPS usually occurs in three stages:

- Stage 1, the acute phase: characterized by pain, swelling, and temperature changes from warm to cold.
- Stage 2, the dystrophic phase: where the pain broadens out and there is progressive degeneration of tissue resulting in possible muscle wasting, osteoporosis, lessened range of motion, etc.
- Stage 3, the atrophic or chronic phase: characterized by atrophy, functional impairment, and permanent damage.

CRPS is managed with physical and/or occupational therapy, pharmacologic or surgical interventions to block the sympathetic nerve system, electrical stimulation of the spinal cord, vitamin C, and drugs like baclofen and bisphosphonates.

Compartment Syndrome

Compartment syndrome is a situation in which pressure within a closed bodily compartment causes muscle and nerve necrosis, swelling, and compromise of the circulation. Its causes include trauma, pressure from casts or dressings, or overuse during exercise. The main sign of compartment syndrome is tight, tender pain that worsens when the area is moved or palpated. Other signs include pastiness and lack of sensation or paralysis. Measurement of compartment pressures is generally used for diagnosis; any pressure $\geq$ 32 mm Hg might cause capillary compression. The patient's leg should be elevated and placed in a position that prevents external compression. The patient can be given mannitol to decrease swelling, and if the compartment pressures are very high (> 37 mm Hg), a fasciotomy, in which an incision is made to release the fascia, is indicated.

Varicose Veins

Varicose veins, a venous disorder, are characterized by persistent dilation of veins. They are initially caused by the deterioration of the venous walls, which is followed by inadequate closure of valve cusps. There are two types: primary varicose veins, which stem from the superficial veins, and secondary varicose veins, which arise in the deep and perforating veins. People are at risk for primary varicose veins if they are female, have familial history of them, have had phlebitis (inflammation of the vein), or are in situations that prolong venous stasis, like pregnancy or occupations requiring prolonged standing. Primary varicose veins are generally bilateral, while secondary varicose veins are typically unilateral. Varicose veins are usually visible externally and may bleed profusely if traumatized. Varicose veins can be treated surgically by ligation and stripping, sclerotherapy, behavioral changes, weight loss, elevation of the feet several times daily, use of support stockings, measured exercise, and/or performance of bathing rituals at night.

Deep Venous Thrombosis and Pulmonary Embolism

In venous thrombosis, blood clots form in the superficial or deep veins (DVT), potentially developing into a pulmonary embolism (PE). DVT is a consequence of venous stasis, damage to the vein's endothelium, and/or hypercoagulability. Risk factors include interventions (surgery, central venous catheters, etc.), cardiac issues (hypertension, varicose veins, heart failure, etc.), obesity, and others. A patient presenting with local pain and swelling, dilated veins, redness, warmth, tightness, and minimal fever should be suspected of DVT. DVT is usually diagnosed with ultrasound, although the most specific and sensitive method is magnetic resonance imaging. A positive Homan's sign, in combination with local swelling, redness, and warmth, is fairly diagnostic for DVT. DVT is initially treated with the anticoagulant heparin or, if contraindicated, an inferior vena cava (IVC) filter placed between the thrombus and the lungs.

Other treatments include thrombolytic drugs (streptokinase, urokinase) and surgical thrombectomy. PE, blockage of a pulmonary artery or capillary, can lead to V/Q mismatch, decreased oxygen pressure and oxyhemoglobin saturation, hypoxemia, and, ultimately, pulmonary hypertension or right congestive heart failure. Physical therapy should not be done without medical clearance for DVT and discontinued if a PE develops.

Chronic Venous Insufficiency and Postphlebitic Syndrome

Chronic venous insufficiency and postphlebitic syndrome are two venous disorders with analogous causes and signs. The origin of each is valvular dysfunction resulting from venous thrombosis destruction and to a lesser extent obstruction of the venous outflow. About half of patients with deep venous thrombosis (DVT) develop one of these disorders within five years. Both are characterized by chronic swollen limbs, ulcerations due to venous stasis, and skin changes. These changes often include hemosiderosis, in which the skin develops a gray-brown hyperpigmentation due to the disintegration of extravasated red blood cells, and/or lipodermatosis, fibrosis or toughening of soft tissues in the lower extremities. Management strategies include elevation of the lower extremities above heart level several times daily for 10 to 15 minutes, the use of compression dressings or stockings, avoidance of pressure sources above the legs, skin hygiene and ulceration care, exercises that assist muscles with pumping venous blood, and surgical ligation of veins.

Anemia

Types Caused by Decreased Production or Increased Destruction of RBCs

Anemia is an erythrocytic disorder in which the numbers of red blood cells (RBCs) are depressed relative to normal due to diminished production, abnormal maturation, or augmented destruction. Types caused by decreased RBC production, increased destruction, or blood loss include:

- Aplastic anemia: This condition is characterized by diminished RBC production (also WBCs and platelets) subsequent to bone marrow damage. RBCs are normal or macrocytic (large). Possible signs include fatigue, dyspnea, evidence of bleeding (petechiae, fecal blood, heavy menses, gums, etc.), pallor, fever, and/or sore throat. Management includes transfusion, bone marrow transplantation, corticosteroids, antibiotics, etc.
- Hemolytic anemia: Patients with this disorder undergo the destruction or premature removal of RBCs; the hemolysis can occur intravascularly or extravascularly. Hemolytic anemia may be caused by a genetic defect related to the RBC structure or membrane or can be autoimmune in nature. Signs include fatigue, nausea, fever, chills, low urine output, jaundice, pain in the abdomen or back, and splenomegaly. The condition is managed with fluids, transfusion, corticosteroids, appendectomy, and elimination of the causative factor.

Posthemorrhagic Anemia and Anemia of Chronic Disease

Red blood cells (RBCs) are depleted (and sometimes abnormal) in anemia. Posthemorrhagic anemia is caused by rapid blood loss from some type of trauma. The symptoms depend on the percentage of blood loss. A 20 to 30% loss presents as faintness, hypotension, and rapid heart rate upon exertion. A person with 30 to 40% blood loss will have additional symptoms, such as dyspnea, clamminess, low urine output, and possibly unconsciousness. When blood loss reaches 40 to 50%, shock and possibly death can occur. Patients with posthemorrhagic anemia are managed with IV and oral fluids, transfusions, bleeding control, and supplemental oxygen.

About half of hospitalized patients and many individuals with inflammatory or neoplastic disorders or chronic infections have anemia of chronic disease (ACD). ACD usually requires no treatment.

Iron Deficiency Anemia

Iron deficiency anemia is an extremely common type of anemia caused by abnormal red blood cell maturation. Other types associated with abnormal maturation include vitamin B_{12} anemia, folic acid anemia, and sickle cell anemia. Iron deficiency anemia occurs when iron storage in the bone marrow is decreased through another cause. The reduction encourages production of abnormal RBCs that are microcytic (small) and microchromic (less colored). Some of the initial causes include blood loss (including menses), pregnancy, a diet deficient in iron, and diminished iron absorption in the gastrointestinal tract. Iron-deficiency anemia can present as fatigue, headache, faintness, difficulty swallowing, softening of the nails, strange cravings, and/or pallid palms, earlobes, or conjunctivae. Management includes identification of the source, iron supplementation, and nutritional advice.

Vitamin B_{12} and Folic Acid Anemias

Vitamin B_{12} and folic acid anemias are two types of anemia that result with decreased levels of nutrients. Both cause production of RBCs that are normal in color but macrocytic (large).

Vitamin B_{12} anemia is caused by poor absorption of that vitamin due to enteritis, iliac disease, Crohn's disease, pancreatic insufficiency, or an associated type of anemia called pernicious anemia in which there is no intrinsic factor to bind vitamin B_{12}. Patients often have icterus, a yellow discoloration in certain areas due to increased blood bilirubin, as well as diarrhea, anorexia, oral ulcers, and/or neurologic changes. Diagnosis includes clinical findings, diminished serum vitamin B_{12} levels, high lactate dehydrogenase and mean corpuscular volume (MCV), and a positive urine Schilling test. This anemia is treated with B_{12} supplementation and nutritional advice.

Folic acid or folate deficiency, due to insufficient intake, presents very similarly to vitamin B_{12} deficiency minus the neurologic issues. It is identified by clinical findings, low serum folate levels, and high lactate dehydrogenase and MCV. Patients are given folic acid supplements.

Sickle Cell Anemia

Sickle cell anemia is an inherited condition in which an individual is homozygous recessive for the hemoglobin S variant (HgSS). The SS variant results in red blood cells that are sickle or crescent-shaped when deoxygenated; the misshapen cells impede blood flow and cause tissue damage. Patients with sickle cell anemia present with symptoms like jaundice, renal failure, retinopathy, leg ulcers, systolic murmur and enlarged heart, and particularly intense pain. The pain can occur in many sites but the most common is the lower back, and it can continue for weeks, often requiring hospitalization. The patient may also develop acute chest syndrome (ACS), characterized by a new infiltrate seen on the chest radiograph and accompanied by symptoms that include cough, fever, sputum, difficulty breathing, high heart rate, or hypoxia. Sickle cell anemia is addressed with rest, hydration, supplemental O_2, exchange of RBCs, analgesics, and counseling. If physical therapy is performed, oximetry is suggested to measure oxygenation and exercise intensity.

Review Video: Sickle Cell Disease
Visit mometrix.com/academy and enter code: 603869

Polycythemia

Polycythemia is a condition where increased production of red blood cells, platelets, and myelocytes results in greater blood volume, viscosity, and hemoglobin. These factors make the heart work harder and cause some organs to become congested. Patients have a high hematocrit. Typical symptoms are headache, faintness, blurred vision, venous thrombosis, bleeding, bruising, tiredness, and paresthesia. There are three types:

1. Primary polycythemia (polycythemia vera): augmented RBCs, WBCs, platelets, and stem cells; prone to bleeding and thrombus formation; possible precursor to myelogenous leukemia or myelofibrosis
2. Secondary polycythemia: augmented production of RBCs due to high erythropoietin subsequent to stem cell changes or continual low tissue oxygenation (from COPD etc.); basically a compensatory mechanism for hypoxia
3. Relative polycythemia: short-term increase in RBCs due to dehydration; reversed with fluids

The primary treatment is phlebotomy in which every few days 0.25 to 0.5 liters of blood is taken out of the vein to decrease blood volume and keep hematocrit levels less than 42% for females and under 45% for males. Polycythemia is also treated with myelosuppressive and antiplatelet drugs (hydroxyurea and aspirin respectively), interferon, and radiophosphorus (primary type).

Neutropenia

Neutropenia is defined as a low absolute neutrophil count (ANC). A neutrophil is one type of white blood cell. Neutropenia is caused by bone marrow anomalies, such as leukemia, chemotherapy, sepsis, and some immunological mechanisms. A patient with neutropenia may have difficulty mounting normal inflammatory responses. Neutropenia is treated with drugs to address the underlying infection (antibiotics, antifungal agents), myeloid growth factor, hematopoietic cell transplantation, and symptomatic therapy for fever. The cutoffs for mild, moderate, and severe neutropenia are as follows:

$$\text{Mild} = \text{ANC } 1000 \text{ to } 1500/\mu L$$
$$\text{Moderate} = \text{ANC } 500 \text{ to } 1000/\mu L$$
$$\text{Severe} = \text{ANC} < 500/\mu L$$

Disseminated Intravascular Coagulation

Disseminated intravascular coagulation (DIC) is a potentially fatal thrombocytic syndrome characterized by both hemorrhaging and blood clot formation. It occurs most often after severe infections, in particular subsequent to gram-negative bacterial sepsis, as well as following some type of trauma or formation of antigen-antibody complexes. The process involved is multifaceted, starting with fibrin deposition in the circulation and associated organ and RBC damage. This is followed by a number of events that encourage bleeding, namely platelet consumption and activation of clotting factors and plasmin. Many symptoms that involve hemorrhage, thrombus formation, and/or organ failure in numerous bodily systems can suggest DIC. These systems include cardiopulmonary, renal, integument, gastrointestinal, and neurologic. Diagnosis includes presence of D-dimer, low platelet counts (thrombocytopenia), prolonged PT and APTT, and low fibrinogen levels. Patients with DIC are typically treated with fluid control, oxygen, transfusion (if there is ongoing bleeding), and measures to sustain hemodynamics and the cardiovascular system. Heparin therapy is sometimes used, but this is controversial.

Hemophilia

Hemophilia is a hereditary disease in which a deficiency in a clotting factor leads to spontaneous hemorrhaging. There are four main types of hemophilia, each involving the lack of one clotting factor. The types, lacking factors, and modes of transmission are:

1. Hemophilia A, factor VIII, X-linked recessive
2. Hemophilia B, factor IX, X-linked recessive
3. Hemophilia C, factor XI, autosomal recessive
4. von Willebrand's disease, factor VIII, autosomal dominant

Bleeding episodes occur sporadically, and sites include mucous membranes, muscles, intracranial (the leading cause of death for hemophiliacs), and joints. Bleeding into joints is referred to as hemarthrosis and occurs in about three-quarters of individuals with hemophilia A. Hemarthrosis is characterized by local warmth and soreness, effusion, and limited range of motion, often flexion. General signs of hemophilia include skin discolorations (petechiae, purpura, ecchymosis), hematomas (including intramuscularly), cardiac issues (rapid heart rate and breathing, hypotension), convulsions, confusion, pain, and intracranial bleeding. Management includes pressure to stop bleeding, joint debridement, replacement therapy for the missing factor, and pain control.

Thalassemia

Thalassemia is an inherited, autosomal recessive, thrombocytic disorder in which synthesis of one of the chains of hemoglobin (Hgb) is defective. The abnormal hemoglobin results in destruction of red blood cell membranes, aberrant RBC production, and hemolysis. The disease is classified in terms of increasing severity as thalassemia minor, intermedia, or major, with the need for chronic transfusion of RBCs increasing with severity. Thalassemia is also defined in terms of the affected hemoglobin chains and number of gene alterations. Hgb is made up of two alpha and two beta chains. If the alpha chain is defective, the person has alpha-thalassemia, which can be further differentiated as alpha trait, alpha-thalassemia minor, or Hgb H disease, depending on whether there are one, two, or three gene changes. Of these, only Hgb H disease leads to chronic hemolytic anemia. Defects in the beta chain manifest as beta-thalassemia minor (one chain, generally asymptomatic) or the much more severe, generally life-shortening beta-thalassemia major, in which beta chains are very reduced or missing and patients present with severe anemia, growth problems, jaundice, etc. Management entails transfusion, supplementation with folate and iron-chelating agents, and splenectomy.

Thrombocytopenia

Thrombocytopenia is characterized by a decreased number of platelets. There are numerous possible causes for this decrease, including the depressed production or increased destruction of platelets and altered platelet distribution subsequent to cardiac surgery. Decreased production can be associated with infections, blood vessel damage, drug reactions, or immune responses. Increased destruction is often triggered by malignancies, the presence of antiplatelet antibodies, or myelosuppressive drugs. The patient may present with evidence of bleeding (nose or gum bleeding, blood in urine or stool, petechiae, etc.), elevated heart and breathing rates, renal failure, spleen enlargement, and/or increased intracranial pressure (if bleeding into the cranium). Patients are treated with immunosuppressive agents, plasma transfusions or plasmapheresis containing anticoagulants, appendectomy, and measures addressing the underlying cause. One frequent type is heparin-induced thrombocytopenia (discussed elsewhere).

Heparin-Induced Thrombocytopenia

The most frequent type of drug-related thrombocytopenia is heparin-induced thrombocytopenia (HIT), which usually manifests about a week after heparin therapy is started in a hospital setting. These patients often have deep vein thrombosis (DVT) in both legs and in upper extremities at venous catheter locations, pulmonary emboli, aortic or ileofemoral thrombus, and skin and systemic reactions. There are two types of HIT: type 1, which is asymptomatic clumping of platelets; and type I, which is immune in nature and involves platelet activation and thrombus formation. Heparin-induced thrombocytopenia is diagnosed by a platelet count less than $100 \times 10^9/L$, positive platelet aggregation, and clinical findings as above. There are also tests to measure associated antibodies called heparin-PF. Patients with HIT should be withdrawn from heparin therapy immediately and started on other types of anticoagulants, such as thrombin inhibitors (argatroban, lepirudin, bivalirudin). Patients are also treated with plasmapheresis, immunoglobulins, and measures to restore skin integrity and relieve pain.

Thrombotic and Idiopathic Thrombocytopenic Purpura

Thrombotic thrombocytopenic purpura (TTP) is the swift amassing of thrombi in small blood vessels subsequent to factors, such as infection, estrogen or drug use, pregnancy, or autoimmune diseases. Thrombocytopenia, low platelet counts, and hemolytic anemia are hallmark clinical and diagnostic signs. Diagnosis is also indicated by elevated lactic dehydrogenase (LDH) but normal coagulation tests. Many clinical symptoms are analogous to other conditions, for example, weakness, fever, paleness, petechiae, headache, and confusion. Other symptoms include paresis on one side, seizures, abdominal tenderness from pancreatitis, and renal failure. Management tools for TTP include antiplatelet, corticosteroid, and immunosuppressive drugs; plasmapheresis; plasma exchange; and spleen removal.

Idiopathic thrombocytopenic purpura (ITP) is an autoimmune disease in which specific IgG autoantibodies attach to platelets. The characteristic features are thrombocytopenia and bleeding or local evidence of it. ITP is typically treated with corticosteroids and, eventually, splenectomy.

Lymph Evaluation Procedures and Lymphedema

Evaluation of the lymph system consists of a relevant history and review of systems. History of infection, trauma, surgery, radiation treatments, and lymphedema should be included. Skin integrity and the edematous site should be examined, and the involved limb should be measured either circumferentially or volumetrically by water displacement. The edema, or swelling, that characterizes lymphedema is due to the accumulation of lymph fluid in tissues or certain regions or nodes. There are two types of lymphedema: the hereditary primary type in which lymph nodes or vessels form atypically, and the secondary type caused by lymphatic system damage and subsequent blockage or destruction. Clinical signs form the basis for diagnosis of lymphedema and include swelling distal or next to the site of impairment, fibrotic skin changes, range of motion loss, fatigue, and local tightness and sensory changes. The edema is pitting at first and non-pitting later, and symptoms are not alleviated with elevation. Lymphedema is primarily relieved by manual lymphatic drainage and lymphedema bandaging (discussed on another card).

Reduce the Risk of Lymphedema

The risk of development of lymphedema can be lowered through tactics such as minimizing long-term sitting or standing, supporting an involved upper extremity, elevating the implicated limb, doing pumping exercises, and avoiding use of the involved limb for vigorous or taxing activities. The individual can wear compressive garments during exercise, refrain from wearing other restrictive clothing or jewelry, maintain a healthy weight, limit sodium intake, and avoid hot environments. Blood pressure measurements and injections should not be performed on the involved limb. Skin care is important, with efforts taken to keep it clean, supple, uninfected, and free of abrasions. Hands and feet should be protected, abrasive chemicals and detergents should not be used, and any situation that can raise the body's core temperature (hot bath, etc.) should be avoided.

Management Techniques for Lymphedema

The basic goal of lymphedema management is to improve drainage and redirect the lymphatic fluids that have built up. All management techniques serve to do this either through external compression of tissues, which increases hydrostatic pressures on the tissues, or through elevation of the limb, which improves lymphatic and venous return. Manual lymphatic drainage is the use of measured, light, repetitive stroking and circular massage in conjunction, if possible, with extremity elevation. First, congestion is cleared in larger bodily areas such as the trunk, and then these movements are repeated moving from distal to proximal to the affected lymph node. The patient usually does exercises in conjunction with receiving manual lymphatic draining, typically active range of motion (ROM), low-intensity resistance, and stretching. Compression as a management technique involves the use of no-stretch, non-elastic or low-stretch elastic bandages or garments on the edematous extremity at rest and during exercise. A pneumatic compression pump is an alternative. Other management techniques include elevation of the limb and scrupulous skin care.

Vascular and Hematologic Disorders Drug Treatments

The drug classifications that might be used for treatment of vascular or hematologic disorders include anticoagulants, antiplatelet agents, thrombolytic agents, and colony-stimulating factors. Anticoagulants are used for the prevention and treatment of deep vein thrombosis and pulmonary embolisms, as well as during atrial fibrillation, acute coronary syndrome, and myocardial infarction. All of these agents can cause excessive bleeding, which the physical therapist should monitor. Deep tissue massage is contraindicated. Anticoagulants include coumarin derivatives, direct thrombin inhibitors, factor X_a inhibitors, and various types of heparin. Coumarin derivatives, mainly warfarin (Coumadin), impede synthesis of vitamin K-dependent clotting factors. Direct thrombin inhibitors, such as lepirudin, directly impede thrombin; note that lepirudin can cause anaphylaxis. Fondaparinux (Arixtra) is a selective inhibitor of factor X_a. It can cause the adverse effect of thrombocytopenia as can heparins. Heparins extend clotting time by inhibiting the conversion of prothrombin to thrombin; they include heparin sodium and low-molecular-weight heparins (LMWHs), such as dalteparin sodium, which lessen the possibility of heparin-induced thrombocytopenia.

Antiplatelet Agents

Antiplatelet agents are indicated for the prevention of coronary heart disease, stroke, peripheral arterial disease, thrombosis associated with stent placement, and during acute coronary syndrome (with anticoagulants). These agents can increase bleeding. There are three classifications of antiplatelet agents: glycoprotein IIb/IIIa inhibitors, calculates, and thienopyridine. Glycoprotein IIb/IIIa inhibitors block the receptors on platelets that bind various associated ligands, ultimately preventing platelet aggregation and thrombus formation. An example of this class is eptifibatide. Salicylates, delivered as aspirin alone or in combination with dipyridamole, act by inhibiting cyclooxygenase and prostaglandin synthetase; this impedes formation of thromboxane A_2 and platelet clumping. Thienopyridine, known as clopidogrel or Plavix, blocks ADP receptors and subsequent fibrinogen binding, lessening the probability of platelet adhesion and aggregation.

Thrombolytics and Colony-Stimulating Factors

Thrombolytics (fibrinolytics) are indicated in situations where clotting is an issue, including acute coronary syndrome, ischemic stroke, critical pulmonary embolism, and catheter use. These drugs promote fibrinolysis by binding to fibrin and transforming plasminogen into plasmin. Examples of fibrinolytics are streptokinase and urokinase. The risk of bleeding at various sites with these agents, especially intracranially, warrants cautious use and generally abstention from physical therapy. Colony-stimulating factors (CSF) are indicated when formation of white and red blood cells is needed. There are two classifications: those that stimulate erythropoiesis and those that stimulate granulocyte production. Erythropoiesis-stimulating factors, such as darbepoetin alpha (Aranesp) and epoetin alpha (Epogen, Procrit), promote division and differentiation of erythroid progenitor cells and encourage bone marrow release of reticulocytes into the circulation where they can mature into erythrocytes. Granulocyte-stimulating factors provoke development and activation of granulocytes, either neutrophils (filgrastim) or eosinophils, monocytes, and macrophages (sargramostim). All CSFs can produce hypertension, edema, and a variety of untoward effects.

Anticoagulation Therapy

The goal of coagulation therapy is the achievement of a specific INR range. INR refers to the International Normalized Ratio for prothrombin time (PT). Typically, the goal range for most cardiac or vascular issues (the prevention and treatment of venous thrombosis, systemic embolisms, atrial fibrillation, etc.) is an INR between 2.0 and 3.0; for acute myocardial infarction or heart valve replacement, the goal INR range is 2.5 to 3.5. However, PT/INR and PTT goals should be determined by the doctor. Low or subtherapeutic values of PT/INR or PTT put the patient at risk for thrombus formation, while high or supertherapeutic ones can result in bleeding. The anticoagulants of choice are usually concomitant warfarin and heparin at first (or heparin alone, as it is fast-acting), followed by discontinuation of the heparin and use of warfarin alone. The physical therapist should always monitor for signs of bleeding.

Types of Blood Transfusion Products

Blood transfusion products, which should always be typed for compatibility, include:

- Whole blood: contains blood cells and plasma; rarely used but may be employed in situations of acute major blood loss accompanied by signs of hypovolemic shock or anemia
- Red blood cells (RBCs): indicated for acute or chronic blood loss, oxygen-carrying deficits, or anemia without hypovolemia; used primarily to resolve anemia
- Platelets: concentrated in plasma; used to reestablish clotting and increase platelet counts after or before anticipated blood loss and to avoid or prevent bleeding
- Fresh-frozen plasma (FFP): used to replenish coagulation factors, to quickly reverse warfarin therapy, and for thrombolytic disorders, such as DIC or TTP
- Albumin or plasma protein fraction (PPF): protein-containing fractions relatively devoid of other proteins or containing albumin, globulins, and plasma proteins respectively; primarily used for volume expansion during shock, intense hemorrhaging, or plasma exchange; should normalize blood pressure and blood volume
- Cryoprecipitate: contains certain clotting factors and fibrinogen in plasma; used for replacement of same for uremic bleeding

Adverse Reactions to Transfusion of Blood Products

Incompatible blood transfusion products can cause immediate anaphylactic reactions mediated by IgA antibodies and manifesting as wheezing, cyanosis, abdominal cramps, mild hives, shock, cardiac arrest, etc. Allergic reactions to blood components mediated by IgE and/or IgG antibodies are apparent within minutes and are signified by symptoms like hives, mild wheezing, hypotension, coughing, and rapid breathing and heart rate. Red blood cell destruction, known as an acute hemolytic reaction, also occurs quickly and is characterized by fever with or without chills; cardiac problems, such as hypotension or cardiac arrest; acute renal failure; cyanosis; etc. If blood components are contaminated with bacteria, an acute febrile, septic reaction will occur within a half-hour, possibly leading to shock. Febrile reactions can also be due to reaction of antileukocyte antibodies to transfused plasma proteins, platelets, or white blood cells; these can occur up to a day after transfusion. Acute lung injury within hours of transfusion can also arise if antibodies reactive to the recipient's granulocytes are given; here, a chest radiograph shows pulmonary edema. Further possible complications include air embolisms, circulatory overload, graft-versus-host disease, and others.

Common Vascular Surgical Procedures

Common vascular surgical procedures include embolization therapy, transcatheter thrombolysis, thrombectomy, peripheral vascular bypass grafting, and endarterectomy:

- Embolization therapy is the deliberate occlusion of a vessel via a catheter, usually because of improper blood flow or hemoptysis.
- Transcatheter thrombolysis is the direct infusion of thrombolytic agents through a catheter into a blood clot in an obstructed vessel; its best use is for acute thrombotic arterial occlusions.
- Thrombectomy utilizes a contact catheter placed against a vessel wall and another non-contact device that dispenses a pressurized fluid to disintegrate the clot, which is then extracted.

- In peripheral vascular bypass grafting, an area of vascular occlusion is bypassed using part of one of the saphenous (major leg) veins or a synthetic material, such as Gore-Tex. Patients need monitoring as they can take up to two days to become hemodynamically stable and are prone to many complications, such as site bleeding, renal failure, and thrombosis.
- In aneurysm repair and reconstruction, the aneurysm is clamped off on either side, excised, and interchanged with a synthetic graft.
- Endarterectomy is the excision of a stenotic region of an arterial wall followed by surgical reunion.

Postural Drainage

Postural Drainage

Postural or bronchial drainage is the mobilization of secretions in lung segments from small to larger airways to be cleared by coughing or endotracheal suctioning. Patients are placed in various positions that use gravity to aid the clearing, and one or more manual techniques are used. Postural drainage is used to prevent the accumulation of secretions in those at risk for pulmonary problems, such as patients with cystic fibrosis or chronic bronchitis, those on lengthy bed rest or ventilation, or postoperative patients whose deep breathing is restricted. It is also used to remove accrued secretions from the lungs in patients with lung diseases (COPD, pneumonia, etc.), those with artificial airways, or anyone very weak. Postural drainage is contraindicated in patients who are coughing up blood, have acute untreated conditions like pulmonary edema or heart failure, are cardiovascularly unstable, or have undergone recent neurosurgery. The manual techniques used are percussion, vibration, and shaking (described on another card).

Manual Techniques Used for Postural Drainage

The manual techniques used for postural drainage include percussion, vibration. and shaking. The most common is percussion, where the therapist mechanically displaces thick or adherent mucus by striking the patient's chest wall rhythmically with cupped hands (or mechanically). Percussion should not be done over local fractures or tumors, nor if the individual has a pulmonary embolus, unstable angina, chest wall pain, or parameters that put them at risk for hemorrhage. Vibration is a gentle compression in the direction of chest movement and pulsation with both hands over the chest during expiration only. Shaking, which is also employed only during expiration, is a more dynamic, bouncy type of vibration in which the therapist locks their thumbs and uses both hands, directly enfolding them around the chest wall.

Postural Drainage Positions for Clearing the Right and Left Upper and Middle Lobes of the Lungs

The seven postural drainage positions for clearing the right and left upper and middle lobes, named according to the area of clearance, are:

1. Anterior apical segments: The patient is seated using a back pillow to recline slightly back; percussion is applied under the clavicle.
2. Posterior apical segments: The patient is seated resting forward inclined with the head on a pillow on the table; percussion is employed above the scapulae with fingers curving over the top of the shoulders.
3. Anterior segments: The patient is supine (head up) on the table with pillows supporting the head, neck, and under the knees; percussion is employed bilaterally over the nipple or just above the breast.
4. Left posterior segment: The patient is lying on the right side, head upward, on a table inclined 30 to 45 degrees above horizontal, with a pillow under the head; percussion is employed directly over the left scapula.

5. Right posterior segment: The patient lies flat on a table (no incline) on the left side, propped by pillows under the head and in front; percussion is applied directly over the right scapula.
6. Lingual (projection of left upper lobe analogous to right middle lobe): The patient is lying on the right with head downward on a table inclined 15° to 30°, supported by pillows; percussion is done just under the left breast.
7. Middle lobe: This position is similar to the lingual except the patient is lying on the left side; percussion is done under the right breast.

Postural Drainage Positions for Clearing the Right and Left Lower Lobes of the Lungs

The five postural drainage positions for clearing the right and left lower lung lobes are (named according to area of clearance):

1. Anterior segments: The patient lies supine on a 30- to 45-degree incline with head downward and pillow support under the knees and head; percussion is employed bilaterally over the lower portion of the ribs.
2. Posterior segments: The patient lays prone, face on the table, and facing downward on a 30- to 45-degree incline with pillow support under the hips; percussion is done bilaterally over the lower part of the ribs.
3. Left lateral segment: The patient lays on the right side facing downward on a 30- to 45-degree incline with pillow support; percussion is employed over the lower lateral aspect of the left rib cage.
4. Right lateral segment: This position is similar to the left lateral segment except the patient is lying on the left side; percussion is applied over the lower lateral portion of the right rib cage.
5. Superior segments: The patient lies prone (head down) on a non-inclined table with a pillow under the abdomen; percussion is done bilaterally, directly below the scapulae (shoulder blade).

Guidelines for Carrying Out Postural Drainage

Postural drainage is done up to four times daily depending on secretion viscosity. It is best performed before or after aerosol therapy for maximum clearance. Good times to do postural drainage are early in the morning to clear up overnight accumulation and early evening to facilitate sleeping but never right after a meal. Sessions should last no longer than an hour as they are fatiguing. Beforehand, the patient should be taught deep breathing and effective coughing. Their clothing should be loose and thin. All needed adjunct equipment should be readily available. Establish which segments need to be drained, and check vital signs, breath sounds, and patient color before beginning. Percussion of each segment is done for 5 to 10 minutes with the patient breathing deeply but not hyperventilating. The patient should be persuaded to take deep double coughs as needed. If he cannot cough instinctively, he should be told to take a number of deep, successive breaths while the therapist applies vibration during expiration. The therapist moves on to the next segment as above regardless of whether there is a productive cough. Afterwards, the patient should sit up and rest while the clinician watches for indications of postural hypotension, checks vital signs and breath sounds, and characterizes secretions produced.

Management of Thoracic Surgery Patients

Patients who have undergone thoracic surgery have substantial chest pain, which makes lung expansion, chest wall mobility, and coughing difficult. Thus, they are prone to accretion of pulmonary secretions and secondary issues, such as pneumonia. In addition, the general anesthesia used during the procedure depresses ciliary action, cough reflexes, and the respiratory center, while the intubation procedure further decreases ciliary action, irritates the mucosal surfaces, and initiates muscle spasms. Pain at the incision depresses chest wall compliance and effective coughing, resulting in shallow breathing and cough. Pain medications given postoperatively also tend to depress the respiratory center and ciliary activity. Post-surgery, the patient is weak and sedentary, leading to pooling of secretions and inefficiency of the cough pump. All of these factors make it essential that a comprehensive program incorporates breathing and coughing exercises, secretion removal, shoulder range-of-motion exercises, posture awareness instruction, and graded aerobic conditioning.

Care Plan for Post-Thoracic Surgery Patients

The patient's status is first determined in terms of vital signs, sputum drainage into chest tubes, etc. The individual should be placed in a semi-Fowler's position, an approximate 30-degree elevation of the bed's head, coupled with slight flexion in the knees and hips, to support relaxation and reduce pain by placing less traction on the incision. Steps to optimize ventilation and re-inflate lung tissue should be initiated to prevent pneumonia or collapsed lung. Deep breathing exercises are initiated on the day of surgery (continuing until the patient is ambulatory), followed by the addition of incentive spirometry or inspiratory resistance exercises. Once the patient is alert, measures to support secretion removal should be instituted, including effective coughing, functional mobility, and modified postural drainage if secretions accrue. Lower-extremity exercises, such as ankle pumping, should be started a day post-surgery to optimize circulation there and prevent DVT and PE. To recoup range of motion (ROM) in the shoulders, shoulder relaxation, active-assistive, and, eventually, active ROM exercises should be initiated. Correct postural alignment (symmetrical) and trunk positioning should be taught. Once chest tubes are eliminated and the patient can get up, progressive graded ambulation or stationary cycling should be started to increase exercise tolerance.

Diaphragmatic Breathing

Diaphragmatic breathing is controlled breathing that maximizes utilization of the diaphragm and reduces the use of accessory muscles (shoulder, neck). This is intended to improve the efficiency of ventilation, make breathing less taxing, increase diaphragmatic movement, augment gas exchange and oxygenation, and facilitate mobilization of secretions during postural drainage. The patient should be in a position that takes advantage of gravity, such as the semi-Fowler's position. If the person instinctively employs accessory muscles, relaxation exercises, such as shoulder rolls or shrugs, should be done first. The therapist places his hand(s) on the patient's rectus abdominis below the anterior costal margin and instructs the patient to breathe in gradually and deeply through the nose and then exhale slowly via the mouth. Shoulders and upper chest should be relaxed, and the individual should refrain from hyperventilation. If necessary, inspiration can be aided by sequential nasal sniffing actions. The patient's understanding of the process can be facilitated by replacing the therapist's hand with his own to feel the movement.

Segmental Breathing

Segmental breathing is the expansion of localized regions of the lungs while keeping other areas quiet. It is useful for expansion of specific areas that are hypoventilated or during postural drainage procedures. One type of segmental breathing is lateral costal (lateral basal) expansion, deep breathing while concentrating on lower rib cage movement, which assists diaphragmatic excursion. This is performed first with the patient supine with legs propped, again with the patient seated, and a final time to teach the patient. The method has several steps. The therapist places his hands on the lateral aspect of the lower ribs and directs the patient to breathe out, during which the clinician applies pressure onto the patient's ribs with the palms. A rapid, downward, inward stretch is then applied. As the patient breathes in, he applies gentle manual resistance to the lower ribs. The patient can use his hands, a towel, or a belt to facilitate the maneuver. Another version is posterior basal expansion, recommended for patients confined to bed after surgery. The patient sits up and bends forward over a pillow. The therapist positions his hands over the posterior aspect of the lower ribs and uses the same type of pressure, stretch, and resistance sequence as for the lateral version.

PREVENT AND ALLEVIATE EPISODES OF DYSPNEA

Dyspnea, or shortness of breath upon exertion or exposure to allergens, commonly occurs in patients with chronic obstructive pulmonary disease (COPD). Episodes of dyspnea can be averted through a combination of controlled breathing techniques, pacing of functional activities within the individual's ventilatory capacity, and awareness. The pursed-lip breathing technique is generally used to relieve episodes of dyspnea that do occur. Pursed-lip breathing is believed to maintain airway patency by creating back pressure in the airways.

The technique for recovery involves having patients sit or stand and bend forward, supporting themselves on a table, in order to encourage diaphragmatic breathing. They then use pursed-lip breathing during expiration, which involves breathing in slowly through the nose and then out gently through pursed or lightly touching lips. Patients should be relaxed, and they should use diaphragmatic breathing, shunning use of accessory abdominal muscles. Patients should be directed to continue this breathing until they are no longer short of breath.

POSITIVE EXPIRATORY PRESSURE BREATHING

Positive expiratory pressure breathing uses a special mouthpiece or mask to control the resistance to airflow, thus increasing patency during exhalation and mobilizing and improving clearance of secretions. The patient is upright, if possible, in a seated position with elbows placed on a table. While wearing the mask or mouthpiece, the patient inhales, sustains the inspiration for 2 to 3 seconds, and exhales aided by active, but not forceful, help from the low (or sometimes higher) pressure of the device. This cycle is repeated 10 to 15 times, after which the patient takes off the device and coughs to discharge secretions. The sequence is reiterated several more times, up to about 15 minutes in total.

GLOSSOPHARYNGEAL BREATHING

Glossopharyngeal breathing is used primarily in patients who are on ventilators due to some sort of neuromuscular damage that influences the innervation of the diaphragm. The main purpose of the technique is to enhance inspiratory capacity. The patient takes a series of up to about 10 gulps of air and then closes the mouth. He then uses the tongue to move air back and trap it in the pharynx. When the glottis opens, the air is propelled into the lungs.

RESPIRATORY RESISTANCE TRAINING

Respiratory resistance training (RRT) is a strengthening of or improvement in the endurance of ventilatory muscles in patients with pulmonary diseases that have damaged these muscles. Most RRT concentrates on training the muscles of inspiration, such as the abdominal muscles and diaphragm. The major types of RRT are:

- Inspiratory resistance training: This is designed to strengthen and improve the stamina of the muscles of inspiration by making them work harder. The patient breathes in through the mouth via a resistive training apparatus (pressure or airflow-based) for an indicated amount of time several times daily. The time of use is increased periodically up to 20 to 30 minutes per session.

- Incentive respiratory spirometry: This is designed to increase the volume of air inspired. It is generally used post-surgically to avert alveolar collapse and atelectasis. The patient is placed in a semi-reclined or other comfortable position and asked to breath normally four times with maximum expiration on the fourth breath. They then put a spirometer (a small device that provides feedback on whether maximum inspiration is achieved) in the mouth and inhale maximally for several seconds through its mouthpiece to a goal setting. This is done 5 to 10 times daily.

Exercises to Mobilize the Chest

Chest mobilization exercises are any drills that mix active movements of the trunk with deep breathing. These exercises are indicated when the lack of mobility of trunk muscles impacts ventilation or postural alignment. Some specific exercises include:

- Mobilization of one side of the chest: The seated patient bends away from the taut side for lengthening and chest expansion. He then uses a fisted hand to push into the tight lateral aspect while bending into that tight side and exhaling. He can also lift the arm on the taut side and bend to the opposite side for further stretch.
- Mobilization of the upper chest and stretching of pectoralis muscles: The patient is seated in a chair with hands clutched behind the head. He pulls the arms back during deep inspiration and forward until elbows touch during expiration.
- Mobilization of the upper chest and shoulders: While seated, the individual lifts both arms directly overhead during inspiration and then bends fully forward, touching the floor during expiration.

Coughing

Normal Cough Mechanism and Issues That Decrease Its Effectiveness

Normally, the cough pump, or cough mechanism, follows a series of steps. In order to cough, a person takes a deep inspiration, after which the glottis closes and the vocal cords tighten. The abdominal muscles contract and the diaphragm rises up, a combination that increases intrathoracic and intraabdominal pressures. Next, the glottis opens, and air is expelled, or expired. Cilia in the epithelial layers of the bronchial tree normally help facilitate the expulsion of secretions.

The cough mechanism is compromised if there is decreased inspiratory capacity due to factors like lung disease, chest trauma, thoracic or abdominal surgery, or injuries that impact neuromuscular control (such as spinal cord injury). Spinal cord injuries above the T12 level or other muscular diseases, such as muscular dystrophy, weaken abdominals, making it difficult to forcibly expel air. Procedures such as intubation and anesthesia, as well as some lung diseases, diminish ciliary action. Similarly, certain procedures (e.g., intubation) and certain conditions (for example, cystic fibrosis) increase or thicken mucus production.

Perform an Effective Cough

After observing the patient's cough, have him assume a relaxed position, preferably seated or leaning forward slightly. The patient is taught controlled diaphragmatic breathing using deep inspirations. The therapist then demonstrates a deep double cough, as well as the correct muscle action of abdominal contraction during coughing. Patients should experience this contraction by placing their hands on their own abdomen and huffing three times upon expiration. Another way to feel a contraction is to make a "K" sound. The patient is then told to take, in sequence, a deep inspiration and a sharp double cough. An effective cough is generally observed after two rounds. Patients with weak inspiratory or abdominal muscles may need an abdominal binder or they may need to use glossopharyngeal breathing. Patients should never be permitted to gasp in air since this can cause fatigue, increased airway resistance, and/or mucus plugging.

Adjunct Techniques for More Effective Coughing or Improvement of Airway Clearance

There are manual-assisted methods (both therapist and self types) to improve coughing and airway clearance. Manual-assisted cough techniques enhance the cough mechanism by applying pressure to the abdominal area, which creates more intra-abdominal pressure and forceful coughing. For therapist-assisted manual cough techniques, the patient is either supine (or semi-reclined) or seated. In the supine method, the therapist places the heels of both hands, one on top of the other, on the patient's abdomen just distal to the xiphoid process (lowest segment of breastbone). The therapist manually aids the patient during the coughing and expiration phase by compressing the abdomen inward and upward, thrusting the diaphragm upward. If the patient is seated, the therapist stands behind the patient and applies similar pressure. In the self-assisted technique, the patient is seated with arms crossed over the abdomen or intertwined hands below the xiphoid process. He should use the wrists or forearms to do the same type of pushing while leaning forward during the coughing phase. Self-assistance may also include splinting (use of pillow or hands over an incision during coughing), humidification, and/or tracheal stimulation.

Exercise Regimens for Lymphedema Management

Exercise regimens for management of lymphedema should target deep breathing and relaxation, flexibility, strengthening and muscular endurance, cardiovascular endurance, and lymphatic drainage exercises:

- Deep breathing exercises are believed to create a continual pumping action that moves lymphatic fluids, while relaxation exercises at the start of a session serve to decrease muscle tension.
- Flexibility exercises, generally self-stretching, increase joint and tissue mobility.
- Strengthening and endurance resistive exercises are only suitable if done with light resistance and minimal muscle fatigue. If performed, lymphedema should be monitored by measuring local circumference changes and skin texture.
- Cardiovascular conditioning exercises (ergometry, walking, etc.) are important components of lymphedema management because they enhance circulation and lymphatic flow. Usually 30 minutes of aerobics are done with the intensity dependent on the presence or absence of edema (approximately 40 to 50% and up to 80% target heart rate, respectively).
- Lymphatic drainage or pumping exercises should be included to improve lymphatic fluid movement, after which the patient should rest with the involved extremity elevated for 30 minutes.

Upper- and Lower-Extremity Lymphedema Management Exercises

The following exercises, which facilitate relaxation and clearance of central channels and nodes, can be used for management of upper- and lower-extremity lymphedema and should be completed first:

- Total body relaxation exercises: The supine patient isometrically contracts and relaxes muscles while deep breathing. The sequence is generally lower trunk (abdominals, erector spinae), hips, legs, feet, toes, upper back, shoulders, upper arms, forearms, wrist, fingers, neck, and face. After relaxing briefly, the sequence is repeated with diaphragmatic breathing.
- Posterior pelvic tilts and partial curl-ups while supine.

- Knee-to-chest movements: While lying on the back, the patient holds one lower leg and pulls the knee to the chest. This is done about 15 times for each leg to target the lingual (lower trunk) nodes.
- Cervical range-of-motion (ROM) exercises: The patient does rotation and lateral flexion exercises, holding each for five counts through five repetitions.
- Scapular exercises: The patient performs active shoulder shrugs, rolls, and retraction and protraction, each for five repetitions of five counts.

Upper-Extremity Lymphedema Management Exercises

After the general exercises discussed on another card, if upper-extremity clearance is the concern, the below movements are done in a proximal to distal manner. Throughout, the patient should occasionally perform self-massage on the uninvolved side, from axilla to chest. The exercises include:

- Active circumfusion of the arm: The supine patient lifts each arm in turn and makes 6- to 12-inch diameter circles in both directions, five repetitions each.
- Foam roll exercises: Lying supine and supported on a foam roll, the patient does shoulder horizontal abduction, adduction, flexion, and extension drills on each side.
- Bilateral hand press: The patient raises the arms to at least shoulder level with palms together in front of the chest. He breathes in for a count of five while pressing the palms together to isometrically contract the pectoralis majors.
- Shoulder mobility: Various exercises, such as the towel stretch, are used to improve shoulder mobility.
- Unilateral arm exercises with involved arm: A series of seated or supine exercises where the involved arm is supported at shoulder level or elevated overhead. These include shoulder rotation, elbow flexion and extension, wrist circumfusion, and hand opening and closure. Two-sided horizontal abduction and adduction of shoulders. Standing overhead (above shoulder level) wall press.
- Wrist and finger exercises (if applicable): These incorporate finger movements in conjunction with a wall press or with hands held above shoulder level. Partial curl-ups. Supine rest: Patient lays supine with the extremity elevated for 30 minutes.

Lower-Extremity Lymphedema Management Exercises

After performing general exercises for lymphedema clearance (de-scribed elsewhere), the patient should perform self-massage of the axillary lymph nodes on the involved side and periodically massage the lower abdominals, moving toward the axilla on the involved side.

Appropriate exercises are:

- Knee-to-chest exercises while supine: Patient should do 15 repetitions with each leg, starting with the uninvolved one.
- Bilateral knees-to-chest while supine: Both knees and hips are flexed and, while grasping the thighs, are brought to the chest together, 10 to 15 times.
- Gluteal setting and posterior pelvic tilts: Patient should perform five repetitions.
- External rotation of hips: The patient lies on the back with legs lifted, supported by a wedge or against the wall, and compresses the buttocks together to externally rotate the hips. Several rotations should be done.

- Knee flexion of involved leg: The supine patient bends the involved hip and knee enough to clear the popliteal area behind the knee and foot from the table, moving the heel back toward the buttocks. The patient should do this approximately 15 times. Active plantarflexion, dorsiflexion, and circumduction of the ankles: Patient performs these exercises while lying on the back with the involved or both legs elevated and propped up against a wall or door frame. Sliding feet down and up wall while in external rotation.
- Cycling and scissor-like movements: Patient performs these while supine with legs in the air.
- Hip adduction across midline: Patient performs this exercise while supine.

Dysfunctions Related to Breast Cancer

Patients with breast cancer commonly undergo removal of at least some portion of their breast(s), as well as excision or irradiation of the nearby axillary lymph nodes. Both surgery and radiation disrupt lymphatic circulation and lead to lymphedema in the arm area, as well as impaired shoulder mobility. Surgical options include mastectomy (complete removal of the breast) and breast-conserving procedures (lumpectomy, segmental mastectomy), but regardless of the procedure used, a lymphadenectomy, or dissection of the axillary lymph node, is a standard adjunct. In addition to lymphedema, postoperatively the patient can experience incisional, posterior cervical, and shoulder girdle pain; vascular and pulmonary complications (particularly DVT and/or pneumonia); chest wall adhesions; and diminished shoulder mobility. The affected upper extremity will be weak, particularly in the shoulder area, and the patient may have depressed grip strength, fatigue, posture problems (for example, rounded shoulders due to pain or tightness), and psychological problems.

Postoperative Breast Cancer Patient Management

The main goals of physical therapy management of the postoperative breast cancer patient are the restitution of shoulder function, recouping a general level of fitness, and the prevention and/or management of lymphedema. General guidelines to achieve these goals include the integration of exercise, as well as massage and compression, into the patient's care plan; the use of shoulder range-of-motion (ROM) exercises as early as possible to preclude mobility impairments; the inclusion of aerobic training; and a gradual increase in the intensity of all exercises to a moderate level. Lymphedema should be specifically addressed through elevation and compression of the involved upper extremity and the use of manual lymphatic drainage massage, if it develops. The probability of restricted upper-extremity mobility should be addressed with active-assistive and active ROM exercises for the shoulder, elbow, and hand and self-stretching once the incision has healed. Upper-extremity ergometry is recommended for strength development, and low-intensity aerobics, such as walking or cycling, are also suggested. The possibility of cardiopulmonary complications should be addressed with patient training in deep breathing, effective coughing, and calf pumping.

Musculoskeletal System

Pain

Systemic, Musculoskeletal, and Other Types of Pain

Systemic pain generally disturbs sleep, while musculoskeletal pain typically diminishes at night. The quality of pain is normally deep aching or throbbing for systemic issues, whereas musculoskeletal problems cause sharp or superficial aches. Systemic pain is constant or comes in waves or spasms; musculoskeletal pain is generally continuous or intermittent. Mechanical stress on the painful area intensifies musculoskeletal pain but not systemic pain, which, in fact, is usually reduced with pressure. Musculoskeletal pain generally lessens once activity ceases. Pain related to muscles, ligaments, and joint capsules is dull and aching, often with muscle cramping. Bone pain is deeper and nagging. Sharp pain is usually associated with issues related to nerves, nerve roots, or fractures, the latter being quite severe and excruciating. If sympathetic nerves are affected, the pain is burning and stinging. Vascular pain is usually throbbing and diffuse. Pain identifiable with specific anatomic pathways and structures is often referred to as neuropathic pain, whereas less identifiable pain is termed somatic pain.

Pain Rating Scales and Questionnaires

There are simple pain rating scales that can be used. These include visual-analog scales, in which the patient marks a line from 0 (no pain) to 10 (most severe pain) where he perceives pain status currently or any time in the past. A thermometer pain rating scale with markings ranging from "no pain at all" up to "the pain is almost unbearable" is a variation of this. The patient can also verbalize the degree of pain or use other types of scales.

There are a number of available questionnaires for patients to use to describe pain. The frequently used McGill-Melzack Pain Questionnaire has sections that ask the patient to mark the location of pain, circle words that describe the pain, evaluate pain change over time, and rate the strength of pain under various conditions. The short-form version asks the patient to evaluate the degree to which he has each of 12 types of pain. These forms both use descriptors that are sensory and affective, meaning words that describe true sensory pain, as opposed to those that might be used when a person just thinks he has pain (affected pain).

Joint Abnormalities

Joints must perform properly for movement and range of motion. Joints that are locking cannot be completely extended and generally cannot go through a full range of motion. Pseudolocking is similar but refers to a lack of extension and flexion at different times. Spasm locking occurs with muscle spasm or quick movement. Another joint problem is giving way due to weak muscles or inhibition of reflexes. Joint laxity is greater than normal range of motion, which can generally be controlled and is not pathological; it is related to ligament function and joint capsule resistance. Joint laxity that is associated with symptoms and pathology and cannot be controlled is called hypermobility. Hypermobility results in various types of joint instability.

Types of Joint Instability

Joint instability is excessive, uncontrollable, pathologically derived joint hypermobility. For assessment purposes, there are two general types of joint instability. The first is translational instability, the loss of small, arthrokinematic joint movements. The other is anatomical instability, which is more excessive and precedent to dislocation or subluxation (partial dislocation). Both types can cause functional instability, or the lack of ability to control joint movement during functional activities. Both can also be initiated voluntarily through muscle contraction or involuntarily due to positioning. When assessing joint stability, the observer should look for injuries on both sides of the joint (the circle concept of instability).

Assessment for Musculoskeletal Problems

The three most important things to observe are the patient's posture, limb position, and skin integrity. Normal standing posture and gait should be observed surreptitiously before the formal assessment. Indications of overt pain include guarding (stiff, rigid movements), bracing weight primarily on one extended limb, rubbing the painful area, grimacing, and sighing accompanied by shoulder movement. The formal assessment is performed in a private area with the patient in underwear. Here, the observer should note whether the patient's body alignment is straight and whether there are any noticeable structural or functional deformities that restrict range of motion, cause malalignment, change bone shape, or cause dislocation. The patient's resting posture should be observed standing, sitting, and supine, including assessment of head, neck, and extremities for alignment, symmetry, atrophy, and deformities. The limb positions should be observed for equality and symmetry, including factors like size, color, position, temperature, etc. The skin should be inspected for integrity, scarring, color changes, bruising, texture, lacerations, edema, pressure sores, and surgical incisions. The examiner should also note crepitus, snapping, or other abnormal sounds in joints during movement.

Examination for Musculoskeletal Issues

Prior to examination, informed consent must be obtained. The normal uninvolved side should be tested first to establish a baseline. The order of movements to be tested is first active, then passive, resisted isometric, and, lastly, painful movements. During active movements, overpressure may be applied carefully in order to feel the joint. All types of movements should be repeated a number of times or sustained for a given amount of time to note differences in degree or type of symptoms, weakness, or precipitate vascular problems. The resisted isometric movements are performed with the joint in a neutral or resting position to avoid stress. Ligamentous tests should be done by applying gentle, repeated stress only up to the point where the patient experiences pain. Myotome testing for muscle groups with common innervation should involve holding the contractions for 5 seconds. The patient should be informed he may have symptoms after the examination. Any findings outside the scope of the therapist's practice indicate the need for referral.

Strains, Sprains, and Tendon Injuries

Strains are tears in the contractile fibers of the muscles and are defined in terms of the degree of tearing (1^0: few fibers, 2^0: approximately half, 3^0: all ruptured). They are due to overstretching, overloading, or sometimes crushing. Sprains are tears in ligaments, which are considered inert tissues as they do contract and are not neurologic. The degree of tearing again defines them, similar to strains; they are also due to overload or overstretch. Both strains and sprains are felt acutely; cause pain on stretching, unless third degree; cause moderate to major weakness and swelling, if second or third degree; and decrease range of motion, unless severe, in which case the response depends on swelling. Some differences observed: muscle spasms are only minor with sprains, but can be much more severe with strains; joint play is only excessive in third-degree sprains; isometric contractions only produce pain if there is a strain; and functional losses present differently. To the latter point, second- and, particularly, third-degree strains or sprains produce reflex inhibition and instability, respectively.

Paratenonitis and tendinosis refer to inflammation and damage to contractile tendons, respectively, as a result of overuse, overstretch, or overload. They tend to be more chronic and may cause crepitus, or popping sounds.

Patient Movement during Examination

Observation of Active Movements for Potential Musculoskeletal Problems

Stated in order, active, passive, and resisted isometric movements are tested during examination for potential musculoskeletal problems. Patients should be asked to perform active or physiological movements, unless a fracture is healing or stress would be put on recently healed soft tissues. The examiner observes and records the point at which pain occurs, whether the movement intensifies the pain, the quality of the pain, the patient's reaction, the extent and nature of restriction, the movement pattern and rhythm, and the movement of associated joints. It is important to note whether the patient uses cheating or trick movements to complete the activity, such as shoulder hiking, and where in the arc of movement the symptoms transpire.

Observation of Passive Movements for Potential Musculoskeletal Problems

Passive, or anatomical, movements are generally observed after active movements. Passive movements involve putting the joint through gentle movements within its range of motion (ROM) while the patient is relaxed. Just as with active movements, the examiner should note when and where during each movement pain is initiated, if the movement increases the intensity and quality of pain, limitations to movement, and movement of associated joints. Measurements of the angles for range of motion are estimated or, preferably quantified, with instruments such as a goniometer or inclinometer. The normal expected joint mobility varies for individuals, but in general, if outside the functional range, it can be classified as limited hypomobility or excessive hypermobility (laxity). Another important observation is the end feel, which is the sensation the examiner feels by applying overpressure at the end of the ROM (differentiated in detail on another card).

Normal End Feels

End feel is the sensation the examiner feels while applying overpressure at the end of a range-of-motion test (passive or, sometimes, active). It is a subjective parameter, but with time should become consistent for the particular examiner. The classification system of Cyriax is often used.

This system identifies three normal end feels:

1. Bone to bone: hard and painless, such as with elbow extension
2. Soft tissue approximation: a spongy compressive feel, such as with elbow or knee flexion
3. Tissue stretch: either elastic (soft) or capsular (hard), depending on the thickness and type of tissue being stretched; due to capsule or ligament issues, such as shoulder lateral rotation or ankle dorsiflexion

Abnormal End Feels

There are many possible abnormal end feels during examination for range of motion (ROM) that are good diagnostic aids for pinpointing the associated problem. Muscle spasms, movement followed by its abrupt halting, can occur early or late in the ROM. Early muscle spasms are generally due to acute injury and inflammation, whereas late muscle spasms are primarily a result of instability. Spasticity, due to upper motor neuron lesions, may feel fairly similar. Tight muscles have a sensation similar to normal tissue stretch but 'mushier.' An abnormal bone-to-bone end feel is one in which the constraint occurs before the normal end of ROM or at an unusual time, usually due to bony growths. Reduced ROM from capsular issues can give a hard capsular end feel, similar to tissue stretch but thicker, or a soft capsular end feel, which is akin to normal tissue stretch but with restricted ROM. Examples of abnormal hard or soft capsular responses include frozen shoulders and synovial inflammation, respectively. Other abnormal types are an empty end feel, which is very painful and indicates no mechanical resistance, such as with acute subacromial bursitis; and springy block type, a tissue stretch in an unexpected place, usually a joint with a meniscus, such as a knee meniscus tear.

Capsular vs Noncapsular Patterns of Limitation

Capsular patterns of limitation, or restriction, are observed when joints controlled by muscles are involved. The possible causes are muscle spasms, capsular contractions, and osteophyte (bony growth) formation. The list of common capsular patterns of joints is extensive, with examples including restricted mouth opening for the temporomandibular joint, limitations of the hip joint (flexion, abduction, medial rotation), restricted knee flexion or extension, side flexion, rotation and extension for the thoracic or lumbar spine, and many others.

Atypical patterns are considered noncapsular, which may be due to an absent capsular reaction, ligamentous adhesion, internal derangement (at knee, ankle, or elbow), or extra-articular lesion, which influences the joint restricted.

Evaluation for Inert Tissue Problems

Inert tissues are those that are not contractile (muscles, tendons, attachments) or nervous tissues. Inert tissues include ligaments, joint capsules, bursae (fluid-filled sacs), cartilage, blood vessels, and dura mater (nervous tissue covering). Evaluations for inert tissue problems should be done after active and passive movements. If there are lesions in inert tissues, one of four typical patterns for range-of-motion (ROM) restriction will be observed:

1. Painless, full ROM: suggesting no lesion on the inert tissues being tested
2. Pain and limited ROM in every direction: indicative of total joint involvement, as seen with arthritis or capsulitis
3. Pain with limited or excessive ROM in some directions but not others: caused by anything that produces a noncapsular pattern of limitation
4. Painless, limited ROM: typically due to osteoarthritis

Isometric Movements

Resisted Isometric Movements

Resisted isometric movements are strong voluntary muscle contractions done with the joint in a resting position. The joint angle and muscle length are kept constant. Characteristic isometric movements involve holding something or pressing against an immovable force. They are performed after other testing. They test primarily for pain elicited in contractile tissues (muscle, tendon), the bone insertion, or associated innervation because extraneous movement that might involve inert tissues is minimalized. Isometric movements are appropriate only with a muscle strength grade between 3 and 5, which is basically some-to-complete range of motion against gravity. The examiner observes the strength of the contraction and whether the contraction causes pain; if so, he notes the intensity and quality of pain. He also identifies the type of contraction triggering the problem. This may require adjunct methods, such as testing for eccentric or concentric contractions. Resisted isometric movements should cause pain in the same direction as active movements if there is some type of contractile (muscle strain, tendinopathies) or associated (nervous system, avulsion, psychological) weakness.

Pain and Movement Patterns Associated with Resisted Isometric Movements

Resisted isometric movements mainly test for pain associated with contractile and nervous system tissues. There are four typical patterns seen:

1. Painless, strong movement: indicates noninvolvement of the area being tested; can be due to first- or second-degree muscle strains, which cause reflex inhibition and weakness or cogwheel contractions
2. Pain and relatively strong movement: implies some sort of local muscle or tendon lesion; can also be caused by avulsion fractures or tendinopathies, including tendinosis (intratendinous degeneration), paratenonitis (inflammation of the external layer of the tendon), a combination of the two, or tendonitis/partial rupture of the tendon
3. Pain and weak movement: indicates a fracture or other severe joint lesion
4. Painless, weak movement: due to contractile or nervous issues; usually caused by neurologic involvement at the peripheral nerve or nerve root level, tendon rupture, or, to a lesser extent, third-degree muscle strains (visible bulge often observed)

Postural vs Phasic Muscles

Theory of postural versus phasic muscles is expounded by Janda, who maintained that muscles are either postural or phasic. Postural, or tonic, muscles are those needed to preserve upright posture, thus making them prone to tightness and hypertonicity. This includes muscles like the gastrocnemius and soleus in the calf, the erector spinae associated with the spine, the pectoralis major, hamstrings, and many others. In addition to postural functions, these muscles are associated with flexor reflexes, generally connect to two joints, are promptly activated during movement, and are resistant to atrophy.

Most other muscles are phasic muscles not directly involved in postural functions, such as the rectus abdominis, external obliques, and gluteus maximus. Phasic muscles are more prone to atrophy, inhibition, hypotonia, and weakness. They are primarily one-joint muscles, generally associated with extensor reflexes, and not quickly activated during movement.

There can be both tight hypertonic postural and weak lengthened phasic muscles at a particular joint. There are generally force couples, or counteracting groups of muscles, around joints that can disrupt balance, stability, or smoothness of movement if one muscle is weak.

Contraction Types

Eccentric contractions are more dynamic and involve generation of a force that is less than the external load, during which muscle fibers lengthen. Eccentric contractions are sometimes used as breaks during resisted isometric movements to distinguish between grade 4 (good) and grade 5 (normal) range of motion.

Concentric contractions are those in which enough force is generated to overcome a resistance and the muscle shortens during the contraction.

Econcentric (also called pseudoisometric) contractions occur in muscles attached to two joints, while the muscle acts both concentrically on one and eccentrically on the other, effectively keeping muscle length constant.

An isometric contraction is one in which the joint angle and muscle length are kept constant, such as holding something or pressing against an immovable force.

Isotonic contractions are those in which the muscle changes length but the tension is kept constant, such as those that occur when the force of contraction exceeds the load on the muscle.

Functional Assessment

Functional assessment is an analysis of the limitations placed on the activities the patient considers important. It is primarily subjective and should be individualized. It evaluates the individual's ability to perform whole-body tasks, rather than move individual joints as examined by other tests. The types of functional activities that should be evaluated, if appropriate, include self-care activities (bathing, eating, going to bathroom, etc.), recreational activities, grocery shopping, work-related activities, walking, sports-related activities, etc.

A good guideline is to evaluate the four areas of human function described by Goldstein:

- Basic or personal activities of daily living (ADLs): including bed, hygiene, eating, dressing, transfer, and walking activities
- Instrumental or advanced ADLs: such as meal preparation, shopping, light housework, check writing, communicating, driving, or having sex

- Work activities: including lifting, carrying, pulling, etc.
- Sport and recreational activities: such as walking, other participatory sports, and drills for agility, reaction time, endurance, etc.

Functional Assessment Tools

There are many functional assessment tools available. The most important consideration with each is that they reliably and inclusively evaluate functions that are important to the patient. Questionnaires ask about daily living skills and mobility. Some use numerical scoring systems that assign different ratings to the extent of each functionality the examiner considers important, as with the Shoulder Evaluation Form, which assigns ratings to the degree of pain, stability, motion, etc., in the shoulder. Some ask the patient to rate the difficulty of performing a particular task or how much he is bothered by certain problems as currently perceived; an example is the Short Musculoskeletal Function Assessment (SMFA) questionnaire. Actual functional tests, such as the upper-extremity function test, timed leg standing, tandem walking, or specific activity tests, are used to simulate activities of daily living to see how well the patient can perform them and, in some cases, provoke symptoms for evaluation.

Special Diagnostic Tests

Special diagnostic tests may be used for musculoskeletal/neuromuscular evaluation to confirm a provisional diagnosis, formulate a differential diagnosis, comprehend unusual or difficult signs or symptoms, or differentiate between structures. Any test used must be reliable, sensitive, and specific. Reliability means the test is dependable and can be trusted to measure what is expected.

Statistically, reliability can be evaluated in terms of parameters, such as the intraclass correlation coefficient (ICC), which is determined by analysis of variance (ANOVA), with a value > 90 indicating enough agreement for reasonable validity; the kappa, or K statistic, if only nominal data is available; and the standard error of measurement (SEM), which indicates the reliability of response over time and should be small. Sensitivity refers to the ability to detect changes and identify true positives. Specificity is the degree to which the test excludes a particular condition and identifies a true negative. Likelihood ratios combine sensitivity and specificity.

Laboratory Tests for Bone Disease or Joint Problems

Bone diseases can often be differentiated by looking in combination at plasma levels of calcium, ionized calcium, inorganic phosphorus, alkaline phosphatase, and phosphorus. Alkaline phosphatase is elevated in most bone diseases, including childhood rickets, adult osteomalacia, Paget's disease, primary hyperparathyroidism, and marked hyperthyroidism. Calcium levels are elevated in primary hyperparathyroidism, multiple myeloma, and Paget's disease (sometimes) but are usually normal in other bone diseases. Samples of synovial fluid can place disease into one of four groups based on appearance:

- Group 1: clear yellow; indicative of noninflammatory conditions or trauma
- Group 2: cloudy; generally due to inflammatory arthritis
- Group 3: brownish with a thick exudate associated with septic arthritis or gout
- Group 4: hemorrhagic; indicates trauma, fractures, bleeding disorders, or tumors

Joint Play and Joint Positions

Joint play, or accessory movement, refers to the involuntary, small range of motion (ROM) that can be achieved through passive movement by the examiner. Joint play, generally 4 mm or more in any direction, is essential for painless voluntary movement of the joint and full ROM.

Therefore, joint play testing is a part of musculoskeletal evaluation. It should be done with both patient and examiner relaxed. The patient is fully supported, and one joint and one movement are evaluated at a time. The uninvolved side is tested first. One particular surface is stabilized while the other is moved. Joint play movements should be assessed with the joint in the loose-packed, or resting, position where there is least stress, not the close-packed, or synarthrodial position, which is more compressed and places joint structures under tension. However, the close-packed position offers maximal joint stability, making it ideal for stabilization of one joint while treating an adjacent one. The resting position should be used for resistive isometric movements.

Palpation in Musculoskeletal Evaluation

Palpation of finger pressure to detect tenderness should be done after identification of the affected tissue. The unaffected side is palpated first, and the palpation is done in a systematic manner. The supported body part is felt for differences in tissue tension, muscle tone, tissue texture, tissue thickness, joint tenderness, temperature disparities, pulses, tremors, fasciculations (inflamed connective tissues), the pathological state of the joint or surrounding tissues, dryness or excess moisture, and any abnormal sensations. The tenderness is graded according to patient complaints as I (pain only), II (pain and wincing), III (wincing and withdrawing of the joint), or IV (palpation not permitted by patient). In particular, tissue thickness can indicate swelling (the abnormal enlargement of a body part due to bone or synovial membrane thickening) or fluid accumulation (edema) in or near the joint. Characteristic feelings of swelling on palpation are acute, hard, warm, tense swelling, suggesting blood accumulation; a boggy, spongy feeling, appearing 8 to 24 hours after occurrence and indicating inflammation and synovial swelling; hard, implying bone swelling; thick and slow-moving with pitting edema; etc.

Resting and Close-Packed Positions for Joints

Each joint has a relatively non-stressed resting position and a compressed, tenser close-packed position. For the major hip and knee joints, the resting position is some flexion, while the close-packed position is full extension with rotation. The foot joints are resting when positioned midway between extremes of range of movement and close-packed when the sole is turned upward. The temporomandibular joint is relaxed with the mouth slightly open and close-packed with clenched teeth. The resting and close-packed positions of each joint are very specific to the joint, and the examiner may need to refer to specific listings for each.

Plain Film Radiography

Two projections using plain film radiography are usually taken: an anteroposterior (AP) and a lateral projection. Others might be taken in special circumstances, such as an oblique view for the lumbar spine. Several projections are needed because of the likelihood of superimposition of structures. Dense structures like metal or bone do not allow penetration of x-rays on the fill and appear relatively white and radiolucent. Less dense structures that allow some penetration like soft tissues (muscles, joint capsules, fat pads, etc.) look grayer, and air spaces that permit complete x-ray penetration are quite black and radiolucent. Fractures, dislocations, and other abnormalities can be visualized. For example, a darker area would be seen where a bone is fractured. Soft tissue injuries are less distinguishable on radiographs and clinical findings are more useful, unless the examiner is extremely adept at interpretation. For musculoskeletal evaluation, the types of things to look for on a radiograph are size, shape, number, alignment, and density of bones; breaks in continuity of the bone; soft-tissue changes, such as swelling or visible fat pads; the width and symmetry of the joint space, etc.

ABCs Search Pattern

The ABCs search pattern is a systematic approach to radiological assessment for potential musculoskeletal problems:

- "A" stands for alignment, which means looking at the general skeletal architecture, bone contours, and alignment between adjacent bones; this can identify missing or extra bones, deformities, fractures, spurs, and joint subluxation or dislocation.
- "B" stands for bone density. General bone density should show significant contrast between soft tissues and bones that, if absent, indicates bone density loss. Texture abnormalities and local bone density changes should also be surveyed.
- "C" denotes cartilage spaces, which should be observed for joint space width, subchondral bone scarring, and changes in thickness of epiphyseal plates that, if abnormal, are generally associated with joint pathology.
- "s" covers soft tissues. Some abnormalities of soft tissues that can be seen are gross swelling or wasting of muscles, radiolucent displacement of fat pads or fat lines, and other areas that are unusually radiolucent or radiopaque, instead of the gray associated with soft tissues.

Diagnostic Imaging Techniques Involving Radiation

One imaging technique involving radiation is arthrography, in which an iodine-containing contrast dye, air, or both are injected into a joint space before taking a radiograph. A variation of this is computed arthrography (CT-arthrography), which merges arthrography with computed tomography (CT), a technique that uses x-ray bombardment from various angles to create a three-dimensional image. Computed tomography can also be used alone and is very useful for assessing cortical bone and identifying spinal stenosis, disc problems, fractures in complex joints, and the like. In myelography, a radiopaque dye is instilled into the epidural space by spinal puncture and a radiograph is taken after diffusion to look at nerve roots and the spinal cord. Venograms and arteriograms use injection of radiopaque dyes into veins and arteries, respectively, to identify conditions, such as blockage after trauma. Discography uses injection of radiopaque dye into the nucleus pulposus of an intervertral disc. Bone scans, or osteoscintigraphy, use intravenous injection of radioactive tracers (usually technetium-99m labeled); this technique is good at identifying the metabolic status of the skeleton, making it especially useful for detecting skeletal metastases, bone disease, and stress fractures with minimal bone loss, etc.

MRI and Diagnostic Ultrasound

Unlike most other techniques that involve radiation, magnetic resonance imaging (MRI) and diagnostic ultrasound utilize electromagnetic radiation and high-frequency sound waves, respectively, to create images of bone and soft tissues. MRI utilizes the fact that a strong magnetic field attracts hydrogen atoms. Depending on the type of image taken, MRI is very good for visualization of the anatomy or pathology of soft tissues like muscles and ligaments. It is now preferred over myelography for interpretation of disc pathology.

Diagnostic ultrasound is based on the principle that high-frequency sound waves (5 MHz to 10 MHz) bombarding tissues have a characteristic echo, or return time, depending on the depth of the structure. Diagnostic ultrasound is primarily used to evaluate soft-tissue injury.

Fractures

Fractures are generally described in terms of whether skin integrity is maintained; the site, configuration, and extent of the fracture; and the relative position of the fragments:

- Bony fractures are referred to as closed, if the skin is not broken, and open, if there are open tears or bony protrusions.
- The site of the fracture refers to its position on the bone, which for long bones would be at the proximal third, distal third, or shaft. Other possible site descriptions include intraarticular and extraarticular, meaning involving or not involving, respectively, the articular surface; and epiphyseal, indicating growth plate involvement.
- The configuration is basically orientation of the fracture. Linear fractures are described as transverse (at right angles to the long axis), oblique (diagonal to the long axis), or spiral (also diagonal but more involved with a circular pattern). Configurations where there are two or more fractures are known as comminuted (usually has wedge-shaped fragments) or segmental (at different levels).
- The extent is either incomplete or complete, depending on whether one portion or all bone cortices, respectively, are disrupted.
- Nondisplaced versus displaced fractures refer respectively to normal or abnormal anatomical alignment of the fracture fragments.

Bone Healing Stages after Fracture

Bones heal in four stages:

1. Hematoma formation: occurs during the first three days after fracture
2. Fibrocartilage: typically forms within two weeks of the break
3. Pro-callus: develops during approximately the same time period, about three to 10 days following the break
4. Remodeling of the bone or permanent callus formation healing: occurs three to 10 weeks after fracture

Here, the term callus refers to a mass of fibrous tissue, calcium, cartilage, and bone. The healing process is encouraged by factors that include early mobilization and weight bearing, preservation of fracture reduction, and patient compliance. It can be deterred by factors, such as comorbidities like diabetes or anemia, osteoporosis, and disruption of the vascular supply to the affected bone. The extent of soft-tissue damage and the type of fracture affect the healing process; for example, comminuted or multiple fragment fractures take longer to heal.

Fracture Management Based on Severity

Depending on factors such as fracture type and homodynamic stability, fractures are treated as elective, urgent, or emergent. Elective management usually applies to any type of nonoperative or operative procedure done within days or weeks in a patient whose fracture is stable and neurovascular system normal. Urgent management, done within one to three days, is a procedure done on a closed but unstable bone in a patient with an intact neurovascular system. Emergent treatments are those done on open fractures, fractures or dislocations where the neurovascular system is damaged or there is compartment syndrome, or spinal injuries with neurological defects. The goal of each is fracture reduction, which is aligning and bringing fragments closer. Methods to achieve fracture reduction are either closed, such as manual manipulation or traction, or open, generally open-reduction internal fixation (ORIF) in which plates, screws, etc., are inserted for immobilization. Otherwise, noninvasive immobilization modalities include casts and splints.

Complications After Fracture

There are many possible complications that can occur shortly after a fracture. Immediate complications within days can include loss of the fixation or reduction, but most are related to other systems and can be critical, including deep vein thrombosis, pulmonary emboli, nerve damage (including paralysis), damage to arteries, compartment syndrome, infection at the incision site, orthostatic hypotension, and shock. Later complications are usually related to the fracture directly, such as its failure to unite within the expected time frame; nonunion; malunion, in which the fracture heals with a deformity; and pseudarthrosis, or formation of a false joint, at the site. Bone-related diseases (such as posttraumatic arthritis, osteomyelitis or inflammation) or myositis ossificans (where there is bone in the muscle) may develop. These complications are considered delayed or late, depending on whether they appear within weeks to months or later, respectively.

Pelvic Ring Fractures

Anteroposterior Compression Pelvic Ring Fractures

Pelvic ring fractures involve the area of the pelvis fashioned by the paired coxal bone, sacrum, sacroiliac joints, and symphysis pubic. There are three possible anteroposterior compression (APC) types of fractures, all of which involve disruption of the pubic symphysis, as well as lateral compression (LC) and vertical shear fractures:

- APC, type 1: shows no other involvement; treated with symptomatic pain management
- APC, type 2: involves more than 2.5 cm tearing of the anterior sacroiliac, sacrospinous, and sacrotuberous ligaments; requires exterior fixation or open-reduction internal fixation (ORIF)
- APC, type III: interrupt completely the pubic symphysis, as well as the posterior ligament complexes, and exhibit hemipelvic displacement; may be managed with external fixation, ORIF, or posterior percutaneous pinning

Lateral Compression and Vertical Shear Pelvic Ring Fractures

Lateral compression (LC) fractures can be of three types:

- LC, type I refers to posterior compression of the sacroiliac joint and oblique public ramus fracture, which can be managed with symptomatic pain relief.
- In LC, type II, the posterior sacroiliac ligament is also ruptured and the hemipelvis is rotated, requiring external fixation or anterior and posterior open-reduction internal fixation (ORIF).
- LC, type III fractures also include an APC or anteroposterior compression injury to the contralateral pelvis, which is managed with anterior and posterior ORIF.

There are also vertical shear fractures, in which a hemipelvis is displaced due to extensive ligament or bone disruption and treated with traction and fixation (percutaneous, external, or anterior and posterior ORIF).

Physical Therapy Interventions for Pelvic Ring Fractures

Appropriate physical therapy interventions depend on the type of pelvic ring fracture. Suitable physical therapy interventions for anteroposterior compression (APC), type I and lateral compression (LC), type I fractures are partial weight bearing (PWB) or weight bearing as tolerated (WBAT) for functional mobility and active/active-assistive range of motion (A/AAROM) of the hip and distal joint.

For APC, type II pelvic ring fractures, appropriate interventions are non-weight bearing (NWB), touch-down weight bearing (TDWB), or PWB mobility; hip and distal joint A/AAROM; and lower-extremity exercise.

For APC, type III fractures, physical therapy is limited to NWB or TDWB on the least-affected side (basically bed transfers) and A/AAROM on distal lower extremities. These restrictions are also appropriate for LC, types II and III and vertical shear fractures. Patients with vertical shear fractures of the pelvic ring should also do positioning, breathing exercises, and uninvolved extremity exercise if they are on bed rest.

Acetabular Fractures

The acetabulum is the concave surface on either side of the pelvis where the head of the femur meets the latter, forming the hip joint. Acetabular, or hip joint, fractures arise as secondary shocks transmitted from high-impact blunt forces elsewhere, such as a foot with extended knee or the posterior pelvis. Patients with these fractures are prone to other complications, such as hematomas, emboli, and DVT. Fractures are defined as either stable or unstable. A stable acetabular fracture is one where the weight-bearing surface is intact and there is less than 2.5 mm displacement of the dome; these are managed with traction and bed rest and/or closed reduction. An unstable fracture is one in which the weight-bearing dome is fractured, which requires percutaneous pinning, open-reduction internal fixation (ORIF), or total hip arthroplasty. Acetabular fractures are also classified in terms of portion severed, i.e. the anterior or posterior column and transverse or complex (T-shaped), involving both columns.

Hip Dislocation

Hip dislocations, or displacements, usually develop in a posterior direction, manifesting as a shortened limb, internal rotation, and adduction in slight flexion. They can occur alone or in conjunction with a femoral or acetabular fracture. If there is no fracture, hip dislocations are managed with closed reduction and muscle relaxation. If these fail, open reduction or traction is used. If there is associated fracture, surgery is necessary.

Intracapsular Femoral Head and Neck Fractures

The femur is the main bone in the human thigh; its head and neck are its highest parts in association with the hip. Thus, these fractures are termed hip fractures. They usually occur in the neck portion. They are subdivided into intracapsular and extracapsular fractures, referring to location within or outside the hip capsule, respectively. Intracapsular femoral neck (i.e. hip) fractures have been classified by Garden as follows:

- A Garden I fracture is impacted but incomplete and can be managed with closed reduction with percutaneous pinning or, rarely, a spica cast.
- A Garden II fracture is a complete fracture without displacement, which is dealt with by closed reduction or open-reduction internal fixation (ORIF).
- Garden III intracapsular fractures are complete with partial displacement but the capsule is partially intact; ORIF is used.
- Garden IV fractures are complete with full displacement and capsule disruption; management options include ORIF and univocal or bipolar arthroplasty.

Extracapsular Femoral Head and Neck Fractures

Femoral head and neck (i.e. hip) fractures that are outside of the hip capsule are termed extracapsular. Within this taxonomy, there are two types of intertrochanteric (between the greater and lesser trochanters) and four types of subtrochanteric (top portion of femoral shaft) fractures.

Intertrochanteric fractures are classified as Evans type I or II, depending on whether the fracture line extends upward or downward from the lesser trochanter. Evans type I is managed with closed-reduction internal fixation or open-reduction internal fixation (ORIF), while options for Evans type II include ORIF, with or without osteotomy and bone grafting, as well as bipolar arthroplasty.

Subtrochanteric fractures are classified as Russell-Taylor types IA, IB, IIA, or IIB. Type A fractures are single, and type B ones have a second fracture line. In types IA and IB, the only or major line is from below the lesser to the distal greater trichinae, whereas for types IIA and IIB, it extends into the greater trichinae. ORIF is a management option for all. Intramedullary rods are used for types IA, IB, and IIA; dynamic hip screws for types IIA and IIB; and bone grafting for type IIB.

Femoral Shaft Fractures

Femoral shaft fractures are generally the result of forceful trauma and can be accompanied by critical complications, such as hypovolemia or shock, hip dislocations, patellar fractures, or abdominal or pelvic injuries. There are three types of femoral fractures:

- Closed, simple or nondisplaced: managed with open-reduction internal fixation (ORIF) or insertion of an intramedullary rod
- Closed, comminuted, impacted, or both: can be treated similarly or with traction and bed rest
- Open, comminuted and displaced: may require irrigation, debridement and wound closure, brief skeletal traction on bed rest, external fixation, and/or an intramedullary rod

Distal Femoral Fractures

Distal femoral fractures are caused by forceful trauma to the femur or some force that pushes the tibia into the intercondylar fossa. They are often accompanied by local soft-tissue injury. There are five possible types. Two are supracondylar, meaning only the femoral shaft is involved: extraarticular, simple, nondisplaced, for which a long leg cast is indicated; and supracondylar: extraarticular, displaced, or comminuted. Management options for the latter include traction on bed rest, open-reduction internal fixation (ORIF), closed reduction with percutaneous plate fixation, some type of knee immobilizer, an intramedullary nail, and/or passive motion. Fractures that involve one or both condyles are classified as unicondylar or intercondylar, which by definition means they are intraarticular. Unicondylar fractures are divided into no displaced types, which are managed with a long cast, and displaced types, which require traction on bed rest, ORIF, a long splint or cast, and/or closed-reduction and percutaneous fixation. Intercondylar fractions are treated with long-term traction, ORIF, or a cast brace.

Patellar Fractures

The patella, or knee cap bone, articulates with the femur. Patellar fractures are generally caused by direct blows or abrupt quadriceps contractions. There are three common types: nondisplaced, displaced, and comminuted. Nondisplaced patellar fractures are treated with closed reduction or with a long leg cast or other immobilizer with the knee in full extension. Displaced patellar fractures, either vertical or transverse, are managed with open-reduction internal fixation (ORIF) and continuous passive motion.

Review Video: Patellar Fracture
Visit mometrix.com/academy and enter code: 140653

Tibial Plateau Fractures

The tibia or shinbone is the larger of two bones in the lower leg. Blows to the tibial plateau at the apex can be critical since they are often accompanied by open wounds, soft tissue damage, dislocation, nerve compression, deep vein thrombosis, and/or infection. There are three common types. The first is nondisplaced, which is treated with closed reduction, immobilization using a cast or brace, and, if necessary, ligament repair; Displaced fractures fall into one of two categories. If the fracture involves a single condyle or split compression, management options are open-reduction internal fixation (ORIF), external fixation, and/or a cast or brace. For displaced fractures that are impacted or significantly comminuted involving both condyles, the management options are skeletal traction with bed rest, ORIF with or without bone grafting, an immobilization brace, and, if necessary. ligament or meniscus repair.

Tibial Shaft and Fibula Fractures

The tibia and fibula are the large and small calf bones, respectively. Fractures occur through direct impact, stress at the knee, or twisting of the ankle. They may be accompanied by ankle fractures, damage to the tibial artery or peroneal nerve, or rupture of the interosseous membrane. There are three classifications of closed tibial shaft fractures and one open type. Closed tibial shaft fractures are described as minimally displaced, which require closed reduction or a long leg cast; moderately displaced, managed with open-reduction internal fixation (ORIF) or a short leg cast; or severely displaced, comminuted, or both, requiring external fixation, ORIF, and/or provisional calcaneal (heel bone) traction. Open tibial shaft fractures are managed with ORIF or external fixation.

Distal Tibial Fractures

Distal tibial fractures generally occur from falls or other vertical loading forces, often in association with ankle fractures. There are three types of closed tibial fractures, based on degree of displacement, and one open type. The closed distal tibial fractures are described as: minimally displaced, which are managed with closed reduction or a short leg cast; moderately displaced, treated with open-reduction internal fixation (ORIF) or a short leg cast; or severely displaced, requiring temporary traction of the calcaneus (heel bone), external fixation, and/or ORIF. Open distal tibial fractures require external fixation.

Ankle Fractures

Ankle fractures are usually due to torque from abnormal loading of the talocrural joint, which connects the tibia and fibula to the talus bone of the foot. There are three possible types:

- Closed, nondisplaced fractures are addressed with closed reduction and a short leg or walking cast.
- Closed fractures that are displaced and/or multifractured are managed via closed reduction, open-reduction internal fixation (ORIF), and a cast or other type of mobilization depending on the amount of edema.
- Open ankle fractures are treated with irrigation and debridement with wound closure, traction, external fixation, and/or ORIF.

Calcaneal Fractures

Calcaneal fractures are those occurring in the calcaneus, or heel bone. They usually occur from high falls or sometimes avulsion, are often bilateral, and may be associated with leg or spinal fractures. There are four types of calcaneal injuries:

- Extraarticular, minimally displaced, which is managed with closed reduction and a short leg cast (SLC)
- Avulsion, with management options of closed reduction, a SLC, and open-reduction internal fixation (ORIF)
- Intraarticular, involving the subtalar joint (foot joint between calcaneus and talus), which is managed with skeletal traction, a SLC, ORIF, closed reduction with percutaneous pinning, and/or arthrodesis, if the fracture is extensive
- Open, which requires irrigation and debridement with wound closure, skeletal traction, and/or external fixation

Forefoot Fractures

The forefoot, or metatarsal bones, includes the five bones connected to the toes. Forefoot fractures are a result of objects falling on the foot, twisting, stress, or avulsion. There are three possible types of forefoot fractures:

- Minimally displaced, which is treated with closed reduction, percutaneous pinning, and/or a short leg or walking cast
- Moderate to severely displaced with fragmentation or angulation, managed with open-reduction internal fixation (ORIF), a short leg cast, and/or percutaneous pinning
- Open, which requires irrigation and debridement with wound closure, skeletal traction, external fixation, and/or ORIF

Spinal Fractures

Causes of Spinal Fractures

Common causes of spinal fractures are vehicle accidents, falls, sports injuries, and violence. Spinal fractures are defined in terms of their location, as involving the anterior column and/or posterior column. The anterior column of the spine includes the vertebral bodies, intervertebral discs, and the anterior and posterior longitudinal ligaments. The posterior column includes the transverse and spinous processes, pedicles and laminae of the vertebral arch, and various ligaments. Spinal fractures are also described in terms of whether they are stable or unstable. A stable fracture involves only one column (anterior or posterior) or is one lacking neurologic insufficiency. Spinal fractures are differentiated in terms of area of the spine affected, as cervical or thoracolumbar. Potential complications of spinal fractures include swelling at the site, hematomas, herniation or dislocation of the intervertebral disc, and spinal cord injury (discussed in detail elsewhere). Therefore, the patient must be closely monitored for other fractures, head and internal injuries, neurovascular parameters, and, in the case of cervical fractures, airway and breathing.

Types of Cervical Spine Fractures

Cervical spine fractures are bone breaks in the neck region. There are basically four types of cervical spine fractures, some of which are further differentiated. Two stable types are vertebral body fractures, which are wedge fractures involving bony impaction and concavity of the vertebral body; and isolated spinous process, or laminal fractures. Both types are managed with a cervical collar. Other categories include bilateral pedicle (Hangman's) fractures of axis C1 and odontoid process fractures. Hangman's fractures can be type I (no angulation, minimal displacement), II (displacement), IIA (minimal displacement, significant angulation), or III (full facet dislocation). Management includes cervical collar immobilization for type I, cervical traction/reduction and later a halo vest for types II or IIA, and posterior open reduction with halo vest or C1-3 fusion for type III. Odontoid process fractures are divided into: type I, oblique avulsion fractures at the tip of the odontoid, simply requiring a cervical collar for immobilization; type II, fractures in the neck of the odontoid, treated with closed reduction, ORIF with halo vest, or C1-2 fusion ± bone grafting and cervical collar; and type III, fractures that extend to C2 vertebral body, managed with closed reduction or ORIF with halo vest.

Thoracolumbar Spine Fractures

Thoracolumbar spine fractures, those occurring below the cervical region, are divided into four types. The first type is a stable, isolated fracture of a spinous process, transverse process, lamina, or facet, which is managed with a cervicothoracic or thoracolumbar orthosis. There are two types of vertebral body fractures: stable vertebral body compression (impacted anterior wedge) fractures, which are managed with temporary bed rest, vertebroplasty, orthoses, hyperextension braces, or, if severe, fusion; and unstable vertebral body burst (axial compression) fractures, which are addressed with short-term bed rest, orthoses, and anterior/posterior decompression and reconstruction, possibly with bone grafting. The last type of thoracolumbar spine fracture is an unstable multidirectional fracture with disc involvement and facet dislocation, which is managed using anterior/posterior decompression and fusion and an orthosis.

Shoulder Girdle Fractures

The areas of possible fracture on the shoulder girdle are primarily the glenohumeral (shoulder) joint, the coracoid process of the scapula, the clavicle (collar bone), and the scapula (bone connecting the arm bone and clavicle). Stable, nondisplaced fractures of the glenohumeral or coracoid regions are treated conservatively with sling immobilization. If there is displacement, they are managed with open-reduction internal fixation (ORIF). Acute management for glenohumeral dislocation is closed reduction to avert neurovascular damage. Clavicle fractures are managed conservatively with a sling unless there are complications, such as neurovascular damage, ligament tears, or a floating shoulder, in which case ORIF is indicated. Scapular fractures are uncommon due to muscular protection, and pain management is usually sufficient.

Proximal Humeral Fractures

The humerus is the long bone of the upper arm. Proximal humeral fractures are due to some type of trauma and primarily occur in the greater tuberosity. Most proximal humeral fractures are nondisplaced or minimally displaced, which would be treated conservatively. Proximal fractures that are displaced are described in terms of the number of parts. One-part displaced proximal humeral fractures are managed with closed reduction or sling immobilization, and two-part ones are managed with closed reduction and percutaneous pinning, open-reduction internal fixation (ORIF), an intramedullary rod, or a sling. If the displaced fracture is three part, the management options are hemiarthroplasty and ORIF; four-part fractures are treated with transcutaneous reduction with fluoroscopy, percutaneous pinning, or ORIF. Another possibility is comminution of the humeral head, which is managed with hemiarthroplasty and sling immobilization.

Humeral Shaft Fractures

Humeral shaft fractures are generally one of three types:

- Closed with minimal displacement: managed with closed reduction, a sling, hanging arm cast, or brace
- Closed, displaced with angulation: requires open-reduction internal fixation (ORIF), an intramedullary rod, or a long arm splint
- Open: necessitates irrigation and debridement with wound closure, external fixation, and/or ORIF

Distal Humeral and Olecranon Fractures

Distal humeral and olecranon fractures are in the elbow region. Distal humeral refers to the portion of the humerus near the elbow, the olecranon (elbow bone) is the upper portion of the ulna (larger forearm bone), and the radial head is the uppermost portion of the radius (smaller forearm bone). Most distal humeral fractures are intercondylar T- or Y-shaped or, for the elderly, transcondylar. Stable distal humeral fractures are managed with immobilization and early range-of-motion (ROM) exercises; comminuted intraarticular ones require open-reduction internal fixation (ORIF) or total elbow arthroplasty (TEA).

Management options for closed olecranon fractures depend on the whether they are nondisplaced (a long arm cast with the elbow in midflexion), displaced (ORIF), or comminuted (ORIF and immobilization). Severely comminuted olecranon fractures are usually found in conjunction with humeral fracture and elbow dislocation.

Radial Head Fractures

The radial head is the uppermost portion of the radius, the smaller forearm bone. Radial head fractures lie in the elbow region. Closed radial head or neck fractures, which are generally associated with elbow dislocation and various soft-tissue disruptions, are managed according to degree of displacement. If the radial head is nondisplaced or minimally displaced, the fracture is managed with closed reduction with early immobilization, a sling or temporary splint, and aspiration of the associated hematoma, if necessary. Treatments for displaced closed radial head fractures include partial or complete excision of the radial head, closed reduction and short-term splinting for those with sufficient range of motion (ROM), and open-reduction internal fixation (ORIF) for people with inadequate ROM. Comminuted closed radial head fractures are managed with ORIF with immobilization and radial head excision with or without a radial head prosthesis and bone grafting.

Forearm Fractures

The larger and shorter bones in the forearm are the ulna and radius, respectively. Most of these fractures are displaced, affecting contiguous articulation; and the humerus or wrist is often fractured as well. Fractures affecting the shaft of either the ulna or radius are managed with casting and, if displaced, closed reduction, or open-reduction internal fixation (ORIF) with a functional brace. Distal radius fractures generally fall into one of three types:

- Extraarticular: treated with closed reduction with percutaneous pinning; ORIF, with or without a functional brace; or a sugar-tong splint or cast
- Intraarticular: managed with options that include ORIF; closed reduction with external fixation and, possibly, percutaneous pinning; or arthroscopic internal fixation
- Intraarticular, comminuted: requires closed reduction with external fixation, ORIF, bone grafting, and/or a splint

Carpal Metacarpal and Phalangeal Fractures

The carpal, metacarpal, and phalangeal (phalanx) bones are located, respectively, just above the wrist crease, in the palm, and in the fingers of the hand. Each term represents a number of bones. Carpal fractures are usually due to compression or hyperextension injuries, and there is generally associated ligament damage or dislocation. The management for nondisplaced carpal fractures is a short arm cast with the wrist held neutral with slight ulnar deviation; for displaced fractures, it is closed reduction and casting or open-reduction internal fixation (ORIF) with a splint or cast. Metacarpal fractures occur subsequent to direct trauma or weight on the long axis, and there may be associated soft-tissue damage. The fracture location determines treatment: ORIF for the articular surface; closed reduction, percutaneous pinning, and/or immobilization, if the fracture is in the neck or shaft; or percutaneous pinning and immobilization for base metacarpal fractures. Phalangeal fractures are caused by crushing, which usually also affects soft tissues. Phalangeal fractures are treated with reduction and splinting, if nondisplaced, or ORIF with splinting, if displaced or intraarticular.

Hip Arthroplasty

Arthroplasty, commonly known as joint replacement, is the surgical repair of a joint or its total or partial replacement with metal (titanium, cobalt alloys, etc.) or plastic (generally polyethylene) parts. Hip arthroplasty is typically total hip arthroplasty (THA), in which the femoral head and the acetabulum are both replaced. THA is done in patients with hip disorders, such as degenerative or rheumatoid arthritis, posttraumatic disorders in the area, a fused hip, bone tumors, etc.

Usually, the components are uncemented, especially in young or active patients; these have sections of porous coated metal, often treated with hydroxyapatite to encourage bony ingrowth and fixation, or press-fit prostheses that are used to attain fixation. Cemented prostheses are generally only used in patients who cannot regenerate bone effectively, such as those with osteoporosis. If the patient has bone or muscle issues that might cause dislocation, a bipolar cup that snaps over the femoral prosthesis might be used. Surgical approaches for THA combine surgery (posterolateral, lateral, or anterolateral) with removal and reattachment of the greater trochanter of the femur.

Joint Resurfacing vs Total Hip Arthroplasty

Joint resurfacing is generally used in patients who have osteonecrosis of the femoral head, instead of total hip arthroplasty (THA). There are two possible joint resurfacing techniques: hemiresurfacing arthroplasty, in which an adjusted cup is implanted, preserving most of the bone; or total joint resurfacing, in which both the femoral head and acetabulum are resurfaced with a double cup.

Knee Arthroplasty

Knee arthroplasty, or replacement, is done to relieve pain or restore joint stability and function. Patients generally have some form of arthritis (rheumatoid, traumatic, or osteoarthritis) or joint disease. There are two types. The first is unicompartmental knee arthroscopy (UKA, also known as unicondylar or partial knee arthroscopy), in which the femoral and tibial articulating surfaces in only one joint compartment (the lateral or medial) are replaced and much of the joint is preserved.

The other is tricompartmental or total knee arthroplasty (TKA), in which prosthetics (metal, plastic, etc.) are used to replace the medial and lateral compartments and resurface the patellofemoral articulation (usually). TKA fixation techniques are comparable to those used in hip replacements: cemented or uncemented porous ingrowth or press-fit. Possible complications include thrombosis or embolism, joint instability, damage to the peroneal nerve, patellar tendon rupture, and others.

Minimally Invasive Hip and Knee Arthroplasties

Minimally invasive surgery (MIS) for a hip or knee arthroplasty is commonplace today for joint replacements or revisions that are less complex. MIS can be done open or arthroscopically using an endoscope. The biggest advantages of MIS hip arthroplasty are that it can be done from the anterior or posterior side and healing is much faster than normal THA. MIS knee arthroscopy involves a much smaller incision than other techniques and minimizes untoward effects like muscle compromise and joint dislocation.

Shoulder Arthroplasty

Shoulder arthroplasty is performed in patients with various types of arthritis (rheumatoid, traumatic, or osteoarthritis), fractures, or avascular necrosis (AVN) to alleviate pain and restore functionality. There are several types of shoulder arthroplasty. The least invasive is proximal humeral hemiarthroplasty, which is prosthetic replacement of the humeral head, if that is the only portion affected. With more damage, some type of total shoulder arthroplasty (TSA) is done, in which the glenoid articulating surface and humeral head are both prosthetically replaced. Most TSA prostheses are unconstrained, and if there is some damage to the rotator cuff or deltoid muscles, they are repaired during the surgery. Some TSA prostheses may be one of two other types: semiconstrained or constrained. Most TSA fixations are cemented or press-fit. Cemented glenoid fixations often lead to loosening, thus requiring revisions. Alternatives include shoulder surface replacement arthroplasty and reverse total arthroplasty (Delta III), which shifts the center of rotation and relies primarily on the deltoid muscles for stability, making it good for situations where there is extensive rotator cup damage.

Total Elbow Arthroplasty

Total elbow arthroplasty (TEA) is used to relieve pain and promote joint range of motion (ROM) and stability, primarily in rheumatoid arthritis patients. Semiconstrained prostheses of metal and polyethylene with a locking pin or snap-fit device are predominantly used. Other TEA procedures include unconstrained and resurfacing arthroplasties. Fixation designs may be cemented, uncemented, or a combination of the two. Potential complications include loosening, joint instability, weakness of the triceps, ulnar nerve palsy, slow wound healing, and infections (addressed elsewhere).

Total Ankle Arthroplasty

Total ankle arthroplasty is infrequently used in patients with unbearable arthritic pain, primarily in relatively healthy older individuals with low physical demands. The most successful prosthetic designs have been two of the semiconstrained type, both of which are made of metal alloy and polyethylene components and use bony ingrowth for fixation. Potential complications of total ankle arthroplasty include loosening, wound infections, and subtler and midtarsal degenerative joint disease. To avert wound complications after surgery, the patient wears a short leg splint before suture removal and does not do any weight bearing until bony ingrowth is complete, which is about three weeks.

Infected Joint Arthroplasty

Infection of the area of a total joint arthroplasty is indicated by fever, wound drainage, unrelenting pain, and abnormally high laboratory values for infection markers, such as white blood cell counts, erythrocyte sedimentation rate, and C-reactive protein. Typically, the joint is aspirated, the fluid is analyzed to isolate the responsible organism, and effective antibiotics prescribed. Irrigation and debridement of the joint area, primary exchange arthroplasty, a two-stage reimplantation or resection, and, possibly, amputation may also be required. A total joint arthroplasty resection involves removal of all previous work, six weeks of IV antibiotics, and then reimplantation of joint components. Two-step resections of the hip or knee include an initial resection of the prosthetic, plus insertion of a cement spacer saturated with antibiotic, and, later, reimplantation.

Total Femur Replacement

Total femur replacement is generally done in patients with advanced malignant sarcoma with extracompartmental involvement. The exact procedure is tailored to the patient, but in general, it entails disarticulation of the hip and knee joints, dissection and ligation of the femoral artery and vein, removal of the entire femur and contiguous musculature, osteotomy of the trochanter bones, insertion of a prosthetic femur secured at the two joints, and wiring of the trochanters into the prosthetic. The procedure permits range of motion at both joints.

Hip Disarticulation and Hemipelvectomy

Hip disarticulation and hemipelvectomy are treatment options for malignant soft-tissue or bone tumors in the hip area. Hip disarticulation entails release of crucial pelvic and hip musculature, dislocation of the hip joint, division of the ligaments, and removal of the extremity. Hemipelvectomy is normally also an amputation of the limb, which is more extensive in that more of the pelvis and, at the end, more of the lower extremity is removed. In young patients with a promising prognosis, a limb-sparing alternative is internal hemipelvectomy, which is usually achieved by additional internal fixation and/or total hip arthroplasty. Patients who have had a leg amputated are potentially plagued by complications, such as infection, phantom pain, orthostatic hypotension, and blood loss. They usually have an attached drain to collect lost blood.

Tibial and Trochanteric Osteotomies

An osteotomy is a surgical procedure in which a bone is divided or sectioned. Tibial osteotomy is a conservative substitute for total knee arthroplasty that maintains the joint by resection of the proximal tibia.

Trochanteric osteotomy is an adjunct to surgical fixation of a hip fracture or total hip replacement. It involves excision of the greater trochanter, leaving intact musculature, and reattachment of the trochanter to the femur with screws after fixation.

Common Types of Spinal Surgeries

Spinal surgeries are indicated for disabling back pain unresponsive to more conservative measures, such as bed rest, anti-inflammatory drugs, lifestyle changes, or physical therapy. Common spinal surgeries include:

- Discectomy or microdiscectomy: removal of the herniated portion or the entire intervertebral disc in patients with herniated nucleus pulpous (HNP)
- Spinal fusion: union of facet joints in the spine with hardware or bone grafting; many types are often done in combination with nerve root decompression surgeries; several indications, including segmental instability, fractures, and arthritis of the facet joints
- Laminectomy: deletion of bone at the interlaminar space to relieve spinal stenosis or nerve root compression
- Foraminotomy: excision of the spinous process and laminae to level of the pedicle; indicated for spinal stenosis, extensive nerve root compression, or HNP; often combined with fusion
- Corpectomy: removal of discs above and below an affected spinal segment, with grafting for fusion of the anterior column; indicated for multilevel stenosis or spondylolisthesis (displacement of the anterior column) with nerve root compression; potential post-operative complications include neurologic damage, infection, dural tears, and nonunion

Vertebroplasty and Kyphoplasty

Vertebroplasty and kyphoplasty are minimally invasive surgeries for progressive osteoporotic vertebral compression fractures, either sudden ones, occurring subsequent to trauma and accompanied by pain and muscle spasm, or anterior wedge compression fractures, in which vertebral height decreases over time with negligible pain. The procedures are inappropriate if there is neurologic damage. In vertebroplasty, polymethylmethacrylate (PMMA) cement is percutaneously injected into the vertebral space for stabilization (but there is no height or deformity restitution). Kyphoplasty is similar, except that the PMMA is more precisely inserted using an inflatable balloon and height deficits and deformities are more likely to be restored because the cement is retained.

Soft-Tissue Repair and Reconstruction Knee Surgeries

Most soft-tissue repair and reconstruction surgeries performed on the knee are done arthroscopically, which means the joint is inspected and repaired using a small incision and an endoscope. There are six common types of knee arthroscopy performed. Two involve a meniscus, or cartilage disc, on either the medial or lateral side. A meniscectomy is the complete or partial removal of a meniscus subsequent to an irreparable tear, while a meniscal repair is resolution of a tear in a vascular region of the meniscus, where healing is likely.

A lateral retinacular release is the freeing of the synovium, capsular and retinacular structures lateral to the patella, and the proximal muscle fibers of the vastus lateralis. The anterior and posterior cruciate ligaments, which form a cross shape in the knee cap area, are reconstructed if insufficient using anterior cruciate ligament (ACL) or posterior cruciate ligament (PCL) reconstruction. These reconstructions utilize autografts or allografts of the patellar or hamstring tendons (ACL) or the patellar or Achilles tendons (PCL). A quadricepsplasty is a separation and/or lengthening of the quadriceps mechanism. Autologous cartilage transplantation is also being done to repair cartilage.

Soft-Tissue Repair and Reconstruction Shoulder Surgeries

Soft-tissue repair and reconstruction surgeries done on the shoulder are usually done arthroscopically, although rotator cuff damage may require open or mini-open repair. There are three main types of shoulder repair. The first is subacromial decompression, or acromioplasty, which is resection of the undersurface of the acromion, a projection on the scapula. Another is a repair of the rotator cuff, a group of muscles and tendons that stabilize the shoulder.

Gait

Normal Gait Cycle

The gait cycle is the time period or series of motions that transpire between two consecutive initial contacts of the same foot. The other foot has its own gait cycle, which is 180 degrees out of phase with it. There are two phases for each foot. The stance phase comprises approximately 60% of the cycle and starts with the foot on the ground, bearing weight. It consists of five instants:

1. The initial contact, or heel strike
2. The load response, where the foot is flat
3. The midstance
4. The terminal stance, where the heel comes off the ground
5. The preswing, when the toe comes off

Initial contact comprises 10% of the gait cycle and is considered a double-limb support or double-leg stance. The load response and midstance combined take up 40% of the cycle and are considered single-limb supports or single-leg stances. The combined terminal stance and preswing portions are approximately 10% of the gait cycle and make up the second double-limb support or weight-unloading period. The foot then enters the swing phase, which comprises about 40% of the gait cycle and consists of three instants: (1) The initial swing, or acceleration forward, during which the knee and ankle flex and the limb swings (2) The midswing, when the swing and other leg are side-by-side (3) The terminal swing, or deceleration, where the leg slows in preparation for the next cycle

FLOAT PHASE OF GAIT

When a person is running or otherwise ambulating quickly, gait cycle changes somewhat. During walking, the stance phase comprises about 60 to 65% of the gait cycle, with the swing phase making up the rest. During running, there are two float phases, or double unsupported phases, in between stance-swing and swing-stance, each making up about 15% of the cycle (for a total of approximately 30%). This, accordingly, shortens the stance and swing phases. Joint movements are similar to those for walking but encompass a greater range of motion; for example, there is considerably more hip flexion during running, particularly in the float phases.

NORMAL PARAMETERS OF GAIT

Normal parameters of gait should be observed in individuals from about 8 to 45 years of age. Many factors are decreased in women compared to men, in older individuals, etc.

Parameters and their normal ranges follow:

- The normal base width between the two feet is 5 to 10 cm (2 to 4 inches).
- The typical step, or gait length, between the contact points of the two feet is approximately 72 cm or 28 inches, although this parameter is affected by many factors, including age, height, sex (less in females), etc.
- The stride length should be double the gait length, about 144 cm, and is the linear distance between similar points of contact on a particular foot (i.e. the gait cycle).
- Lateral pelvic shift or list, which is pelvic side movement during walking, should be minimal, only 2.5 to 5.0 cm, as should vertical pelvic shift.
- Normal pelvic rotation is 8 degrees (4 degrees each, forward on the swing leg and posteriorly on the stance leg), with the thorax moving in the other direction simultaneously.
- The center of gravity shifts in a figure eight pattern within a 5 cm square area, which makes the head descend or ascend during weight-loading or weight-unloading periods, respectively.
- A customary cadence is 90 to 120 steps per minute, with women usually taking 6 to 9 steps a minute more and older people taking fewer. An average gait speed is 1.4 meters per second or 3 mph.

INITIAL CONTACT PORTION OF THE STANCE PHASE OF THE GAIT CYCLE

The stance phase of the gait cycle is considered the closed kinetic chain phase of gait because the foot is fixed and joints must adjust. If gait is normal, each instant or portion of the stance phase produces characteristic kinematic motion regardless of force. There are also typical kinetic motions, both external reaction forces and internal forces of muscles.

For the initial contact or heel-strike portion of the stance phase, the expected kinematic motions are: 20- to 40-degree flexion of the hip moving toward extension, plus minor adduction and lateral rotation; the knee in full extension prior to heel contact and flexing during the heel strike; the tibia in slight lateral rotation; the foot in rigid supination (sole upward) at the point of heel contact; and the ankle moving toward plantar flexion.

Abnormal responses to look for include increased knee flexion or early plantar flexion, indicating pain; tactics to extend the knee, suggesting some sort of weakness there; and touching down of other parts of the foot before heel strike, generally suggestive of some muscular or neurological issue.

Load-Response Portion of the Stance Phase of the Gait Cycle

The load-response or foot flat portion of the stance phase is also called the weight acceptance instant because it is the point at which the person chooses to bear weight on the limb. Expected normal kinematic motions during the load-response portion of the stance phase are: the hip moving into extension, adduction, and medial rotation; the knee flexed approximately 20 degrees moving toward extension; the tibia in medial rotation; the foot in pronation (rotated somewhat inward with weight born on the inside); and the ankle in plantar flexion to dorsiflexion over the fixed foot. Excessive or absent knee motion during this phase suggests weak quadriceps, plasticity, or contractures of the plantar flexor.

Midstance Portion of the Stance Phase of the Gait Cycle

During the midstance or single-leg support instant, the trunk should be above the supporting foot with evenly distributed weight and the pelvis should drop somewhat to the swing leg side. The normal expected kinematic motions at each joint are: the hip moving through a neutral position, with the pelvis rotating posteriorly; the knee flexed 15 degrees, shifting toward extension; the tibia in medial rotation; the foot neutral; and the ankle in slight (3-degree) dorsiflexion. Any painful joint pathology, such as arthritis, fallen arches, or plantar fasciitis, will cause the individual to shorten this phase. Rolling off of this phase is a positive Trendelenburg's sign caused by weakness of the gluteus medius nerve root.

Weight-Unloading Periods of the Stance Phase of the Gait Cycle

During the heel-off or terminal-stance portion of the weight-unloading period, the trunk moves toward the stance leg and the pelvis is posteriorly rotated. The normal joint kinematic movements are: a 10- to 15-degree extension of hip abduction with lateral rotation; the knee flexing 4 degrees, moving toward extension; the tibia in lateral rotation; the foot in supination as it stiffens for push-off; and the ankle in 15-degree dorsiflexion toward plantar flexion. During the toe-off or preswing instant while acceleration is initiated, the hip is normally moving toward a 10-degree extension in abduction and lateral rotation; the knee moves from close to full extension to 40-degree flexion; the tibia is in lateral rotation; the foot is in supination; and the ankle is in 20-degree plantar flexion. Indications of pain during the preswing period suggest some sort of pathology related to the hallux (great toe), often in the metatarsophalangeal joint. Inability to push off indicates weak plantar flexors and sacral nerve root issues.

Swing Phase of the Gait Cycle

During the swing phase of the gait cycle, the involved lower extremity is said to be in an open kinetic chain because the foot is not fixed to the ground and the limb and joints are less stressed than during most of the stance phase. During the initial swing or acceleration instant of the swing phase into the midswing, the hip is slightly flexed (up to 15 degrees) and medially rotated. The knee increasingly flexes up to 30 to 60 degrees, with lateral rotation of the tibia moving toward neutral. The foot and ankle are in an approximate 20-degree dorsiflexion with some pronation. Excessive hip flexion during midswing indicates drop foot. Moving from midswing into the terminal swing or deceleration portion, the hip flexes more, to approximately 30 to 40 degrees; the knee should be almost fully extended with slight lateral tibial rotation; the ankle is normally neutral; and the foot is in slight supination.

Muscle Groups Involved in the Various Phases of Gait

The muscle groups involved during gait are reflective of the mechanical goals of each portion. During the initial-contact instant of the stance phase, the goals are positioning the foot, initiation of deceleration, and use of the ankle dorsiflexors, hip extensors, and knee flexors. During the loading-response phase, the objectives are acceptance of the weight, stabilization of the pelvis, and deceleration, which uses the knee extensors, hip abductors, and ankle plantar flexors. The midstance serves to stabilize the knee, while maintaining momentum; and the goal of the terminal-stance portion is mass acceleration. Both use ankle plantar flexors but differently, namely isometrically for midstance and concentrically for terminal stance. The preswing serves as preparation for the swing phase and employs the hip flexors. The beginning of the swing phase, the initial swing, is used to clear the foot and change cadence, which necessitates use of the ankle dorsiflexors and hip flexors. Clearing of the foot and use of the ankle dorsiflexor continues during midswing. The goals of the terminal swing are deceleration of the shank and leg, positioning of the foot, and preparation for contact, utilizing knee flexors and extensors, hip extensors, and ankle dorsiflexors.

Gait Assessment Observation

During observation, male patients should wear shorts, females should wear shorts and a bra, and all should usually be barefoot. The examiner observes the patient's posture, degree of symmetry, and general gait parameters (utilizing aids if necessary). He observes the patient's gait from the front, side, and back, each directionally, which means that for the stance phase, the direction is from the foot up to the pelvis and lumbar spine and vice versa for the swing phase. The movement pattern of the upper limbs is also noted. The salient observation points from the anterior or posterior views are undesired presence of pelvic tilt or rotation; presence of reciprocal arm swing, as desired; rotation of the trunk and upper limb in opposition to the pelvis, as expected; muscle atrophy of the thigh or leg; the positioning at various gait phases; toe angling (should be 5 to 18 degrees outward); and normal behavior of hip, knee, ankle, and foot joints, as well as the tibia (described elsewhere). The anterior and posterior views are superior for observation of the weight-loading and weight-unloading portions of gait, respectively. The lateral view is good for observation of shoulder and thorax rotation, spinal posture, joint movements, gait parameters (such as step or stride length), and coordination of movement.

Gait Assessment Examination

The examination portion of gait assessment consists of measurement of the parameters of gait to compare left and right gait cycles; measurement of each leg to look for differences; and often, the use of locomotion scales, grading systems, or other functional tests. These locomotion scales are often tailored to the population the patient falls into, for example, people with rheumatoid arthritis or the elderly. Gait-related parameters beyond the amount and type of joint movement are generally included, for example, the ability to climb stairs or the degree of guardedness during portions of the gait cycle. An important aspect of the examination portion is determination of whether the patient is employing compensatory mechanisms.

Antalgic Gait

Abnormal gait patterns have three sources: joint pathology or injury, compensation for these in joints on the same side of the body, or compensation on the opposite side. Antalgic gait is abnormal painful gait due to injury to the pelvis or any of the major joints from the hip down. It is seen with various forms of arthritis, osteomyelitis, tumors, foreign bodies in the foot, and various other conditions. The patient tries to take weight off the affected limb as rapidly as possible, making the stance phase for that leg relatively short, reducing the step length on the uninvolved side, and decreasing walking velocity and cadence. The individual often supports the painful area with a hand or arm and may transfer body weight over a painful hip.

Gluteus Maximus and Gluteus Medius Gaits

Gluteus maximus and gluteus medius gaits are two abnormal gait patterns. Gluteus maximus gait has a distinctive backward lurch of the trunk on initial contact, which compensates for a weak gluteus maximus muscle, allowing hip extension.

Gluteus medius, or Trendelenburg's gait, is excessive lateral list toward the stance leg, compensating for weak abductor muscles in the buttocks, the gluteus medius, or the gluteus minimus. If gluteus medius muscles on both sides are weak, there is noticeable side-to-side movement. The pattern is called Trendelenburg's gait because there is a positive Trendelenburg's sign, which is drooping on the contralateral side. This gait can also be seen with congenital hip dislocation and deformities.

Arthrogenic and Contracture Gaits

Arthrogenic and contracture gaits are two abnormal gait patterns generally due to previous prolonged immobilization. An arthrogenic (stiff knee or hip) gait, also caused by fusion at the joint, is a pattern whereby the individual uses plantar flexion of the opposing ankle and circumduction of the stiff extremity to lift the entire affected leg higher than usual for clearance.

In contracture gaits, the person uses compensatory mechanisms to counteract contractures for clearance. There are several patterns depending on the site of contracture. For example, increased lumbar lordosis combined with trunk extension and knee flexion is indicative of a hip flexion contraction.

Abnormal Gait Patterns in Patients with Congenital Deformities

One abnormal gait pattern observed primarily in patients with congenital deformities is equinus gait of toe walking. This pattern is associated with children that have congenital talipes equinovarus, or clubfoot, which is internal rotation of the foot at the ankle. These children rotate their pelvis and femur laterally for compensation, bear weight during gait on the dorsolateral or lateral portion of the foot, limp, and exhibit a shortened weight-bearing phase.

Short leg, or painless estrogenic, gait occurs when a person has differing leg lengths or a deformity in a leg bone. The patient shifts laterally toward the affected side, tilting the pelvis and walking with a limp.

Possible additional abnormalities of gait include supination of the foot on the involved side, increased flexion in the uninvolved limb, and hiking of the hip during the swing phase.

Abnormal Gait Patterns Neurologic in Origin

Abnormal gait patterns that are generally neurologic in origin include:

- Ataxic gait: seen in patients with poor sensation or lack of muscle control; characterized by poor balance, wide base, staggering or exaggerated movements, slapping of the feet, and looking downward
- Hemiplegic or hemiparetic gait: also known as neurogenic or flaccid gait; characterized by outward swinging or pushing of the paraplegic leg and use of upper limb across the trunk for balance

- Parkinsonian gait: distinguished by flexion of neck, trunk, and knees, shuffling or short steps, and absence of normal arm movement
- Scissors gait: also known as neurogenic or spastic gait; due to spastic paralysis of the hip adductors; patient draws knees together during gait
- Steppage or drop foot gait: due to loss of control of dorsiflexor muscles as a result of muscle or nerve damage; compensatory pattern in which the individual lifts the knee too high and then slaps the foot on the floor

Abnormal Gait Patterns from Muscle Weakness

Gluteus maximus and gluteus medius gaits are discussed elsewhere. Other common abnormal gait patterns due to muscle weakness include:

- Quadriceps avoidance gait: compensatory gait reflective of quadriceps muscle injury of some kind; characterized by forward flexion of the trunk, forceful plantar flexion of the ankle, and knee hyperextension
- Plantar flexion gait: compensatory gait due to plantar flexor deficit; distinguished by absent or decreased push-off, shortened stance phase, and short step length on uninvolved side
- Psoatic limp: observed in patients with inhibition of the psoas major muscle due to a hip condition like Legg-Calve-Perthes disease; characterized by difficulty in swing phase, limping, and overstated trunk and pelvic movement

Lordosis

Lordosis is a common spinal deformity in which there is abnormal forward curvature of the spine in the lumbar and cervical regions. Among its causes are postural or functional deformities, compensation for another deformity like kyphosis (described elsewhere), and lax abdominal or other muscles in combination with tight muscles (particularly the hip flexors or lumbar extensors). People with pathological lordosis have postural abnormalities developed as compensation to maintain the proper center of gravity, such as drooping shoulders, medial rotation of the legs, hyperextended knees, slight plantar flexion in the ankle joints, and forward thrusting of the head. Their pelvic angle is increased from the normal 30 to about 40 degrees, putting them in an anterior pelvic tilt; they develop stress on many joints; many of their muscles are elongated and weak, particularly the deep lumbar extensors; and other muscles are tight, such as the hip flexors. Swayback deformity is similar in that there is a 40-degree pelvic inclination, but there is posterior spinal curvature in the thoracolumbar region and the hip joint is pushed forward. People with swayback generally have weak hip flexors, lower abdominals, and lower thoracic extensors; and tight hip extensors, upper abdominals, and lower lumber extensors.

Kyphosis

Kyphosis is exaggerated posterior curvature of the spine in the thoracic region. Causes of kyphosis include vertebral compression fractures, osteoporosis, tumors, congenital defects, and compensation for lordosis, paralysis, and Scheuermann's vertebral osteochondritis. The latter is a common disease in which there is inflammation of bone and cartilage in the ring epiphysis of the vertebral body. There are four varieties of kyphosis:

- Round back: a long, rounded, curved back
- Flat back: a mobile lumbar spine, making the spine appear very flat
- Humpback (also called gibbus): a sharp posterior angulation in a small portion of the thoracic spine
- Dowager's hump: the degeneration of thoracic vertebral bodies due to osteoporosis

People with round, flat, or humpback all have decreased pelvic inclination (approximately 20 degrees). Dowager's hump manifests as loss of height, forward flexion of the head, and protruding abdomen, resulting from the attempt to maintain normal center of gravity. Each of these types is associated with stress on certain joints, poor body alignment, and characteristic elongated, weak and short, strong muscles. Abnormal thoracic and lumbar spine curvatures can result in kypholordotic posture.

Scoliosis

Scoliosis is abnormal curvature of the spine in a lateral direction. If found in the cervical spine, it is termed torticollis. Depending on the cause, scoliosis is considered either nonstructural (functional), due to things like postural issues, inflammation, nerve root irritation, or compensation; or structural, due to bone deformities or muscle weakness. The vast majority of structural scoliosis cases are idiopathic, in which there is rotation and distortion of the vertebral bodies. Other causes of structural scoliosis include upper or lower motor neuron lesions, muscular diseases, trauma, and conditions responsible for bone destruction. Nonstructural scoliosis is not progressive, and the individual can flex forward, reducing the abnormal curvature; whereas structural scoliosis is progressive, the person is relatively inflexible, and side bending is asymmetrical.

Neuromuscular & Nervous Systems

Components of a Neurologic Examination

The first component of a neurologic examination is a detailed patient history, which in this case may be obtained from the patient but is often relayed by a family member or witness. It should include relevant questions related to issues, such as whether the patient lost consciousness, whether he fell, and whether he has deficits like vision problems, memory loss, or speech changes. The patient should be observed for things such as degree of alertness, body position, posture, movement patterns, presence of involuntary movements like tremors, etc. A mental status examination should be done, including describing and quantifying level of consciousness with measures like the Glasgow Coma Scale, evaluating cognitive function, and assessing emotional state, memory, and speech and language ability. Level of consciousness and cognitive function tests are described further elsewhere. The patient's vital signs should be measured and regularly monitored. Cranial nerve testing and vision testing are recommended. Motor function testing, including strength testing, tests for muscle tone, reflex testing, sensation testing, and coordination tests, should all be done (described further elsewhere). There are also a number of diagnostic tests that may be performed.

Review Video: The Nervous System
Visit mometrix.com/academy and enter code: 708428

Level of Consciousness

Level of consciousness is an indication of a person's mental status and is potentially predictive of severity and prognosis. A normal awake, attentive, interactive level of consciousness is described as "alert." A person who needs various increasing levels of arousal and experiences increasing states of confusion can be described in order as "lethargic," "obtunded," or in "stupor" (semi-coma). A patient who cannot be aroused and may have missing reflex responses is defined as being in a "coma" or "deep coma." Other abnormal states of consciousness include "delirium," disorientation accompanied by irritation, misperception, and offensive behavior, and "dementia," an altered mental state due to organic disease but not involving altered arousal.

Glasgow Coma Scale

The Glasgow Coma Scale (GCS) is a commonly used scale that quantifies a patient's mental status in terms of three important parameters: best eye opening (E), motor response (M), and verbal response (V). Each parameter is rated on a scale from 1 to 5 and the total score added up (range 3 to 15). A patient with a score of 8 or less is considered to be in a coma. The scale uses the following guidelines:

- The eye-opening response is rated from nil, where the eyes do not open in response to any type of stimulus, to spontaneous, eye opening without stimulation.
- The motor response is rated from nil, where there is no motor movement, to the maximal, where the patient obeys and follows commands.
- The verbal response portion ranges from nil or no vocalization to maximal, where the patient is oriented and can carry on a normal conversation.

Cognitive Functions Evaluation

Appropriate cognitive functions to evaluate during a mental status examination are attention, orientation, memory, calculation, construction, abstraction, and judgment:

- Attention, the ability to mentally focus on a stimulus or task, can be tested by asking patients to repeat series of numbers or letters or spell words.
- Orientation, the facility to understand in terms of person, place, and time, can be assessed by asking patients questions such as their name, age, address, etc.
- Memory has three components: immediate recall, short-term memory, and long-term memory, which can each be addressed by asking patients to recount words after a few seconds, words after a few minutes, or past events.
- Calculation is the ability to solve mathematical problems, which can be assessed by asking them to perform simple calculations involving whole numbers.
- Construction is the capacity to construct a multidimensional shape, which can be tested by having patients draw a figure.
- Abstraction is the capacity for abstract as opposed to literal reasoning, which can be assessed with object comparison.
- Judgment is the ability to reason, which can be determined by having patients demonstrate common sense and safety.

Cranial Nerves Involving Smell or Vision

Cranial nerve testing is indicative of the neurologic status of the patient. There are 12 cranial nerves (CN). The following are associated with sense of smell or vision:

- CN I, the olfactory nerve: originates in cerebral cortex; controls sense of smell; tested by having patient sniff something with one open nostril
- CN II, the optic nerve: originates in the thalamus; related to central and peripheral vision; patient should be tested in all quadrants for acuity and field of vision
- CN III, the oculomotor nerve: derived from the midbrain; serves several functions related to vision, including upward, inward, and inferomedial eye movement; eyelid elevation (ask patient to open eyes wide); pupil constriction (shine light into eye); and visual focusing (ask patient to follow object with a complete gaze)
- CN IV, the trochlear nerve: comes from midbrain; controls inferomedial eye movement
- CN VI, the abducens nerve: originates in the pons; controls lateral eye movement and proprioception

Cranial nerves III, IV, and VI are evaluated at the same time in terms of different aspects of eye movement, which should be tested with eye movements both saccadic (looking in particular directions) and pursuit (following a moving finger).

Cranial Nerves Originating in the Pons

The four cranial nerves (CN) originating in the pons are:

1. CN V, the trigeminal nerve: has four functions, which are control of facial sensation (perform sensory testing on patient's face for touch, pain, and temperature); mastication (look for deviation of the jaw); the corneal reflex (brush cotton lightly against cornea); and the jaw jerk (press masseter muscle in the cheek as patient clamps the jaw).
2. CN VI, the abducens nerve: controls lateral eye movement and proprioception; tested in conjunction with CNs III and IV by assessing saccadic (looking laterally) and pursuit (following a moving finger) eye movements.
3. CN VII, the facial nerve: has three purposes, which are control of facial expression (ask patient to assume expressions like smiling, pursing lips, etc. to check for muscle paralysis); taste on anterior two-thirds of the tongue (apply cotton swabs with saline or sugar to check ability to differentiate them), and autonomic control of lacrimal and salivary glands (introduce a stimulus that should produce tearing).
4. CN VIII, the vestibulocochlear nerve: the vestibular branch is involved with sense of equilibrium (test oculocephalic reflex by rotating patient's head and watching to see if eyes move in opposite direction as expected, and assess balance or vestibulospinal function); the cochlear branch controls the sense of hearing (tests include auditory acuity and the Weber and Rinne tests, utilizing vibration of a tuning fork at forehead or mastoid bone).

Cranial Nerves Originating in the Medulla

There are three cranial nerves originating in the medulla plus the spinal accessory:

1. CN IX, the glossopharyngeal nerve: multiple functions include regulation of gag reflex (provoke gag with tongue depressor), superior pharyngeal muscle (test phonation, voice quality, and pitch), taste in posterior one-third of tongue (have patient differentiate between saline and sugar on cotton swab), salivary gland autonomic functions; sensations from external auditory meatus and skin in posterior ear; and blood pressure
2. CN X, the vagus nerve: involved in swallowing (test along with CN IX), the soft palate (have patient say "ah" and see if it elevates), and parasympathetic control of heart, lungs, and abdominal organs
3. CN XII, the hypoglossal nerve: controls movement and proprioception of the tongue during mastication and speech (observe tongue for midline and lateral movement and listen for articulation problems)
4. Spinal accessory: a complex of CN XI and CI to C5 that is involved with motor control of the trapezius and sternocleidomastoid muscles (instruct patient to rotate head or shrug shoulders while applying gentle resistance to look for weakness)

Vision Testing During Neurologic Examination

Vision testing as part of a neurologic examination should include cranial nerve testing (as discussed elsewhere) and further examination of the pupils by the physician for size and similarity, shape, and reactivity. Normally, the pupils of both eyes should be the same size (maximal 1 mm difference) and that size should be 2 to 4 mm in light and 4 to 8 mm in darkness. Normal pupils are round, but if the person has neurologic dysfunction, they may appear oval or irregular. Reactivity is tested by shining a light into the eye, which normally constricts the pupil but produces no or some other type of reaction in people with neurologic conditions. On the other hand, moving into darkness should normally dilate the pupils. The clinician also observes for nystagmus, involuntary rhythmic movement of the eyes, which can indicate equilibrium problems; cerebellar lesions; or disparity between reflexes coordinating the two eyes. During transfers or ambulation, the therapist can help patients with nystagmus by having them focus on a point or object in front of them.

Strength Testing during Motor Function Assessment

Strength testing is part of motor function assessment. Strength is broadly defined as the force output of a contracting muscle, which is a function of the amount of tension it can produce. There are different ways of evaluating strength. Muscle strength can be graded from 0 to 5 or 0 to N (normal) using manual muscle testing, strong or weak when describing ability to do resisted isometrics, or in terms of proportion of available range of motion. Functional strength, the ability of the neuromuscular system to control functional activities in a smooth and coordinated manner, is another way to grade strength.

Muscle Tone Testing During Motor Function Assessment

Changes in muscle tone are related to the presence of neurologic lesions or other factors, such as stress, pain, medications, and arousal of the central nervous system. The common abnormalities are: hypertonicity, or increased muscle contractility, possibly accompanied by spasticity or rigidity; hypotonicity, or decreased muscle contractility, usually with flaccidity (less muscle resistance); and dystonia, disordered tone with involuntary movements. There are various ways of grading abnormal muscle tone. It can be rated passively as mild, moderate, or severe in terms of resistance; actively in terms of whether the person can perform functional mobility and voluntary movement; or either way as in whether or not they can achieve full range of motion. The Modified Ashworth Scale is a numeric grading system for abnormal tone that rates it from 0 (no increase in muscle tone) to 4 (affected parts are rigid for extension and flexion). For a neurologic exam, a good method is whether the patient has abnormal decorticate (flexion) posturing indicative of corticospinal tract lesions and/or abnormal decerebrate (extension) posturing indicative of brain stem lesions.

Reflexes

Deep Tendon Reflexes

Reflexes are tested if there is suspected neurological involvement associated with musculoskeletal pain. Deep tendon reflexes are investigated by placing the patient in a relaxed supine or sitting position, with the tendon to be tested in a slight stretch, and then striking the tendon with a reflex hammer to see whether a normal response occurs.

Deep tendon reflexes are graded from 0 to 4 as follows:

- 0: absent, areflexia
- 1: diminished, hyporeflexia
- 2: average, normal
- 3: exaggerated, brisk
- 4: clonus, very brisk, hyperreflexia

Each reflex is tested five or six times to see whether the reflex response diminishes, which indicates nerve root issues. Responses can be enhanced using the Jendrassik maneuver (clenching teeth, squeezing hands) when testing the lower limbs or squeezing the legs during upper limb testing.

Deep Reflexes with Corresponding Nerve Root Sections

Beginning at the top, the common deep tendon reflexes tested and the corresponding central nervous system segments are:

- Jaw: cranial nerve V
- Biceps: C5 to C6
- Brachioradialis: C5 to C6
- Triceps: C7 to C8
- Patella: L3 to L4
- Tibialis biceps tendon: to elicit contraction
- Brachioradialis tendon: to get elbow flexion and/or forearm pronation
- Distal triceps tendon: to trigger elbow extension and muscle contraction
- Patellar tendon: for leg extension
- Tibialis posterior tendon: to get plantar flexion of the foot with inversion
- Semimembranosus tendon and biceps femoris tendon: to elicit knee flexion and muscle contraction
- Achilles tendon: for plantar flexion

Superficial Reflexes

Superficial reflexes are triggered by superficial stroking of a skin area with an object that is sharp but will not break the skin. Common superficial reflexes tested include the upper and lower abdominal, cremasteric, plantar, gluteal, and anal areas. The normal expected responses and the relevant central nervous system segments for each are:

- Upper abdominal reflex: should move the umbilicus up and toward the area being stroked; T7 to T9
- Lower abdominal reflex: should shift the umbilicus down and toward the area being stroked; T11 to T12
- Cremasteric reflex on the upper, inner part of the male's thigh: should elevate the scrotum; T12, L1
- Plantar reflex on the lateral side of the sole of the foot: should produce flexion of toes; S1 to S2
- Gluteal reflex: should tense the skin in that buttock region; L4 to L5, S1 to S3
- Anal reflex: should contract the anal sphincter muscles; S2 to S4

Other superficial reflexes commonly evaluated as part of cranial nerve (CN) testing are corneal, gag, and swallowing.

Pathological Reflexes

Four reflexes elicit the same response and are associated pathologically with pyramidal tract nervous system lesions. These are the Babinski reflex, stroking of the lateral aspect of the sole of the foot; Chaddock's reflex, stroking of the lateral side of the foot under the lateral malleolus; Oppenheim's reflex, stroking of the anteromedial tibial surface; and Gordon's reflex, firm squeezing of the calf muscles. These trigger extension of the big toe and fanning of the four small toes if there are pathological lesions. The Babinski is a normal response in newborns and can be indicative of organic hemiplegia. Other pathological reflexes involving the lower limbs include Piotrowski's, dorsiflexion and supination of the foot upon percussion of the tibialis anterior muscle, seen with organic CNS disease; Brudzinski's, flexion of the other leg upon passive flexion of one leg, suggesting meningitis; Rossolimo's, flexion of toes when their plantar surface is tapped, indicating pyramidal tract lesions; and Schaeffer's, flexion of toes and foot after pinching the center of the Achilles tendon, indicative of organic hemiplegic. Hoffman's reflex, elicited by flicking the end of the index, middle, or ring fingers, will cause the thumb or other non-flicked finger to flex, indicating tetany or pyramidal tract lesions.

Sensory Examination

A sensory examination should start with a cursory scan of sensation, in which the assessor runs his hands firmly over the patient's skin bilaterally. This can be done with the patient's eyes open, while the patient indicates disparities in sensation between affected and unaffected sides. The patient then closes the eyes for detailed sensory testing, in which the examiner outlines the specific area of altered sensation and associates it with known dermatomes and peripheral nerves, keeping in mind that referred pain can confuse the picture. Other common sensory tests are superficial tactile sensation testing, using cotton or a brush, and superficial pain testing (pin prick), which uses light tapping with a sharp object. The latter tests the responses of group II afferent nerve fibers, which respond to pressure, touch, or vibration. Other group II tests include placing a tuning fork against bony protuberances (vibration) and squeezing the Achilles tendon (deep pressure). Group III fibers that are associated with temperature sensation and fast pain can be evaluated by touching the patient with hot- and cold-water-filled test tubes. There are a number of tests for proprioception (sense of position) and other sensations.

Sensation Testing During Neurologic Examination

Sensation testing should be done in a dermatomal pattern, meaning all the dermatomes or skin areas innervated by the different spinal nerves should be included. The sensations to be covered and means of testing are:

- Pain: evaluated by asking patient to distinguish between dull and sharp stimuli, typically a pen cap or pin
- Pressure: done by applying firm finger pressure to see if patient feels it
- Light touch: is similar to pressure except light pressure (finger, cotton ball, cloth) is applied
- Proprioception: evaluated by gripping the distal interphalangeal joints in hand or foot and asking patient to identify whether the joint is moving up or down
- Vibration: done by placing activated tuning fork on bony prominence and having patient indicate when vibration slows and stops
- Temperature: uses test tubes filled with warm or cold water placed against the body
- Stereognosis: employs a familiar object placed in patient's hand for identification
- Two-point discrimination: uses a caliper or drafting compass on the area
- Graphesthesia: done by tracing a letter or number in patient's palm for identification
- Double simultaneous stimulation: evaluated by asking patient to identify two points being touched simultaneously

Scanning Examination

A scanning examination is a combination of a scan of peripheral joints, myotome testing, and a sensory scan. Both upper limb and lower limb scans are done. A scanning examination is useful for differentiating between spinal-derived referred pain and pain specific to a peripheral joint. The examination involves doing a few strategic movements at each joint, including those likely to exacerbate symptoms based on history, followed by testing of key myotomes or muscles related to specific nerve roots, and then sensory scanning. Possible parts of the sensory scan are tests for reflexes, determination of the distribution of dermatomes and peripheral nerves, and neurodynamic tests. A scanning examination is a normal part of cervical and lumbar spinal assessment, but here it is used as part of peripheral assessment. Tests specific to the peripheral joint (reflexes, sensory tests) are performed for clarification as opposed to tests for specific spinal areas if spinal involvement is suggested.

Upper and Lowers Quarter Screens

Nerve Root Dermatomes, Myotomes, Reflexes, and Paresthesias Found on an Upper-Quarter Screen

Upper- and lower-quarter screens are short evaluations for bilateral range of motion, muscle strength, sensations, and deep tendon reflexes. An upper-quarter screen is the evaluation of one side down to generally the T1 nerve root, roughly equivalent to an upper limb scan. For lesions in each nerve root in this area, the following might be observed:

Nerve root	Myotome	Dermatome
C1	cervical rotation	vertex of skull
C2	shoulder shrug	posterior head
C3	shoulder shrug	neck
C4	shoulder shrug	acromioclavicular joint
C5	shoulder abduction	lateral arm
C6	wrist extension	lateral forearm,
C7	elbow extension,	palmar distal phalanx of triceps
C8	thumb extension,	palmar distal part of tricep
T1	finger abduction	medial forearm

This list does not thoroughly examine all possibilities.

Nerve Root Dermatomes, Myotomes, Reflexes, and Paresthesias Found on an Lower-Quarter Screening

A lower-quarter screening is roughly equivalent to a lower limb scan and involves evaluation on one side from nerve roots L1 to S1or lower. Most thoracic nerve root involvement is hard to localize. For lesions in each nerve root in this area, the following might be observed:

Nerve root	Myotome	Dermatome
L1	hip flexion	back and thigh near groin
L2	hip flexion	back, front of thigh to knee
L3	knee extension	middle third of front thigh
L4	knee extension	patella, medial malleolus
L5	great toe extension	fibular head, dorsum of foot
S1	ankle plantar flexion	lateral malleolus, plantar surface

This list does not thoroughly examine all possibilities. S2 lesions have similar effects as S1, and S3 and S4 lesions mainly involve the groin and genital areas, respectively.

Classifications of Nerve Injuries

The most frequently used classification of nerve injuries is Seddon's system which grades them into three categories:

- Neurapraxia is a temporary (minutes to days) physiological block initiated by pressure or stretch of the nerve. There is no axonal injury and, therefore, no wallerian degeneration. The individual experiences pain, numbness, muscle weakness, and some loss of proprioception.

- Nerve injuries that significantly damage the axons and cause wallerian degeneration but preserve the internal structure of the nerve are known as axonotmesis. This person experiences pain, muscle weakness, and a complete loss of motor, sensory, and sympathetic nerve functions. Sensation returns before motor functioning, and total recovery takes months.
- Neurotmesis occurs when the structure of the nerve is actually destroyed because it has been severed, severely scarred, or significantly compressed at length. The person with neurotmesis experiences no pain as there is anesthesia, but otherwise symptoms are similar to axonotmesis, namely muscle wasting and complete loss of motor, sensory, and sympathetic functions. Recovery requires surgery and takes months.

Damage to Peripheral Nerves vs Contractile Tissues

Pain, weakness, and other symptoms in an area could be due to damage to the contractile tissues or the peripheral nerves associated with them. Thus, it is important to recognize signs of peripheral nerve damage. Neurapraxia, axonotmesis, and neurotmesis (defined on another card) are all associated with muscle weakness or muscle wasting but are neural in origin. Axonotmesis and neurotmesis can result in motor losses, such as reflex loss, joint instability, decreased range of motion, and others; sensory deficits, such as loss of vasomotor tone, depressed or abnormal sensations, skin and nail changes, and ulcerations; and sympathetic losses like dryness due to depression of sweat glands and loss of the pilomotor response. If a patient has combined sensory and motor loss, nervous tissue lesions should be suspected and the areas of loss should be examined to determine the origin.

Neurodynamic Tests

Neurodynamic, or neural tension, tests are exercises that put neural tissue under tension to potentially duplicate symptoms a patient may be experiencing. They are done to pinpoint whether a particular mechanical malfunction is due to stretching of a specific peripheral nerve or nerve root. Examples of these neurodynamic tests are the straight leg raise, the slump test, and the upper limb tension test. The basic operating principle of these tests is that neural tissue shifts toward the associated joint at the start of elongation, creating tension points. If there is nerve damage, the patient will experience tension and discomfort. The test is deemed positive if the patient's symptoms are mimicked during performance, if there is an asymmetric response, or if the patient's reaction is changed with movement of a distal body part.

Diagnostic Lumbar Puncture

A lumbar puncture (LP) is a procedure in which cerebrospinal fluid (CSF) is collected using a needle inserted into the subarachnoid space at lumbar level L1 or lower in the vertebra, usually between L3 and L4. The patient lies on the side during the collection. Numerous tubes of CSF are collected to test for characteristics like color, pH, cytology, and certain substances. Results of CSF testing are used to differentiate potential causes of neurologic dysfunction, including issues such as CNS metastases from tumors, cerebral hemorrhage, meningitis, encephalitis, demyelinating disorders like multiple sclerosis, etc. LP is also used to dispense spinal anesthetic, drain CSF in patients with hydrocephalus, and instill therapeutic or diagnostic agents. Potential complications of lumbar puncture include headache, backache, high temperature, site bleeding, and trouble voiding.

Mechanical Diagnosis of Neurological Problems

Electroencephalography, Evoked Potentials, Electromyography, and Nerve Conduction Velocity Studies

Electroencephalography (EEG), evoked potentials (EP), electromyography (EMG), and nerve conduction velocity studies all involve electrical responses in some way:

- In EEG, electrodes are attached to a patient's scalp to record electrical brain activity. EEG shows characteristic patterns for certain neurologic conditions, for example, seizures in epilepsy show rapid, spiking waves.
- EPs involve placing electrodes over parts of the brain or brain stem, applying an appropriate stimulus, and looking for conduction delays of the generated electrical responses, which can indicate lesions or tumors along that sensory pathway.
- In EMG, muscles are electrically stimulated and their activity documented.
- In nerve conduction studies, the conduction times and amplitudes of electrical response along peripheral nerves are quantified.

EMG and nerve conduction studies are generally combined to distinguish muscle diseases from peripheral nerve injury.

Imaging Techniques Used to Diagnose Neurologic Problems

Most post-traumatic imaging done for assessment is computed tomography (CT) and/or magnetic resonance imaging (MRI). A brain or head CT is useful for identifying intracranial hemorrhage, cerebral aneurysm, etc. It is considered by many to be the definitive test for distinguishing between hemorrhagic and ischemic processes due to a cerebrovascular accident (CVA) to determine whether tissue plasminogen activator (tPA) should be administered. Other variations include CT scanning of the spine and xenon CT, in which xenon gas is inhaled and cerebral blood flow measured. Some prefer MRI for imaging, as it provides better contrast, or a variation called magnetic resonance angiography. Simple radiography may be used as well. Other techniques are cerebral angiography, in which a radiopaque contrast medium is instilled via catheter and a radiograph taken; positron emission tomography (PET), in which radioactive chemicals are injected; digital-subtraction angiography (DSA), using contrast dye, radiography, and computer subtraction; myelography; and transesophageal or transthoracic echocardiography. Ultrasound is used to look at blood flow, either low frequency in transcranial Doppler sonography or high frequency in carotid duplex ultrasound.

Traumatic Brain Injuries

Traumatic Brain Injuries

Traumatic brain injuries (TBIs) are generally described in terms of their location, extent, and severity and the mechanism of injury:

- The location of a TBI is the cranium alone, the cranium and brain structures, or brain structures alone. TBI location is often differentiated as closed, in which protective mechanisms are maintained; open, where they are altered; coup, meaning the lesion is deep relative to the impact site; contrecoup, where the lesion and impact site are on opposite sides; or combined coup-countrecoup.
- Ways of classifying the extent include primary versus secondary (direct brain changes alone versus further complications) or focal versus diffuse, meaning specific or gross lesions.

- Severity is usually defined in terms of cognitive deficits or the Glasgow Coma Scale and diagnostic tests.
- The mechanism of injury refers to the type of force causing the damage, which is generally either acceleration-deceleration, rotational, or direct impact.

Secondary Acceleration-Deceleration Traumatic Brain Injuries

Common types of traumatic brain injuries (TBIs) due to secondary acceleration-deceleration forces are:

- Cerebral concussion: This is a shaking of the brain. It is characterized clinically by a transitory loss of consciousness or state of confusion, headache, faintness, irritability, inappropriate laughter, nausea, diminished concentration and memory, amnesia, and/or altered gait.
- Cerebral contusion: This is a slight hemorrhage to the brain. It can also occur after a skull fracture. Symptomatically, it resembles a cerebral concussion except there may be a lag period before presentation.
- Postconcussive syndrome (PCS): This is a syndrome in which clinical findings are consistent with cerebral concussion, persisting for weeks or months, also including sleep disturbances and depression.
- Cerebral laceration: This is a tear of the cortical surface. It is usually found in association with cerebral contusion near bony surfaces. Clinical signs are variable depending on area implicated, intracranial pressure, and mass effect.
- Diffuse axonal injury (DAI): This is pervasive shearing of white matter, usually after a motor vehicle accident. Its severity is defined in terms of how long the person remains in a coma, its main clinical finding. Severe DAI also presents as abnormal posturing.

Hematoma After Traumatic Brain Injury

A hematoma is a semi-solid mass or accumulation of blood in tissues. There are three common types of hematomas that occur after a traumatic brain injury. Each is defined by the area of the brain where the blood has accumulated:

1. The first is epidural hematoma (EDH), in which blood accumulates in the epidural space after tearing of meningeal arteries usually due to cranial fractures.
2. Another is subdural hematoma (SDH), blood accretion in the subdural space due to tears in cerebral veins, intracranial hemorrhage, or excessive bleeding from a cerebral contusion. SDH can occur acutely or as late as several months after the precipitating event.
3. Lastly, intracerebral hematoma (ICH) is blood accumulation in the brain tissues. ICH can be caused by acceleration-deceleration forces after injury, shearing of cortical blood vessels, fractures, hypertension, or delayed bleeding.

All three of these types of hematoma present similarly, with possible clinical findings of headache, altered consciousness, contralateral hemiparesis, posture issues, etc. With EDH or SDH, the patient may have a lucid period between two bouts of loss of consciousness.

Secondary Complications from Traumatic Brain Injuries

Common secondary complications from traumatic brain injuries (TBI) include increased intracranial pressure (ICP), anoxia, and seizures:

- ICP occurs in the majority of TBI patients because the skull cannot adapt to the large fluid volumes resulting from edema or hemorrhage. Possible sequelae from ICP include compression of brain tissue, decreased blood flow to brain tissues, herniation, unresponsiveness, impaired consciousness, headache, high blood pressure, low heart rate, and others.
- Neurons in the hippocampus, cerebellum, and basal ganglia are susceptible to the effects of anoxia, or inadequate oxygenation; thus, disorders like amnesia and movement problems that are associated with these areas of the brain are common.
- Posttraumatic epilepsy or seizures usually occur in TBI patients who had open head injuries or subdural hematoma or who are older, and events are usually set off by some type of trigger, such as stress, infection, or electrolyte imbalance. Common seizure medications include phenytoin, phenobarbital, and carbamazepine.

Clinical Problems Associated with Traumatic Brain Injuries

Traumatic brain injury patients often have a decreased level of consciousness. They also generally have various cognitive deficits, such as memory loss or disorientation. The most common motor deficits seen are abnormal postures, either decerebrate or decorticate rigidity. Other possible motor deficits include generalized weakness, tonic and primitive reflexes that cannot be controlled, balance problems, ataxia, and impaired motor sequencing. Certain senses may be impaired or lost. Communication is difficult due to abnormal tone or posturing. Many patients develop personality or psychological problems. In addition, many TBI patients have other injuries that need to be considered.

Spinal Cord Injuries

Spinal Cord Injuries

A spinal cord injury (SCI) is generally described in terms of its location, mechanism of action, and, often, severity. The location is the level of the spinal cord lesion in the cervical, thoracic, or lumbar spine. Functional deficits associated with the different lesion levels are spontaneous breathing (C4), shoulder shrugging (C5), elbow flexion (C6), elbow extension (C7), finger flexion (C8 to T1), use of intercostal and abdominal muscles (T1 to T12), hip flexion (L1 to L2), hip adduction (L3), hip abduction (L4), dorsiflexion of foot (L5), plantar flexion of foot (S1 to S2), and rectal sphincter tone (S2 to S4). Possible mechanisms of injury include forward hyperflexion, hyperextension, axial compression, rotation, contusion, laceration, and transection. Forward hyperflexion and hyperextension can both cause disc herniation and vertebral dislocation or fracture, plus discontinuity in posterior or anterior spinal ligaments, respectively. Severity is classified on another card.

American Spinal Injury Impairment Scale

Spinal cord injuries from trauma or impingement usually result in some level of paraplegia or quadriplegia, the inability to move the lower body or all four limbs, respectively. Spinal cord injury (SCI) severity is usually classified according to the American Spinal Injury Association Impairment Scale in terms of motor and sensory function retained. The classifications are:

- **A**: complete, no sensory or motor function in S4 to S5
- **B**: incomplete, maintenance of sensory function but no motor function below neurologic level, including S4 to S5

- **C**: incomplete, motor function preserved below neurologic level with majority of key muscles functioning at < 3/5
- **D**: incomplete, similar to C except most key muscles function ≥ 3/5
- **E**: normal, intact sensory and motor functions

Secondary Spinal Cord Injury

Secondary spinal cord injury is the collection of pathological problems that can occur subsequent to a spinal cord injury (SCI). Much of secondary SCI is vascular in nature, including possible vasospasm in spinal blood vessels, intraparenchymal hemorrhage, and breakdown of the barrier between blood and the brain and spinal cord. The patient goes into neurogenic shock and loses the ability to autoregulate functions. Other complications include increasing calcium levels, which stimulate free radicals, leading to further tissue damage. The neurologic substances catecholamines and opioids are discharged, and microglia and macrophages accumulate. Immediately after a SCI, the injured person experiences spinal shock, hypotension, bradycardia, and hypothermia. Later, physiological sequelae can include autonomic dysreflexia, orthostatic hypotension, impaired functions (respiratory, bladder, bowel, sexual), deep venous thrombosis, diabetes insipidus, SIADH, etc.

Incomplete Spinal Cord Injury Syndromes

Incomplete spinal cord injury syndromes include:

- Central cord syndrome: impingement of the central cord through a hyperextension injury, presence of a tumor, rheumatoid arthritis, or a cyst within the spinal cord (syringomyelia); lesion applies pressure to anterior horn cells, causing bilateral motor paralysis primarily in the upper extremities, sensory losses, and sometimes bowel and bladder dysfunction
- Anterior cord syndrome: damage to anterior cord via a hyperflexion injury, disc herniation, or damage to an anterior spinal artery; causes damage to the anterolateral spinothalamic and cortical spinal tracts and the anterior horn, resulting in bilateral loss of pain and temperature sensations and most motor functions
- Brown-Sequard syndrome: damage to half of the spinal cord due to things like stab wounds, epidural hematoma, cervical spondylosis, etc.; patient loses sensations of pain and temperature on the opposite side, and on the same side, losses include sensations of touch, proprioception, and vibration and motor function.
- Dorsal column or posterior cord syndrome: compression of posterior spinal artery from tumor or infarct; bilateral deficits in senses of vibration and proprioception
- Cauda equina injuries: due to fracture or dislocation below L1; may cause flaccidity, areflexia, loss of excretory functions

Management of Spinal Cord Injuries

Medically, a patient with a spinal cord injury (SCI) is stabilized, including ventilatory support and treatment for secondary injuries as needed. The patient is immobilized, using a collar, orthosis, traction, halo vest, and/or surgical fusion of fragments, and generally given methylprednisolone promptly to enhance blood flow and decrease possible tissue damage.

For symptoms of autonomic dysreflexia (in injuries above T6), such as significant hypertension, pounding headache, etc., patients are given medications to lower blood pressure (nitroglycerin patch, vasodilators, nifedipine).

Patients with postural hypotension are managed with fluids, abdominal binders, or appropriate drugs. Associated pain is usually dysesthetic (phantom) pain, addressed with NSAIDS, antiepileptics, anticonvulsants, tricyclic antidepressants, or psychological techniques. Pressure ulcers are addressed with pressure-relief techniques. Heterotopic ossification of nearby bones is managed with etidronate, range-of-motion exercises, and, sometimes, surgical resection. If contractures develop, a good stretching program is indicated. Patients may be given oral warfarin or IV heparin to prevent deep vein thrombosis. The significant complications of respiratory compromise, bladder and bowel dysfunction, sexual dysfunction, and spasticity are discussed elsewhere.

Respiratory Compromise in Spinal Cord Injury

Patients with high cervical spinal cord injuries often cannot breathe independently because they are paralyzed or their diaphragm, usually innervated by nerve roots C3 to C5, is weak. Lower level injuries can also cause respiratory compromise as other breathing-related muscles may be affected, such as the external intercostals innervated starting at the T1 level, upper abdominals at T7 to T9, and lower abdominals at T9 to T11. Injuries below T12 should not affect respiration. If there is respiratory compromise, possible interventions include use of abdominal binders, upright positioning, assisted cough techniques, diaphragmatic strengthening exercises, and incentive spirometry.

Bladder, Bowel, and Sexual Dysfunctions in Spinal Cord Injury Patients

The bladder is innervated by spinal nerves at the S2 to S4 sacral. It is flaccid or areflexic during the initial spinal shock after injury and remains so in patients whose injury is to the cauda equina or conus medullaris, the terminal end of the spinal cord. These patients have a flaccid or non-reflexive bladder, which necessitates manual emptying. However, if the injury is above the S2 level, the patient will have a reflex or spastic bladder, which they can induce to empty through external stimulation. Bladder training is a key component of therapy. The anal sphincter is innervated at the S2 level, and patients may have bowel problems as well. Correspondingly, a regular bowel program, high-fiber diet, fluids, stool softeners, and/or manual stimulation are generally indicated. In terms of sexual dysfunction, the main problem for males is limitation of the ability to ejaculate, which makes them less fertile. Women can become pregnant but cannot feel uterine contractions during labor. The therapist's role is basically informational in this case.

Spasticity as a Complication of Spinal Cord Injuries

Spasticity, or muscle hypertonicity, is a common complication in spinal cord injuries. It is probably due to lingering effects of supraspinal centers and inadequate modulation of spinal pathways. The presence of spasticity is both good and bad because while it is annoying to the patient and others, it also facilitates muscle bulking, prevents muscle atrophy, and helps circulation. Appropriate physical therapy interventions for spasticity include weight bearing, static stretching, correct positioning, cryotherapy, electrical stimulation, and aquatic exercises. A common drug given for spasticity is baclofen, administered orally or via an intrathecal pump. Other pharmacologic agents include botulinum toxin A injections into the muscle (causing its temporary paralysis); injectable phenol as a nerve block; and oral diazepam, clonidine, or dantrolene sodium. Spasticity can also be addressed surgically. Surgical procedures include neurectomy, excision of a portion of the nerve; rhizotomy, resection of a dorsal or sensory nerve; myelotomy, cutting of spinal cord tracts; and tenotomy, tendon release.

Cerebrovascular Accidents

Cerebrovascular Accidents

A cerebrovascular accident (CVA), or stroke, is the sudden onset of neurologic signs resulting from blockage or rupture of a blood vessel in the brain. It is often preceded days or months in advance by a transient ischemic attack (TIA), a focal brain or retinal disturbance of short duration.

The majority of strokes are ischemic CVAs, meaning there is decreased oxygenation to the brain due to a poor blood supply. This type of CVA is further characterized as either thrombotic, due to blood vessel constriction (for example, atherosclerosis), or embolic, due to a clot lodged in a cerebral blood vessel. Cerebral tissue in the area undergoes infarct or death, adjacent neurons are injured, and other substances are released that cause additional cellular damage.

The other common type of CVA is a hemorrhagic CVA, in which there is excessive bleeding due to rupture of a cerebral blood vessel, again causing cerebral hypoperfusion. Hemorrhagic CVAs are caused by factors such as hypertension and vessel malformations. A rarer type observed is a lacunar CVA, which is an infarction in a small vessel in regions like the basal ganglia and thalamus; this type is seen primarily in patients with diabetes and hypertension and does not cause cognitive or visual deficits.

Neurologic Signs of a Cerebrovascular Accident for Different Arteries Affected

Arteries in the brain affected by a cerebrovascular accident and the corresponding neurologic signs are the:

- Internal carotid artery: blindness on one side; hemiplegia and hemianesthesia on the opposing side; significant aphasia (inability to produce and understand speech)
- Middle cerebral artery: altered speech, cognition, mobility, and sensation; contralateral hemiplegia or hemiparesis; motor and sensory loss; and visual field losses
- Anterior cerebral artery: amnesia, personality changes, confusion; bladder incontinence; contralateral hemiplegic or hemiparesis
- Posterior cerebral artery: hemianesthesia; ataxia; tremors; memory loss; aphasia; vision problems; hemiplegia on opposite side
- Posterior inferior cerebellar artery: difficulty swallowing and speaking; anesthesia for pain and temperature in face and cornea on ipsilateral side and trunk and extremities on contralateral side
- Anterior inferior and superior cerebellar arteries: articulation and gross movement problems; nystagmus
- Vertebral or basilar arteries: signs dependent on amount of occlusion, ranging from weakness and other sensory and motor deficits to coma; if in anterior portion of the pons, "Locked-in" Syndrome occurs, characterized by complete lack of movement, except for eyelids

Diagnosis and Acute Management of a Cerebrovascular Accident

The patient experiencing a cerebrovascular accident (CVA) should be hospitalized. The doctor performs a physical examination that includes neurological tests for motor and sensory functions, reflexes, and speech. Imaging is done to determine whether the brain vessel damage causing CVA is ischemic or hemorrhagic. Common imaging techniques used are magnetic resonance imaging or computed tomography. Acute medical management is directed at regulating the person's blood pressure, cerebral perfusion, and intracranial pressure. Patients are usually given the anticoagulant heparin, diuretics, calcium channel blockers, prophylactic anticonvulsants, and the antithrombolytic tissue plasminogen activator (tPA), if the stroke is ischemic. Patients with hemorrhagic CVAs often require surgical procedures, such as evacuation of the hematoma, removal of a blood vessel, or placement of a metal clip at the base of an aneurysm. Unproven treatment options include administration of cytoprotective drugs like calcium channel blockers, injection of fibrinolytic agents via a catheter, use of mechanical clot removal devices, and application of mild to moderate hypothermia to preserve neurologic function.

The Brunnstrom Stages of Recovery Following a Cerebrovascular Accident

S. Brunnstrom identified seven stages of motor recovery by patients who have had a cerebrovascular accident:

1. Stage I is flaccidity, in which the patient has no voluntary or reflex activity in the involved extremity.
2. The next 4 stages involve some degree of spasticity or hypertonicity.
3. Stage II is the period when spasticity and synergy patterns begin to develop. In Brunnstrom's view, synergy patterns involve characteristic groups of muscles that work together to create movement patterns, for example, flexion versus extension of the same region.
4. Stage III of recovery is the period where spasticity increases and peaks, during which movement synergies of the involved extremity can be executed voluntarily.
5. Spasticity then begins to decline during stages IV and V.
6. During stage IV, the patient can deviate from characteristic synergy patterns and perform some combined movements.
7. During stage V, synergy patterns are less evident and the patient can perform more complex combined movements.
8. By stage VI, spasticity has vanished and the individual can perform isolated and combined movements.
9. The final stage VII is characterized by a return to normal function and renewed ability to perform fine motor skills.

Impairments Found in Patients Who Have Undergone a Cerebrovascular Accident

After a stroke, patients usually have flaccid muscles, followed by a period of spasticity, before recovery of motor skills (see card on Brunnstrom Stages of Recovery). Spasticity is often developed at first in the shoulder and pelvic girdles, resulting in characteristic posturing. Patients have difficulty with processes requiring strength, such as gripping, and may exhibit apraxia, the inability to perform complex movements. They have sensory, communication, and/or orofacial impairments. Aphasia occurs in about 30% of stroke patients as Broca's aphasia, where they have trouble with expression; Wernicke's aphasia, where they cannot understand what is being said; or global aphasia, which encompasses both. Orofacial deficits include facial asymmetries, dysphagia (difficulty swallowing), and inability to coordinate eating and breathing. Patients usually have respiratory problems, in particular decreased lung expansion and volumes due to lessened ability to control respiratory muscles. Primitive spinal and brain stem reflexes are recalled, and patients may have associated reactions (all discussed elsewhere). Deep tendon reflexes may be absent or exaggerated, depending on whether they are in a flaccid or spastic phase. Common initial problems are bowel and bladder dysfunction.

Primitive Spinal and Brain Stem Reflexes Recalled After a Person Has a Cerebrovascular Accident

Patients revert to use of primitive, non-voluntary spinal and brain stem reflexes when their central nervous system is damaged. Common spinal level reflexes are:

- Flexor withdrawal: extension of the toes with ankle dorsiflexion when a stimulus is applied to the bottom of the foot
- Cross-extension: flexion followed by extension of opposing extremity after application of stimulus to ball of foot when leg is extended

- Startle: extension and abduction of the upper extremities in response to an unexpected loud noise
- Grasp: flexion of the toes or fingers when pressure is applied to the ball of the foot or palm of the hand, respectively

Primitive brain stem reflexes include:

- Symmetric tonic neck reflex: where flexion or extension of the neck results in similar response in arms but opposite in legs
- Asymmetric tonic neck reflex: where rotation of the neck to one side results in extension of the same side arm and leg, and flexion of the arm and leg on the opposite side
- Tonic labyrinthine reflex: in which lying prone or supine encourages flexion or extension, respectively
- Tonic thumb reflex: in which elevation of the involved extremity causes thumb extension with the forearm in supination

Associated reactions are automatic movements in other parts of the body in response to active or resisted movements.

Complications Observed Following a Cerebrovascular Accident

Development of contractures and deformities is one of the most common complications of cerebrovascular accident, due primarily to the spasticity present after a stroke. The vast majority of patients with hemiplegia develop shoulder pain and, often, loss of function caused by either muscle weakness or spasticity. Complex regional pain syndrome (CRPS) often occurs. CRPS is a three-stage process developing over the course of six months to a year, in which initially the person has burning and aching pain, edema, warm skin, and fast hair and nail growth; which develops into joint stiffness, brittle nails, and cool skin; and eventually, into irreparable skin changes and contractures. Patients who have had CVA are also prone to falls, thrombophlebitis, joint and muscle pain, and depression.

Cerebral Aneurysm, Arteriovenous Malformation, and Subarachnoid Hemorrhage

A cerebral aneurysm is a localized ballooning or dilation of a cerebral blood vessel due to weakness in its wall. Causes include congenital defects, high blood pressure, atherosclerosis, and trauma. An arteriovenous malformation (AVM) is an abnormal connection between arteries and veins without capillary interface. AVM is usually congenital and can cause signs like headache, paralysis, epilepsy, and sensory deficits. Both cerebral aneurysms and AVMs can lead to bleeding complications in the brain, making them primary mechanisms (along with tumors, trauma, and infections) for subarachnoid hemorrhage (SAH), one type of hemorrhagic cerebrovascular accident in which blood accumulates in the subarachnoid space. Low-grade SAH may be asymptomatic or present simply as headache and neck rigidity, but increasing severity is characterized by further neurological deficits and the possibility of coma. Management of SAH may include surgical intervention, such as aneurysm repair with blood evacuation, and various measures to stabilize the patient. Common complications are further bleeding, hydrocephalus, seizure, and vasospasm, which can lead to tissue damage and sensory alterations.

Dementia

Dementia is the serious loss of cognitive ability in a heretofore unimpaired individual in areas such as memory, attention span, language, and problem solving. There are many conditions that directly cause or factor into development of dementia. The most widespread cause is Alzheimer's disease (AD), characterized by gradual cognitive losses and the presence of amyloid plaques in the brain in place of white matter. Lewy body dementia (LBD) is a form of dementia characterized by fluctuating cognition, visual hallucinations, and motor features of parkinsonism. It has been associated with presence of Lewy bodies in neurons, clumps of alpha-synuclein and ubiquitin protein. Parkinson's disease itself is a contributor to dementia. Another type that appears more abruptly is vascular dementia, due to multiple cortical or subcortical infarctions or deep ischemic injury. In this case, the deficits are generally confined to emotional lability, depression, body preoccupation, and nighttime confusion. AIDS, alcoholism, and metabolic disorders have been associated with dementia as well. Physical therapy considerations include reduction of distractions, simplification of instructions, and completion of transfers in a manner that will reduce the patient's fear of falling.

HYDROCEPHALUS

Hydrocephalus is the abnormal accumulation of cerebrospinal fluid (CSF) in the ventricles or cavities of the brain. This usually causes increased intracranial pressure, head enlargement, headache, convulsions, and/or altered consciousness. There are two types. The first is noncommunicating, or obstructive, hydrocephalus, which is caused by an obstruction to CSF flow in the ventricular system. The other is communicating hydrocephalus, in which the obstruction is at the border of the subarachnoid space. Hydrocephalus is managed by addressing the underlying cause, if possible, or using shunts to divert the accumulating CSF. Some communicating hydrocephalus is a subset called normal-pressure hydrocephalus (NHP), in which there is no increase in intracranial pressure. NHP is characterized by confusion, gait changes, and urinary incontinence; it is usually improved with a lumbar puncture to remove surplus CSF or placement of a ventriculoperitoneal shunt.

SEIZURES

A seizure is an abrupt-onset, aberrant neurologic functioning due to excessive neuronal activation in the cerebral cortex or deep limbic. Epilepsy is a recurrent form. Underlying causes of seizure include cerebrovascular accidents, head trauma or surgery, and meningitis. Seizures are classified as partial, if they occur focally in one hemisphere, or generalized, if they derive from both hemispheres or at deep midline. Partial seizures are further divided into simple partial (no loss of consciousness), complex partial (transitory loss with motionless staring), and partial with secondary generalization (moving toward both hemispheres). Generalized seizures are categorized as tonic (abrupt flexor or extensor rigidity), clonic (rhythmic, jerky muscle movements), tonic-clonic (sudden extensor rigidity, then flexor jerking), atonic (no muscle tone), absence (transitory unresponsiveness and blank staring), and myoclonic (rapid, nonrhythmic jerking). Possible signs of seizure include aura, tremors, visual changes, hallucinations, and faintness. The definitive diagnostic tool is EEG. Management includes addressing the cause, prescribing antiepileptic drugs, resectioning the focal point, and embedding a vagal nerve stimulator. Status epilepticus, where seizures continue, is an emergency necessitating life support.

Review Video: Seizures
Visit mometrix.com/academy and enter code: 977061

SYNCOPE

Syncope is the brief loss of consciousness and postural tone due to cerebral underperfusion. It is usually accompanied by slow heart rate and hypotension. Syncope has four types of origins: cardiogenic, due to drug toxicity or various types of cardiac abnormalities; neurologic, with causes like seizure, vertigo, and cerebral atherosclerosis; reflexive, due to carotid sinus syndrome or some type of vasovagal response; and orthostatic, caused by things like protracted bed rest or drug side effects. Syncope is confirmed through history, event recorders, tilt-table testing, and CT or MRI, if there is new neurologic evidence. Its management is highly dependent on the underlying cause.

Poliomyelitis and Postpoliomyelitis Syndrome

Poliomyelitis is a neuroinfectious disease, meaning it is of infectious origin, in this case caused by polioviruses spread via the fecal-oral route or through drinking contaminated water. Poliomyelitis is preventable with administration of inactivated poliovirus vaccine (IVP). There is a wide range of clinical presentation for poliomyelitis. Milder cases can be asymptomatic, a general illness without fever, or aseptic meningitis. However, more severe poliomyelitis usually presents as asymmetric paralysis of respiratory, throat, and leg muscles, along with fever and muscle pain. This paralysis may go away, have lingering effects, or lead to death. Polio is managed with administration of analgesics and fever reducers, bronchopulmonary hygiene, bed rest, and techniques to prevent contractures, such as positioning and range of motion.

Postpoliomyelitis syndrome (PPS) is a condition that occurs decades after paralytic poliomyelitis. It is due to overuse or aging of originally involved motor units and is characterized by fatigue, pain, cold intolerance, and, sometimes, muscle atrophy or inflammation. Short bouts of exercise interspersed with rest periods are suggested; aquatic exercise is a good option as it decreases stress on joints, bones, and muscles.

Meningitis and Encephalitis

Meningitis and encephalitis are two neuroinfectious diseases in which there is inflammation of the meninges or brain tissues. respectively. Meningitis is spread through inhalation of infected airborne mucous droplets. Bacterial meningitis can be caused by meningococci, pneumococci, or Haemophilus and affects many parts of the brain, leading to high intracranial pressure, hydrocephalus, headache, neck rigidity, and, potentially, a number of other primarily neurologic complications. There is also a milder viral form. Meningitis is addressed with antibiotics, anti-infective agents, immunologic agents, analgesics, IV fluids and vasopressors to maintain blood pressure, measures to regulate intracranial pressure, and use of ventilators, if indicated.

Infectious encephalitis is mainly transmitted by herpes simplex type I virus-containing respiratory droplets. Other modes of encephalitis transmission are through bites from mosquitoes infected with another virus and nasal intake during swimming of an ameba. Symptoms of encephalitis include fever, altered consciousness and other neurologic abnormalities, severe frontal lobe headaches, hyperthermia, weakness, etc. It is treated with anti-infectives, IV fluids and electrolytes, management of intracranial pressure, mechanical ventilation, and nasogastric feeding.

Review Video: Meningitis
Visit mometrix.com/academy and enter code: 277418

Vestibular Disorders

The vestibular system is made up of various canals and organs in the inner ear, as well as parts of the brain and spinal cord. Normally, it stabilizes visual images on the retina during movement, preserves postural stability during head movements, and maintains spatial orientation. If the system is disrupted, the patient may experience vertigo, or the sensation that the surroundings are moving or spinning. Widespread conditions associated with vestibular dysfunction include:

- Benign positional paroxysmal vertigo (BPPV): brief, severe vertigo occurring with head position changes; due primarily to some type of trauma; Hallpike-Dix test often used to pinpoint affected canal by observing for nystagmus and vertigo with head in different positions; later, Epley maneuver is used to right the patient, who should sleep that night in a semirecumbent position
- Acute vestibular neuronitis: sudden-onset, longer-lasting vertigo; usually due to viral infection; treatment mainly supportive
- Meniere's disease: episodes of vertigo due to end lymphatic fluid in the inner ear; management includes salt restriction, diuretics, vestibular reducing medications, endolymphatic shunt, etc.
- Bilateral vestibular hypofunction (BVH): generally, permanent oscillating vision and unsteady gait; caused by aminoglycoside drugs

Measure Vestibular Dysfunction Tests

The majority of the tests to measure vestibular dysfunction are some type of vision test. One is the dynamic visual acuity test (DVA), in which the patient reads the low line on the eye chart while the professional oscillates his head to look for declining visual acuity. Several vision tests look for presence of nystagmus, or involuntary eyeball movement, including static ocular observation and head shaking, followed by clinician observation. Other vision tests include examination saccades, the head thrust test, the rotary chair test, caloric testing, and the Hallpike-Dix test (discussed elsewhere). Absent or slowed nystagmus is indicative of pathology in many of these tests. Another somewhat different assessment is the Romberg test, in which the patient stands with feet together, first with eyes open and then closed, and increased sway or balance loss with the latter is suggestive of vestibular dysfunction. The sensory organization test is a six-part assessment, during which the patient stands either on a fixed or moving platform with eyes open, closed, or in front of a moving screen and sway is noted for each condition.

Amyotrophic Lateral Sclerosis

Amyotrophic lateral sclerosis (ALS or Lou Gehrig's disease) is a progressive, degenerative central nervous system disorder involving upper and motor neurons. The causative agent is unknown. Symptoms include hyperreflexia and muscle atrophy, inflammation, and weakness with resultant functional problems (difficulty speaking, swallowing, breathing, walking, etc.). A diagnosis of ALS is made through observation of clinical signs, EMG, nerve conduction velocity studies, imaging techniques, and biopsies. Management is primarily supportive, including bronchopulmonary hygiene, limitation of spasticity, and psychosocial measures. The patient may be given the drug Rilutek. The role of the physical therapist with ALS patients is to find ways for the patient to cope as well as possible with his disability, including use of adaptive equipment.

Review Video: Amyotrophic Lateral Sclerosis (ALS)
Visit mometrix.com/academy and enter code: 178603

Guillain-Barre Syndrome

Guillain-Barre syndrome (GBS) is a degenerative central nervous system disorder. It is triggered by an antibody response to a viral infection that destroys Schwann cells forming the myelin sheath. GBS presents as lumbar pain, symmetric weakness, unusual skin tingling, and autonomic nervous system dysfunction, possibly leading to respiratory muscle paralysis. It is confirmed by testing cerebrospinal fluid for increased protein levels and looking at electrical activity via EMG. Initial hospitalization is imperative. Prognosis is variable, ranging from full recovery to death. Patients are often on a ventilator at first. Management strategies include immunosuppressive drugs, IV immunoglobulins, plasma exchange, respiratory assistance, pain management, and physical therapy. Acute phase therapy includes things like postural drainage, passive range of motion, and massage. As respiratory and autonomic functions improve, acclimation to upright posture should be started, and as they recover muscle strength, short episodes of non-fatiguing exercise should be initiated.

Multiple Sclerosis

Multiple sclerosis (MS) is a degenerative disorder in which white matter of the central nervous system and optic nerve is demyelinated. It is felt that the underlying cause is an autoimmune reaction triggered by a viral or other infection.

There are six categories of MS based primarily on disease course:

1. Relapsing-remitting
2. Primary progressive: from onset
3. Secondary-progressive: initially relapsing-remitting, then progressive
4. Progressive-relapsing: progressive from onset, but may include periods of recovery
5. Benign or mild
6. Malignant: Marburg's variant, rapidly progressive

MS is confirmed by presence of two or more plaques at demyelination areas observed on MRI, elevated myelin protein and IgG in a cerebrospinal fluid sample, evoked potentials, and clinical symptoms. The latter include double and blurred vision, focal weakness, vertigo, paresthesias, urinary incontinence, and, in later phases, a variety of additional neurologic problems (primarily spasticity and ataxia). Pharmacologic agents used for management include corticosteroids, interferons, immunosuppressants, and muscle relaxants. Physical therapy is an important part of management (discussed further elsewhere).

Parkinson's Disease

Parkinson's disease (PD) is a progressive, degenerative neurologic condition characterized by bradykinesia (slow movement), rigidity, tremor, and postural instability. The underlying cause of PD is presence of lesions in the substantia nigra of the basal ganglia of the midbrain, which leads to decreasing levels of the neurotransmitter dopamine. A PD patient typically has a characteristic shuffling gait, stooped posture, rigidity in trunk and extremities, tremors in head and extremities (all making them prone to falls), and other neurologic difficulties (speech problems, blank starring, dementia, etc.). Patients are staged from I to V using the Hoehn and Yahr Classification of Disability. Diagnosis is confirmed by presence of at least two of the four characteristic features indicated above and the exclusion of other syndromes that mimic PD. Medical management consists primarily of administration of antiparkinsonian drugs that replace dopamine, primarily levodopa (L-dopa). With long-term use of L-dopa, patients may still have periods of involuntary dyskinesias. There are also surgical options, such as a pallidotomy (removal or disconnection of globus pallidus), placement of a deep brain stimulator, and stem cell implants. Physical therapy is discussed elsewhere.

Rancho Los Amigos Scale of Cognitive Functioning

The Rancho Los Amigos Scale of Cognitive Functioning describes levels of cognitive functioning. It is useful for evaluating traumatic brain injury and other patients with various levels of cognitive ability. There are 10 levels. Characteristic behavior is described for each. Patients at levels I, II, and III (No Response, Generalized Response, Localized Response, respectively) require total assistance. Those at levels IV (Confused/Agitated) and V (Confused, Inappropriate Nonagitated) require maximal assistance. A level VI patient is Confused, Appropriate, needing moderate assistance; and one at level VII is Automatic, Appropriate, needing minimal assistance for performance of daily living skills. Levels VIII and IX (both Purposeful, Appropriate) necessitate only standby assistance, the latter upon request; an individual at level X is also Purposeful, Appropriate, but independent with modifications.

Cerebral Palsy

Cerebral palsy (CP) is a neurologic disorder characterized by delayed motor development, poor muscle tone, impaired movement patterns, and postural problems. CP is caused by damage to the brain early in the developmental process, before, during, or shortly after birth. It is not progressive. Among the risk factors for development of CP are certain prenatal maternal infections, asphyxia of the child during birthing, and brain infection or trauma during infancy. CP cases are generally classified in terms of the distribution of involvement (quadriplegia, diplegia, and hemiplegia), type of abnormal muscle tone, and severity. Spasticity, or hypertonus, is the most commonly observed type of muscle tone. Many CP patients have dyskinesia (disordered movement), athetosis (postural instability), and/or ataxia (in this case, loss of coordination). Other deficits associated with CP include feeding, speech, visual, and hearing impairments; intellectual disability; and seizures.

PT for a Child with Cerebral Palsy

The physical therapy examination for a person with cerebral palsy (CP) identifies his impairments and functional limitations within the context of the specific type of cerebral palsy in order to institute appropriate physical therapy. With the most common type, spastic cerebral palsy, typical impairments are increased muscle stiffness; slow movement, impacting balance and posture; decreased trunk rotation, making movement transitions difficult; decreased range of motion, affecting reaching and ambulation; skeletal malalignment and deformities; muscle weakness; and erroneous muscle recruitment. Physical therapy should focus on increased movement, righting and equilibrium exercises, protective reactions, movement transitions, skeletal positioning, use of orthoses, and muscle sequencing exercises. CP patients with athetosis or ataxia have postural instability due to low or fluctuating muscle tone, as well as uncoordinated movements; lack of midrange control, impacting reaching and walking; difficulty using their hands for support during transitions; a lack of graded movement, making it difficult to grasp or change positions; and emotional lability. Treatment should focus on holding postures, control of movements, holding midrange movements, upper-extremity weight bearing, stabilization, and behavior modification.

Myelomeningocele

Myelomeningocele (MMC) is a congenital disorder primarily involving the nervous system in which there is defective development of the spinal cord during gestation. The defect for MMC, also known as spina bifida cystica, is an incomplete vertebral closure with a cyst containing a malformed spinal cord. The MMC is generally removed and closed surgically within the first day of birth. The main defects neurologically are motor paralysis and sensory loss below the level of the MMC. The children tend to develop certain lower-extremity deformities, particularly foot deformities, such as clubfoot. They are also prone to osteoporosis, neuropathic fractures, spinal deformities, and hydrocephalus. The hydrocephalus, or increased levels of spinal fluid in the brain, is usually but not always found in association with a prevalent associated malformation in the cerebellum, medulla, and cervical portion of the spinal cord, called Arnold-Chiari type II malformation. Thus, most MMC patients have some sort of shunt to drain the cerebrospinal fluid. MMC patients may have central nervous system deterioration, hydromelia (excess CSF in the spinal cord) or a tethered spinal cord leading to scoliosis, various sensory impairments, bowel and bladder problems, and, interestingly, latex allergies.

Neurological Genetic Disorders in Children

Some important genetic disorders involving the neurologic system are: Down Syndrome: presence of extra 21st chromosome in bodily cells, resulting in intellectual disability, developmental delays, musculoskeletal deficits (such as instability at the atlanto-axial joint involving the two upper cervical vertebra), hypotonicity, flat facial features, a variety of neurological deficits, etc.

Arthropyosis multiplex congenital: a nonprogressive neuromuscular syndrome inherited on chromosome 9 (or 5 in neurogenic form); characterized by multiple contractures

Osteogenesis imperfecta: autonomic dominant disorder affecting collagen synthesis and bone metabolism, making individual prone to bone fractures; Spinal muscle atrophy (SMA): autonomic recessive, progressive neurologic disorder destroying anterior horn cells and lower motor neurons; Type I acute infantile SMA occurs shortly after birth and is characterized by respiratory and other oral issues and a frog-leg posture; Type II chronic SMA starts at approximately 2 to 18 months of age characterized by muscle weakness and scoliosis; later-onset Kugelberg-Welander SMA is similar

Duchenne muscular dystrophy (DMD): X-linked recessive trait in which muscle protein dystrophin is absent; symptomatic only in boys, presenting as progressive weakness (including cardiac and respiratory muscles), diminished range of motion, and contractures

Fragile X syndrome: presence of fragile site on X chromosome; signified by intellectual disability and other neurologic defects

Integumentary System

Burns

Basic Pathophysiology of Burns

When heat energy is absorbed causing a burn, the skin and sometimes subcutaneous tissue below develops a zone of coagulation in the center. This zone of coagulation, or eschar, is basically a scab of dead cells. Surrounding the zone of coagulation is a zone of stasis containing partially viable cells, and around that is a zone of hyperemia that is less damaged and capable of healing. Burns are classified in terms of how deep the zone of coagulation extends, reaching only the epidermis in a superficial burn, into the dermis for a partial-thickness burn, and into subcutaneous tissue for a full-thickness burn. Vasoactive substances are released after a burn injury, which can lead to increased vascular permeability and cell membrane damage. Increased vascular permeability can result in edema and associated sequelae, such as muscle damage, hypovolemia, and diminished intravascular volume. It can also impact a number of hematologic factors ultimately, resulting in increased blood viscosity. The effects of cell membrane destruction cause electrolyte changes. The eventual systemic effects of burn injuries can include a variety of respiratory, cardiovascular, gastrointestinal, genitourinary, and renal complications.

Review Video: Integumentary System
Visit mometrix.com/academy and enter code: 655980

Types of Thermal Burns

The four possible types of thermal burns, starting with the most common are:

- Scald burns: result from contact with hot liquid; generally partial- or full-thickness; often cover large areas
- Flame burns: caused by flame contact from fire, flammable liquids, ignition of clothing, or subsequent to carbon monoxide poisoning; most often superficial or deep partial-thickness
- Flash burns: occur when flammable liquids, such as gasoline, detonate; often partial-thickness and widely dispersed; usually coupled with upper airway thermal injury
- Contact burns: due to contact with hot objects, such as coal or hot glasses; often deep partial- or full-thickness; frequently occur in association with crushing incidents, such as car accidents; common in the elderly

Electrical Burns and Potential Complications

The actual burn caused by exposure to electrical current is generally superficial, but further tissue damage takes place along the pathway of the current. Muscles, nerves, bones, and other tissues are affected. Electrical burns are actually wounds, as they have an entrance and an exit point. The entrance wound is a hollow, necrotic area found where the current entered, and the exit wound is located at the point of grounding. Wound severity is dependent on factors like length of contact, voltage, and pathway. Electrical burns can cause a variety of cardiovascular complications, such as cardiac arrest, dysrhythmias, myocardial infarction, and heart muscle damage. They can also cause a number of neurologic problems, such as transitory loss of consciousness, seizures, and paralysis; secondary fractures due to muscle contractions or falls; ruptures; and later psychological problems. Lightning emits a very high electrical current, which can cause electrical burns through a direct strike to the grounded individual, a flash discharge, ground current, or a shock wave from associated static electricity.

Chemical Burns and Ultraviolet and Ionizing Radiation Burns

Chemical burns alter body tissue, changing its pH and metabolic characteristics. There may or may not be allied thermal injury. Chemical burns can cause critical pulmonary and/or metabolic complications.

Ionizing radiation burns include sunburns, which are superficial to partial-thickness burns from too much exposure to UV rays, and ionizing radiation burns that are due to the formation of free radicals from any type of electromagnetic or particulate radiation.

Ionizing radiation burns or acute radiation syndrome can be accompanied by a variety of gastrointestinal, hematologic, and/or vascular problems. Some of the most critical complications are hematologic as ionizing radiation depresses the numbers of all major types of blood cells and can lead to hemorrhage.

Burn Classifications

Burns are classified in terms of their extent and depth. Extent is defined as the total body surface area (TBSA) affected. TBSA is important to know because it is used to determine the volume of fluid needed for therapy and is predictive for the possibility of mortality. There are two methods of calculating TBSA:

- Rule of nines: the sum of assigned percentages in nine bodily regions, if burned; the front, back, and each leg are assigned 18%, the head and each arm are each assigned 9%, and the genitalia are designated as 1%; provision is made for partial regional burning

- Lund and Browder formula: a calculation that more accurately assigns percentages to specific regions and accounts for age differences; requires a corresponding chart to add up percentages for the calculation of TBSA

Burns that are irregularly shaped may be estimated using the person's palm as representative of 1% of TBSA. Burn depth is generally visibly estimated as superficial, moderate- or deep-partial thickness, or full thickness. There are also investigational ways of assessing depth, such as laser Doppler flowery, ultrasound, MRI, etc.

American Burn Association's Guidelines for Admission to a Burn Center

The American Burn Association advocates that a patient be admitted to a burn center for medical treatment if he meets any of the following criteria:

- The diagnosis is a partial-thickness burn covering more than 10% of TBSA (total body surface area).
- The burns occur on the face, hands, feet, genitalia or surrounding area, or any larger joints.
- The patient has third-degree burns.
- The patient has electrical or chemical burns and/or inhalation injury.
- The patient has preexisting medical problems that would present complications.
- The patient presents with both trauma and burns, but the latter is more critical.
- The patient is a child currently in a center without adequate facilities.
- The patient has special needs or requires long-term rehabilitation.

Inhalation Injury and Monoxide Poisoning During the Resuscitative Phase of Treating Burns

Assessment and management of inhalation injury and monoxide poisoning are some of the most important strategies during the resuscitative phase of burn management because the oropharynx and tracheobronchial tree can be damaged considerably by thermal injuries and chemical inhalants can harm lung tissue. Indications of inhalation injury include altered mental status, burns on or near the facial area, laryngeal edema, blood gases in a hypoxic range, etc. People with inhalation injuries often need to be intubated to keep the airway patent. Typically, inhalation injury occurs within the first 26 hours, followed by pulmonary edema and then bronchopneumonia, if not managed properly. Carbon monoxide (CO) inhalation usually causes asphyxia due to replacement of oxygen with CO molecules in hemoglobin, producing carboxyhemoglobin as well as increased pulmonary secretions. The patient develops disorientation, visual problems, and often coma unless the poisoning is reversed with 100% oxygen administration.

Essential Aspects of Burn Care During the Resuscitative Phase

The essential aspects of resuscitative burn care are repeated fluid resuscitation, infection control, maintenance of proper body temperature, pain management, and initial burn care (discussed further elsewhere). Changes in vascular pressure, permeability, mediator release, and protein concentrations cause fluids to move outside the intravascular spaces. This fluid shift, especially when greater than 20% TBSA is burned, is potentially fatal as it can cause hypovolemia, burn shock, and renal failure.

Therefore, IV fluid replacement with plasma or solutions is essential during the first two to three days. The affected skin no longer provides a protective barrier against microorganisms, thus making infection control imperative. The patient should be observed for signs of sepsis, aseptic techniques must be applied, a tetanus shot is indicated, and topical antimicrobial agents or antibiotics should be used as required. Compromised thermoregulation and the potential for hypothermia should be addressed with dry dressings to reduce heat loss and placement of the patient in a warm environment. The patient should be given IV analgesia (for example, opioids) that can exceed normal dosages.

Initial Burn Care

During the resuscitative phase, the burn itself needs to be counteracted. Initial burn care entails removing clothing and jewelry, rinsing or lavage, debridement, cleaning, dressing with topical antimicrobial agents, and, possibly, covering the burn. Debridement is the removal of dead, damaged, or infected wound tissue. There are two types of surgical procedures that might be indicated if there is an inflexible eschar, edema, and decreased arterial blood flow, the combination of which could eventually lead to limb loss. Both involve making an incision that releases pressure, through the eschar in an escharotomy or through the fascia in a fasciotomy.

Surgical Procedures Used During the Reparative Phase of Burn Management

Currently, burn management during the reparative phase generally involves early excision, grafting, and non-surgical procedures (discussed elsewhere). Excision entails surgical removal of the eschar to uncover the viable tissue. There are two types of excision performed: tangential, in which the eschar is removed in layers as far as the dermis; and full-thickness, where one thick layer down to the subcutaneous tissue is taken off.

Grafting is the transplantation of skin or skin substitutes onto a readied wound bed. There are many possible types of grafts, most being autografts, which are grafts in which the patient's skin from a different part of the body is taken (the donor site) and grafted permanently onto the new recipient site. Autografts are done either as split-thickness skin grafts (STSG), encompassing the epidermis and some of the dermis, or as full-thickness skin-grafts (FTSG), which extend further to the entire dermis. Types of permanent autografts are mesh, sheer, cultured epidermal, composite, and allogenic; the last three involve laboratory culture of cells. Temporary grafts include homografts (cadaver skin), heterografts (other animal species), and amnion (placental membrane).

Skin Substitutes for Temporary or Permanent Grafts for Burned Areas

There are currently at least three types of skin substitutes used as temporary graft options:

1. Biobrane is made of nylon mesh saturated with porcine collagen and silicone; it is appropriate for early use on smaller superficial to partial-thickness burns and spontaneously disengages from the wound within two weeks.
2. Dermagraft TC is made of a material containing biological wound-healing and growth factors; it is used for partial-thickness burns.
3. TransCyte is a polymer membrane containing cultured human fibroblast cells, which secrete substances involved in skin regeneration; it is used both for partial-thickness burns and deeper ones prior to autografting.

There are at least two permanent options:

1. AlloDerm is made of cadaver dermis and epidermis rendered immunologically inert; it is generally used in combination with a thin autograft on top for full-thickness burns or in post-burn reconstruction after contracture release.
2. Integra is the permanent option of choice for potentially fatal situations in which there are full- or deep partial-thickness burns. It is composed of an inner layer of bovine collagen and chondroitin-6-sulfate and an outer barrier, one of Silastic, which is later replaced with a thin autograft.

Non-Surgical Procedures During the Reparative Phase of Burn Management

During the reparative phase of burn management, the wound is generally cleaned and debrided several times daily to curtail infection and promote tissue healing. Debridement, the removal of dead or infected tissue, is discussed in detail elsewhere. Note that some burn units allow physical therapists, not only doctors and/or nurses, to do the debridement. The burn wounds, skin grafts, and donor sites used to procure grafts are commonly covered with dressings. Nonbiologic types of dressings include petrolatum, silver, polyurethane, foam, silicone, and negative pressure therapy. Negative pressure therapy—for example, the wound VAC system—is only appropriate for use on skin grafts. All of the other nonbiologic dressings can be used on partial-thickness burns, and most are also utilized on the graft or donor site as well. The other dressing category is biosynthetic and biologic. The modalities here are all appropriate for partial-thickness burns. They include oat (Glucan II, also used on grafts and donor sites), collagen and fibroblasts with or without keratinocytes, cadaver allografts, and xenografts, the latter two being grafts from other species.

Preferred Positioning of Affected Areas for Burn Patients

It is crucial to correctly position the joints at risk for contracture formation after burns. Proper positioning decreases the possibility of tightening and reduces edema. The burn injury areas and their proper positioning are the:

- Neck: in extension without rotation
- Shoulder: in abduction (90-degree angle) with external rotation and slight horizontal flexion
- Elbow and forearm: in extension with palm upward
- Wrist: neutral or slightly extended
- Hand: in functional position if the burn is on the back of the hand; with fingers and thumb extended if burn is on the palm
- Hip: in neutral extension/flexion and rotation with slight abduction
- Knee: extended
- Ankle: neutral or slightly bent without inversion; toes neutral

Three Types of Burn Scars

After burns undergo healing, the area becomes scarred. There are three types of burn scars that might develop, which are:

- Normotrophic scars: These are relatively normal looking because dermal collagen fibers are assembled in an organized parallel fashion.
- Hypertrophic scars: These have an aberrant appearance as dermal collagen fibers are assembled in a disorganized fashion but within the margins of the original wound.
- Keloid scars: These extend outside the margins of the original wound and are usually red or pink, raised, fibrous scars caused by excessive collagen accumulation. They are more common in, but not limited to, people of color.

Wounds

Types of Possible Wounds

The possible types of wounds include:

- Trauma wounds: injuries brought about by some sort of external force; Surgical wounds: enduring skin defects subsequent to surgical incision
- Vascular insufficiency wounds, further broken down as: Arterial insufficiency wounds: injuries sustained secondarily to arterial insufficiency, usually from tissue damage subsequent to atherosclerosis; typically found in distal lower extremities, exhibiting as intermittent claudicating, well-defined, and deep wounds, decreased pulsation and temperature there, and cyanosis; the patient has pain that is alleviated with rest and increased with elevation
- Venous insufficiency wounds: ulcerations caused by poor venous function, inadequate supplies to surrounding tissues, and subsequent tissue death; wounds are shallow, irregular, hot, and edematous with draining; clinically, patient has localized limb pain, which is relieved with elevation and increased upon standing
- Pressure wounds: ulcerations due to continued localized pressure, resulting in external and, eventually, internal tissue damage; occur often in bed- or chair-ridden patients
- Neuropathic or neurotropic ulcers: ulcers that result from secondary neurologic and skin complications of diabetes (and, to a lesser extent, spina bifida, syphilis, etc.); diabetic ulcers are generally deep wounds often located at pressure points (plantar, hammer toes, etc.), which are painless themselves but result in generalized lower-extremity pain

Venous Insufficiency Wounds

One theory as to why venous insufficiency wounds develop expounds that venous hypertension produces widening of the capillary pores. The long saphenous vein becomes dilated, allowing large macromolecules, such as fibrinogen, into the interstitial areas with resultant edema. Fibrin builds up in the dermis, fashioning a fibrin cuff that forms a mechanical barrier to oxygen and nutrient transport. This ultimately leads to cell dysfunction and death and skin ulcers.

Another theory is the white blood cell-trapping hypothesis, which asserts that periodic elevations in venous pressures depress capillary blood flow, leading to local trapping of white blood cells, obstruction, the release of various proteolytic and chemotactic substances, and, ultimately, tissue death and ulcerations.

How Wounds Heal

More superficial wounds heal by a process called reepithelialization, in which fresh epithelial cells simply propagate and mature within a day or two of wounding. Deeper wounds, however, undergo a three-step process. First, there is an inflammatory phase in which platelets aggregate to form a clot and various types of leukocytes are recruited for phagocytosis and wound healing. Next is a fibrinoplastic phase in which granulation or healing tissue is formed. Granulation occurs because fibrocytes and other undifferentiated cells proliferate and migrate to the site, forming fibroblasts, collagen, and new pink-colored scar tissue. The last phase is remodeling, in which the scar tissue matures, which can take months depending on the wound. Wounds that do not heal in a timely manner (general healing within six weeks, remodeling within a year) are considered chronic wounds and typically suggest some further underlying condition.

Factors That Can Delay Wound Healing

Older individuals tend to have more delayed wound healing, primarily due to diminished collagen production and/or the presence of comorbidities, such as diabetes or vascular problems. Lifestyle choices can impact wound healing, particularly if they increase the possibility of venous compromise. Nutritional habits are significant factors because tissue regeneration requires all of the major macronutrients and some micronutrients. Injuries make added demands on nutritional stores, particularly glucose and protein components. Stress during recovery can delay wound healing. If the person has any medical condition that compromises health (for example cancer, AIDS, or CHF), wound healing will be delayed. Certain medications (like steroids, NSAIDS, etc.), radiation therapy, and chemotherapy can impede wound healing. Patients on anticoagulants can bleed during dressing removal or debridement. In addition, patients who are cognitively or physically impaired, and thus may have difficulty performing wound care upon discharge, can experience delayed wound healing.

Wound Patient's History

A wound patient's history should include information about specifics regarding the wound itself, the patient's possible risk factors, and psychosocial aspects that could affect recovery. Wound history should address the time and circumstances of the wound, previous wound history, and the diagnostic tests, laboratory work, and interventions that have been or are scheduled to be performed. Risk factors for poor wound healing or associated complications should be noted. They include things like amount of weight bearing on the wound site or standing in general, cigarette use, nutrition level, age, recent weight changes, medications (particularly anticoagulants), and the presence and control of certain comorbidities, such as diabetes, immunodeficiency disorders, or anything that can cause altered sensation. It is also important to find out about the patient's potential support system and mobility issues.

Physical Examination of a Wound Patient

The physical examination of a wound patient should include tests that evaluate the patient's ability to sense touch, temperature, and motion variations. The pain associated with the wound should be characterized by common parameters, as well as component analysis. Wound pains are usually described as having a non-cyclic acute component (lone episode in conjunction with treatment), a cyclic acute component (recurring pain during repeated treatments), or a chronic wound pain component (unrelated to external management). Goniometric angle measurements should be made if a wound traverses a joint line, the joint is edematous, or range of motion is otherwise impacted. The therapist should assess whether the patient's needed strength or ability to be functionally mobile is affected and address this in the treatment plan. One of the most essential components of the physical examination is to observe for evidence of edema and lymphedema. Edema points to deficient tissue oxygen perfusion and increased risk of infection, while lymphedema is indicative of conditions, such as cellulitis and venous insufficiency.

Wound Evaluation

Wounds are usually photographed and documented in terms of location, orientation, size, depth, color, and drainage. A wound culture is taken as well. Location is described in terms of the wound's relationship to anatomical landmarks. Since wounds are often irregular in shape, orientation is frequently illustrated in terms of a clock, with 12 o'clock representing the individual's head. Size is documented in terms of vertical length and horizontal width, while depth is calculated using a sterile cotton-tip applicator inserted at right angles into the wound. Measurements should be consistent for all wounds, and centimeters are suggested. If the wound continues underneath the skin, known as tunneling or undermining, it should also be documented using a sterile applicator. The wound colors present and their percentages should be noted. Possible colors and the associated types of tissue are pink (newly epithelialized tissue), red (healing), yellow (necrotic or infected), and black (eschar). Wound drainage is clarified in terms of its type, amount, and odor (described further elsewhere).

Wound Drainage

Wound drainage is expressed in terms of its type, amount, and odor. The types of wound drainage include:

- Serous: transparent, thin, indicative of healing
- Serosanguineous: containing blood
- Purulent: viscous, white, and pus-like; potentially infectious, necessitating wound culture
- Green: potentially infectious with Pseudomonas; also requiring culture

The amount of drainage is usually described in increasing amounts as absent, scant, minimal, moderate, large, or copious. Large amounts of drainage generally suggest infection, while declining amounts suggest resolution. Odors are generally described as absent, mild, or foul, with the latter again pointing to infection. Any drainage situation suggestive of infection means that a wound culture should be taken. Wound cultures should also be taken if there is local inflammation, edema, erythematic, high temperature, cellulitis, significant pain, or delayed healing. Wound culturing from the internal wound bed is done by performing a tissue biopsy, needle aspiration, or swab cultures, the latter of which can be legally procured by the physical therapist.

Wound Classifications

Wounds that are not pressure ulcers are classified as superficial (epidermis only), partial-thickness (penetrating the dermis), or full-thickness (continuing deeper to the muscle and possibly bone). Pressure ulcers, on the other hand, are staged as follows:

- Suspected deep tissue injury: confined areas of discoloration under the skin or a blood blister, indicating underlying soft tissue injury
- Stage I: reddened skin area, generally over a bony protuberance
- Stage II: superficial open ulcer with a reddish pink wound bed or a serum-filled blister; equivalent to partial-thickness loss
- Stage III: equivalent to full-thickness loss; subcutaneous fat, tunneling, and slough often present but no revealing of muscles, tendons, or bones
- Stage IV: full-thickness damage with exposed muscles, tendons, or bones and possible tunneling, slough, and/or eschar
- Unstageable: full-thickness loss hidden by eschar and/or slough

Wound Cleaning

Wound cleaning is performed to detach loose cellular debris and microorganisms from the wound bed to promote healing and deter infection. Depending on facility and state policies, it may be performed by the physical therapist. Generally, wound cleaning should be done using the most neutral solution possible, considering the type of wound. Clean technique is generally satisfactory for most wound care, but sterile technique (sterile instruments, gloves, and solutions) is indicated during surgical interventions or acute traumatic incidents. The solution of choice for most wound cleaning is sterile saline, although there are no studies indicating that plain tap water cannot be used. Other means of wound cleaning are wound cleansers containing surfactants, irrigation devices, and scrubbing equipment, such as sponges or cloths. Topical antiseptics are contraindicated, except for acute trauma wounds as they are cytotoxic.

Selective Wound Debridement

Wound debridement, the removal of dead, damaged, or infected tissue from the wound bed, serves to promote reepithialization and healing, prevent infection, allow topical agents to work, and rectify any abnormal wound repair. Debridement can be either selective, in which only nonviable tissue is removed, or nonselective, which gets rid of both viable and nonviable tissues. Approaches to selective debridement include sharp, autolytic, and enzymatic debridement:

- In sharp debridement, some sort of sharp instrument, hydrosurgery device, or laser is used to remove the tissue. There is risk of bleeding and infection, but this technique is quite effective for excision of large, thick eschars. Physical therapists must check local policies to see whether they are permitted to perform sharp debridement.
- Autolytic debridement utilizes the body's own enzymes to lyse dead tissue. A moisture-preserving topical dressing is applied, and the body is allowed time for the autolysis. There is risk of infection, making this technique implausible for immunocompromised patients.
- With enzymatic debridement, enzymes that break down collagen, fibrin, or elastin are topically applied to the wound (i.e., collagenases, fibrinolytics, or proteolytics).

Nonselective Wound Debridement

Nonselective wound debridement refers to the removal of both viable and nonviable tissues in the wound area. It usually involves some type of mechanical debridement, including the use of wet-to-dry dressings, a whirlpool, or pulsed lavage:

- With the dressing method, a saline-wetted gauze is applied, allowed to dry, and then pulled off, removing adhered tissue with it. This method is only appropriate for pressure ulcers. Soaking the affected area in a whirlpool accomplishes mechanical debridement via agitation of the necrotic tissues.
- Whirlpools should only be used in patients with large area stage III or IV wounds and at temperatures that are tepid up to normal body temperature. Sometimes antibacterial agents are added if the infectious potential far outweighs their possible cytotoxic effects.
- In pulsed lavage, the wound is mechanically debrided by irrigation with saline through a pulsed, pressurized system, usually in conjunction with later suction. This method is very good for stimulating granulation and can be used in patients who generally cannot use the whirlpool (such as those with venous insufficiency).

Negative Pressure Wound Therapy

Negative pressure wound therapy uses localized uninterrupted or intermittent negative pressure through a permeable dressing to heal wounds. The commercially available system is called Vacuum Assisted Closure (V.A.C.). The dressing distributes the applied negative pressure and helps eliminate some of the interstitial fluid. The negative pressure encourages propagation of the epithelial cells and granulation tissue, liberates biochemical mediates from cell plasma membranes, and may cause growth of new blood vessels. All of these effects aid wound healing. Normally, the patient receives local negative pressure continuously for the first two days, which mostly decreases edema, followed by intermittent negative pressure to assist development of granulation tissue. This technique is applicable to any wound, except if significant dead tissue or eschar (30%), cancerous cells, or exposed blood vessels are present at the site. Patients with untreated osteomyelitis should not receive V.A.C.

Dressings Used for Partial- or Full-Thickness Wounds with Minimal or Moderate Drainage

There are many types of wound dressings. Those that are appropriate for partial- or full-thickness wounds with minimal or moderate drainage include:

- Gauze: very porous; used for all types of wounds; not necessarily the most effective; can be put on dry or wet (to be removed wet or after drying)
- Hydrocolloids: contain particles that react with moisture to form a gel, act as an impermeable barrier, reduce surface pH (thus reducing bacterial growth), and provide a moist and autolytic wound environment
- Hydrogels: gels made of water and glycerin that can be shaped to the area; used only in conjunction with other dressings on full-thickness wounds
- Foams: polyurethane foams with inner hydrophilic (water-compatible) and outer hydrophobic (water-resistant) surfaces; advantages include permeability to oxygen and lack of adhesion to the skin
- Transparent films: polymer sheets with adhesive backs; primarily used for superficial wounds or in conjunction with foams or gauze; highly conformable and waterproof

Dressings Used for More Serious or Special Types of Wounds

Dressings for more serious or special types of wounds include:

- Calcium alginates: fibrous sheets developed from seaweed, the main constituent being alginic acid, which ultimately forms a viscous gel when in contact with wound exudates; appropriate for partial- or full-thickness wounds with considerable drainage; afford a moist wound environment and facilitate autolysis
- Collagen matrix dressings: sheets, particles, or gels made from bovine collagen; appropriate for problematic wounds as they facilitate granulation and epithelialization
- Small intestine submucosa dressings: sheets containing collagen tissue from pig submucosa; utilized for partial- or full-thickness wounds, at autograft donor sites, and for second-degree burns; promote cell migration with little scarring and no rejection
- Topical dressings: gels or ointments containing water or petrolatum, antimicrobials, and/or other reagents; used for any wounds requiring topical medications, particularly antimicrobials, as a way of circumventing systemic administration

Other Systems

Metabolic and Endocrine Systems

Thyroid Hormone Tests

Available thyroid tests include:

- Serum thyroxine (T_4) and serum triiodothyronine (T_3): both radioimmunoassays (RIAs) for major systemically released thyroid hormones; respective normal values are 4 to 12 µg/dl and 40 to 204 ng/dl
- Free thyroxine index: indicative of unbound thyroxine as about 99% is bound to thyroxine-binding globulin (TBG) or other proteins; normal values with direct RIA [radioimmunoassay] are 0.8 to 2.7 ng/ml; indirect normal values fall between 4.6 and 11.2 ng/ml
- Thyroid-stimulating hormone (TSH): normal values by radioisotope or chemical labeling techniques are 0.4 to 8.9 µIU/ml (U = units)

- Thyrotropin-releasing hormone (TRH): measured at baseline and after IV administration of TRH; normally, administration of TRH increases its level 6 μIU/ml and should increase TSH as well in patients with hypothyroidism, but not in those with hyperthyroidism

Thyroid Function Tests

Tests for thyroid function include uptake assays, imaging techniques, and needle biopsy. The triiodothyronine resin uptake (RT_3U) test involves the use of radioisotopes to calculate bound versus unbound serum T_3 and T_4 (thyroxine) by indirectly measuring unfilled binding sites; uptake is high with hyperthyroidism and low in hypothyroidism. The thyroidal 24-hour radioactive iodine uptake test involves administration of radioactive iodine and measurement of the iodine after 24 hours. This test is indicative of the metabolic activity of the thyroid gland, with hypothyroidism suggested if the uptake is less than the normal 5% to 30%. In thyroid imaging or scanning, radionuclides are given intravenously to visualize the thyroid gland and the amount of uptake that has occurred. Other diagnostic tools include ultrasound imaging and fine-needle aspiration biopsy of thyroid cells (to check for malignancy).

Possible Causes of Hyperthyroidism

Hyperthyroidism is the overproduction of thyroid hormones. Most hyperthyroidism is caused by Graves' disease, an inherited autoimmune disorder characterized by thyroid enlargement, double vision, prominent eyes, pretibial myxedema, atrial fibrillation, hand quivers, and weak quadriceps. Hyperthyroidism can be caused by the presence of neoplasms in the gland, which can include benign thyroid adenomas and several types of malignant thyroid carcinomas (papillary, follicular, anaplastic. or medullary).

Hyperthyroidism can also be due to thyroiditis, or inflammation of the gland, due to infection or some other etiology. Goiter, enlargement of the thyroid gland, often as a result of iodine deficiency, can cause certain areas of the gland to function independently and overproduce thyroid hormones. Hyperthyroidism can be exogenous, meaning it is due to the ingestion of too much iodine or thyroid hormone. Rarely, it can also be caused by production of ectopic thyroid hormone in the ovaries or from follicular carcinomas that have metastasized.

Management of Hyperthyroidism

Hyperthyroidism, the overproduction of thyroid hormones, causes excessive stimulation of the sympathetic nervous system and decreased parasympathetic tone. Individuals with hyperthyroidism are nervous and irritable, fatigued, and heat intolerant. They are prone to perspire; they often have cardiac issues, such as palpitations, atrial fibrillation, and/or tachycardia; and they may have diarrhea, menstrual dysfunction, tremors, goiter, thyroid bruits on auscultation, nail damage or loss, and/or eyelid lag or retraction. Hyperthyroidism is managed mainly with drugs that inhibit the syntheses of thyroid hormones (methimazole or propylthiouracil) or with iodides (Lugol's solution or SSKI), which work by blocking hormone release or inhibiting their synthesis. A surgical subtotal-thyroidectomy is indicated in patients that cannot take these medications (primarily children), individuals with large goiters or thyroid carcinoma, and pregnant women.

Possible Causes of Hypothyroidism

Hypothyroidism is the inadequate exposure of peripheral tissues to thyroid hormones, usually as a result of diminished thyroid hormone production. There are two types of hypothyroidism: primary, in which there is a glandular dysfunction, and secondary, which is really a pituitary malfunction when low levels of thyroid-stimulating hormone (TSH) in turn produce low levels of thyroid hormones. With either type, causes of the hypothyroidism include incomplete or maldevelopment of the thyroid gland, inherited deficiencies in hormone synthesis or activity, autoimmune types of thyroiditis (inflammation of the gland), insufficient levels of iodine, hypopituitarism, hypothalamic dysfunction, ablation of the thyroid gland, and certain drug toxicities.

Management of Hypothyroidism

People with hypothyroidism tend to be lethargic, sleepy, constipated, weak, and hoarse. Their skin is usually pale with a yellow tint, rough, dry, cool, and edematous in certain areas (eyelids, feet, hands). Patients may experience paresthesia (tingling), decreased ability to hear, and cardiac issues, such as bradycardia (slow heart rate), high blood pressure, cardiac failure, and/or pericardial effusion. In severe instances, they may experience respiratory failure and/or coma. The presence of hypothyroidism is also indicated by low glucose and serum sodium concentrations, anemia, and proteinuria. A number of proteins are usually elevated, including cholesterol, lactate dehydrogenase, liver enzymes, creatinine phosphokinase, myoglobin, homocysteine, and prolactin. People with hypothyroidism generally need constant thyroid hormone replacement, usually with some brand of levothyroxine (Synthroid, Levothroid, etc.) or desiccated thyroid, liothyronine, or liotrix.

Pituitary and Growth Hormone Tests

Three pituitary hormones are most frequently quantified, often in conjunction with some sort of stimulation or other test to confirm functionality: growth hormone (GH), adrenocorticotropic hormone (ACTH), and antidiuretic hormone (ADH). Serum growth hormone (GH) levels are measured by radioimmunoassay (RIA). Normal values are 0 to 5 ng/ml for males and 0 to 10 ng/ml for females. Children suspected of having pituitary dwarfism or tumors are commonly given a growth hormone stimulation test in which GH is measured at baseline and after administration of arginine or insulin.

If the patient is normal, this causes a GH rise; if the patient is afflicted, no increase is seen. Another GH test used for suspected childhood gigantism or adult acromegaly is the glucose load or growth hormone suppression test. With this technique, GH is measured at baseline and after intake of a glucose solution, which in a normal person should reduce GH secretion but in afflicted individuals does not.

Adrenocorticotropic and Antidiuretic Hormone Tests

Along with serum growth hormone levels, adrenocorticotropic hormone and antidiuretic hormone are the major pituitary hormones measured. Plasma adrenocorticotropic hormone (ACTH) levels are quantified by radioimmunoassay (RIA). Generally, normal levels are higher in the morning (25 to 100 pg/ml) than at night (0 to 50 pg/ml). Primary and secondary adrenal insufficiency is identified by the ACTH-stimulation test in which Cosyntropin (Cortrosyn), a synthetic version of ACTH, is given to the patient. Baseline and subsequent plasma levels of cortisol are measured; normal individuals experience an increase of >20 μg/dl within 30 minutes to an hour.

Plasma antidiuretic hormone (ADH, vasopressin) levels should normally be 2 to 12 pg/ml or less than 2 pg/ml, depending on whether serum osmolality is greater or less than 290 mOsm/kg. One test associated with ADH is the water deprivation test, a diagnostic for diabetes insipidus (DI). The patient is denied fluids, and urine osmolality is serially measured; osmolality changes in normal individuals but not in DI patients. The patient may be simultaneously given ADH to distinguish between pituitary and renal dysfunction. The water loading test is diagnostic for SIADH, syndrome of inappropriate antidiuretic hormone. During this test, water is ingested, and plasma and urine osmolality are measured over time. SIADH patients show none of the normal osmolality changes.

Hyperpituitarism

Hyperpituitarism Caused by Growth Hormone or Adrenocorticotropic Hormone Overproduction

Hyperpituitarism is the hypersecretion of pituitary hormones, usually as a result of benign anterior lobe adenomas (tumors). The most prevalent type is growth hormone (GH) overproduction. GH overproduction is associated with gigantism in children, clinically distinguished by disproportionately long limbs. It is also linked to acromegaly in adults, in which the individuals may have enlarged hands and feet, rough facial features, joint pain, hand tremors, carpel tunnel syndrome, infrequent or absent menstrual periods (women), impotence (men), diabetes, and/or hypertension. The preferred treatment is surgical removal of the adenoma; GH suppressive agents are also choices.

Overproduction of adrenocorticotropic hormone (ACTH) results in increased serum and urine cortisol and, primarily, a disease called Cushing's syndrome. Cushing's syndrome is distinguished by obesity in the trunk area, thin extremities, osteoporosis, susceptibility to bruising, a round and red moon face, menstrual abnormalities (women), muscle weakness, and glucose intolerance. It is managed with ablation of the pituitary lesion, steroidogenic inhibitors, or resection of the adrenal glands.

Hyperpituitarism Caused by Antidiuretic Hormone Overproduction

Antidiuretic hormone (ADH) overproduction results in the syndrome of inappropriate ADH secretion (SIADH) in which the patient has fluid and electrolyte imbalances (specifically hyponatremia) due to too much water readsorption. There are many conditions that can cause SIADH, the most common being small cell or oat cell lung carcinomas, as well as other malignancies, other lung diseases, side effects from drugs, and head trauma. Patients with severe SIADH have interstitial edema due to hyponatremia and low serum sodium levels, causing headaches, nausea, disorientation, and possible seizures and coma from cerebral edema. Treatment usually focuses on restoring the electrolyte and fluid balance (via fluid restriction, use of diuretics, IV sodium chloride) or addressing the primary cause.

Hypopituitarism and Diabetes Insipidus

Hypopituitarism refers to insufficient secretion of pituitary hormones. It can be primary subsequent to pituitary neoplasms or tissue damage during pregnancy (Sheehan's syndrome), or it can be secondary to some sort of damage to the hypothalamus or adjacent structures (tumors, trauma, etc.). Complete pituitary hormone deficiency is known as panhypopituitarism, which has many possible manifestations depending on the hormone affected, the target, and severity. One manifestation is diabetes insipidus (DI), in which abnormally large amounts of dilute urine are excreted. There are many versions of DI depending on the etiology. For example, in pituitary DI, vasopressin is not synthesized or released, and in nephrogenic DI, there is a renal dysfunction due to lack of vasopressin receptors in renal ducts. Whatever the cause, signs usually include excessive urination, hypernatremia, dehydration, thirst, dry skin, and, possibly, nervous system effects. If the etiology is neurogenic, DI is treated with vasopressin or similar drugs, and if it is nephrogenic, diuretics in conjunction with restricted sodium intake are indicated. Other manifestations of hypopituitarism include hypogonadism, short stature, reproductive issues, etc. Treatments include various pituitary or other hormones.

Adrenal Function

Glucocorticoid levels are usually taken to diagnose Cushing's syndrome or Addison's disease. Normal serum cortisol levels (by RIA) should be 5 to 23 μg/dl in the morning and 3 to 16 μg/dl in the evening. Urine levels over 24 hours are also measured and should be in the range of 20 to 90 μg/dl. Cortisol release depends on pituitary release of adrenocorticotropic hormone, which is also generally measured. Serum or urine androgen levels may be determined in women who exhibit hirsutism (male pattern excessive hair growth), amenorrhea (inappropriate lack of menstruation), voice changes, and/or increased muscle mass. Mineralocorticoids, usually aldosterone, are measured in the morning while supine and about four hours later; normal serum levels should be between 2 and 50 ng/dl depending on position. Electrolyte levels provide good indirect screening methods for mineralocorticoids. Increased potassium levels can be indicative of a disorder as aldosterone secretion is regulated by the renin-angiogenesis system. Catecholamines (epinephrine, norepinephrine) may be measured in the urine over 24 hours; alternatively, their precursor dopamine or their major metabolite vanillylmandelic acid (VMA) during the same time period may be quantified.

Glucose Tolerance Test

A glucose tolerance test is a metabolic test for adrenal gland function. It is the main diagnostic test for gestational diabetes mellitus and is used to corroborate some diagnoses for diabetes mellitus. The test is completed after the patient has fasted for approximately 10 hours; the clinician administers 75 or 100 grams of glucose and then periodically measures blood glucose levels. Within two hours of glucose administration, blood glucose levels should return to baseline amounts; if they do not, diabetes is suggested. A normal blood glucose level after fasting should be in the range of 70 to 110 milligrams per deciliter. This test is useful because the mineralocorticoid cortisol normally secreted by the adrenal cortex affects carbohydrate (as well as protein and fat) metabolism.

Review Video: Glucose Tolerance Test
Visit mometrix.com/academy and enter code: 539108

Common Adrenal Disorders

Adrenal disorders include adrenal hyperfunction, adrenal insufficiency, and pheochromocytoma:

- Adrenal hyperfunction, or Cushing's syndrome, is caused by the increased secretion of glucocorticoids from the adrenal cortex subsequent to adrenocorticotropic hormone (ACTH) overproduction by the pituitary (discussed further on other cards).
- Primary adrenal insufficiency or Addison's disease is an autoimmune disorder in which the adrenal cortex is destroyed, leading to reduced levels of glucocorticoids, mineralocorticoids, and androgens. Secondary adrenal insufficiency is the withering of the adrenal cortex subsequent to ACTH deficiency, leading to similar hormone deficiencies. Patients are hypoglycemic, do not respond well to stress, and have fluid and electrolyte imbalances. Their symptoms include fatigue, weight loss, gastrointestinal issues, muscle and joint pain, hypotension, and hyperpigmentation. Adrenal insufficiency is managed with steroids like hydrocortisone.
- Pheochromocytoma is an uncommon disorder in which a tumor in the medullar portion causes surplus secretion of catecholamines. Signs include hypertension and other cardiac issues, nervousness, and high blood and urine glucose levels. The tumor is usually excised.

Insulin Resistance and Metabolic Syndromes

Insulin resistance syndrome and metabolic syndrome are two pancreatic disorders that generally precede development of type 2 diabetes and, often, cardiac disease. Insulin resistance syndrome is characterized by compensatory hyperinsulinemia (high blood levels of insulin) and hyperglycemia, and is more common in (but not limited to) the overweight or obese. It may or may not be found in conjunction with metabolic syndrome.

Metabolic syndrome is defined as the presence of at least three of the following parameters: a fasting glucose > 110 mg/dl, blood pressure > 135/85 mm Hg, plasma triglycerides > 150 mg/dl, low HDL cholesterol (< 45 mg/dl for men and < 50 mg/dl for women), and a large waist circumference (> 102 cm for men and > 88 cm for women). The combination of these risk factors increases the probability of development of type 2 diabetes and cardiovascular disease, which can be offset somewhat by lifestyle changes and exercise for weight loss.

Diabetes

Type 1 Diabetes Mellitus Management

Diabetes mellitus is a disorder in which either not enough insulin is produced or cells are resistant to insulin. Because insulin aids glucose storage in the form of glycogen in muscles, diabetics are glucose intolerant and hyperglycemic (high plasma glucose levels). Individuals with type 1 diabetes (also known as insulin-dependent or juvenile-onset diabetes) inherit an autoimmune state that destroys the pancreatic beta cells responsible for insulin secretion, resulting in low or nonexistent levels of insulin. Signs appear early in life, usually before 40 years of age. These symptoms are the same for both types 1 and 2, namely a fasting plasma glucose ≥ 126 mg/dl, a glucose level ≥ 200 mg/dl two hours after glucose loading, and/or any glucose reading of ≥ 200 mg/dl in conjunction with excessive urination and thirst, weight loss, and blurred vision. Type 1 diabetics are managed with some combination of insulin administration [oral, intramuscular, or continuous subcutaneous insulin infusion (CSII) pumps], blood glucose monitoring, proper diet and meal planning, various hypoglycemic agents, and exercise.

Review Video: Diabetes Mellitus: Diet, Exercise, & Medications
Visit mometrix.com/academy and enter code: 774388

Glucose Monitoring Tests

Glucose monitoring tests for diabetics are either self- or medical-monitoring. Self-monitoring tests include blood glucose finger-stick types and urine testing. For blood glucose finger-stick samples, capillary blood is taken via needle stick from a finger or earlobe, put on a reagent strip, and then evaluated against a color chart or read in a portable electronic meter against a reference of between 60 and 110 mg/dl. Samples can also be taken on inpatients from an indwelling arterial line. Urine testing is done by placing a reagent strip into a urine sample and reading it against a color chart. Finger-stick tests produce dynamic results and can be used to determine management changes, while urine tests are only appropriate in stable patients.

Medical-monitoring tests do not directly measure blood glucose. One type, done typically every three to six months, determines the percentage of glycosylated hemoglobin (GHB) in the blood, which should be in the range of 7.5 to 11.4% in patients with controlled diabetes. Another type (done approximately every three weeks) quantifies fructosamine or glycated protein, which should be near 300 mmol/liter if diabetes is under control. These medical-monitoring tests are performed because hyperglycemia saturates both hemoglobin molecules and serum proteins.

Insulin Pump Therapy

In continuous subcutaneous insulin infusion (CSII) pump therapy, patients wear a small, light, battery-driven pump attached to an infusion catheter that is inserted subcutaneously on the abdomen. The catheter is changed every two or three days and can be disconnected for activities like bathing. The pump can be set to deliver insulin either as a bolus dose or at a basal rate. Human-buffered insulin, which is short acting, or an insulin analog, which is rapid, is infused. CSII therapy is used in both type 1 and type 2 diabetics. The ideal candidates are diabetics who have shown their facility for self-monitoring. Specific indications include patients who often undergo glycemic variations, those who experience hyperglycemia in the morning, those with erratic schedules, pregnant type 1 diabetics, and adolescents who get diabetic ketoacidosis. Insulin pump therapy is also suggested for nocturnal use in children.

Type 2 Diabetes Mellitus Management

In type 2 diabetes mellitus, the patient usually has increased cellular resistance to the effects of insulin. The body compensates by secreting excess insulin, initially from the pancreatic beta cells, which eventually results in failure to produce enough insulin or the body's inability to use it. Type 2 diabetes is significantly associated with obesity and aging and, therefore, often called adult-onset or non-insulin dependent diabetes. It is found more often in those over 40 years old but is now being seen in younger obese individuals. In addition to glucose parameters seen in type 1 diabetics (fasting ≥ 126 mg/dl, two-hour post-load ≥ 200 mg/dl, and/or random ≥ 200 mg/dl in association with polyuria, polydipsia, weight loss, and blurred vision), type 2 diabetics may also present with recurrent infections, delayed wound healing, genital itching, other visual changes, and/or paresthesia (skin tingling, burning). As with type 1 diabetics, they are managed with some combination of insulin administration [oral, intramuscular, or continuous subcutaneous insulin infusion (CSII) pumps], blood glucose monitoring, proper diet and meal planning, various hypoglycemic agents, and exercise.

Hypoglycemic Agents used for Treatment of Hyperglycemia in Patients with Diabetes Mellitus or Drug-Induced Hyperglycemia (other than Insulin or Agents that Augment its Secretion)

Hypoglycemic agents used for treatment of hyperglycemia in patients with diabetes mellitus or drug-induced hyperglycemia include:

- Alpha-glycosidase inhibitors: delay hydrolysis of complex carbohydrates and disaccharides, as well as glucose absorption by inhibiting pancreatic alpha-amylase and intestinal alpha-glycosidases; examples include acarbose and miglitol; possible gastrointestinal side effects
- Amylin analogs: use a synthetic version of amylin that protracts gastric emptying time, reduces glucagon secretion after meals, and suppresses appetite; pramlintide (Symlin) is an example; given subcutaneously at mealtime; often causes nausea or hypoglycemia if given with insulin
- Biguanides: augments insulin sensitivity by promoting peripheral glucose uptake and utilization; depresses hepatic glucose production and its intestinal absorption; an example is metformin (Glucophage); gastrointestinal side effects and potentially fatal lactic acidosis possible
- DPP-IV (dipeptidyl peptidase IV) inhibitors: increase the presence of active peptide incretin hormones, which normalize glucose levels; sitagliptin (Januvia) is an example; given orally to type 2 diabetics with few side effects
- Thiazolidinediones: improve target cell responses to insulin; examples are pioglitazone (Actos) and rosiglitazone (Avandia); can cause heart failure, edema, and hepatotoxicity

Insulin Products and Other Hypoglycemic Agents

Insulin is normally secreted by the pancreas beta cells and targets various tissues via membrane receptors in order to regulate carbohydrate, protein, and lipid metabolism. It is given in various forms to both type 1 diabetics, who cannot produce sufficient amounts, and type 2 diabetics, who are relatively insensitive to it. Recombinant DNA insulin products are administered. These are defined in terms of their rapidity and duration as: ultra-rapid acting (e.g., insulin inhalation, lispro), rapid acting (regular preps, such as Humulin R), intermediate (e.g., NPH or Humulin N), intermediate to long-acting (e.g., detemir or Levemir), or long-acting (e.g., glargine or Lantus).

Insulin administration can cause subcutaneous fat changes, hypoglycemia, weight gain, and respiratory issues.

Sulfonylureas and meglitinides are two classes of agents that promote insulin release. Both also potentially cause hypoglycemia and/or weight gain; sulfonylureas can cause photosensitivity. Examples of sulfonylureas are glimepiride, glipizide, and various preparations of glyburide. Nateglinide (Starlix) and repaglinide (Prandin) are meglitinides. The incretin mimetic analog exenatide (Byetta) also augments insulin secretion (plus slows gastric emptying); it is given subcutaneously at mealtime.

Diabetic Ketoacidosis

Possible complications of diabetes mellitus are diabetic ketoacidosis and a variety of pathological conditions linked to lesions in small and large blood vessels. Diabetic ketoacidosis (DKA) is an advanced complication in which continuing ineffective concentrations of circulating insulin lead to extremely high plasma glucose levels (> 500 mg/dl), unrestrained fat breakdown, and high levels of tissue ketone bodies. Ketone bodies are acidic and, thus, cause acidosis, highly acidic blood. People with diabetic ketoacidosis are lethargic, dehydrated, and thirsty; lack muscle tone and proper reflexes; and have numerous gastrointestinal problems, an acetone-smelling breath, difficulty breathing, dilated pupils, and/or hypothermia. Treatments for diabetic ketoacidosis include administration of insulin, fluids, electrolytes, and/or supplemental oxygen; mechanical ventilation is also a possible option.

Diabetic Dermopathy and Foot Care for Diabetics

Patients with diabetes often develop diabetic dermopathy, or skin lesions from vascular damage. Vascular complications in diabetes include microangiopathy (microvascular), macroangiopathy (macrovascular), and neuropathy, all of which can contribute to diabetic dermopathy. The most important part of management of diabetic dermopathy is good foot care as it can prevent poor wound healing and other complications. Proper foot care for patients with diabetes includes frequent medical or podiatric assessments, proper removal of corns and calluses, daily inspection of the feet (using a mirror if necessary), daily cleansing with lukewarm water and soap, meticulous drying of the feet (especially between the toes), and use of hand cream or lanolin in dry areas. Patients should always wear clean socks and comfortable shoes, and they should cut their nails straight across and file them with an emery board. They should not expose their feet to extremes of heat or cold, wear compressive garments, or walk barefoot or without socks.

Diabetic Neuropathy

Diabetic neuropathy is a potential complication of diabetes in which damage to the myelin sheaths of nerve cells impedes nerve conduction. The most common diabetic neuropathies fall into the category of symmetric polyneuropathies. Symmetric polyneuropathies, in which the main deficits are sensory (such as paresthesias, numbness, and pain), are classified as peripheral sensory polyneuropathy; these patients present with foot ulcers and an inability to do an ankle jerk or adequately feel vibrations there. If motor deficits predominate, the patient has a peripheral motor neuropathy, characterized by weakness, muscle atrophy, decreased strength, and claw or hammer toes. Another type is autonomic neuropathy, which generally presents as gastrointestinal and/or cardiac problems. Another category is focal and multimodal neuropathies, which target specific nerves and bodily areas, such as cranial (headaches, facial pain), trunk and limb (cramping, constriction), or proximal areas (lower back, thighs). Diabetic neuropathy is managed with stringent glycemic control, pain relievers (antidepressants, anticonvulsants, etc.), aldose reductase inhibitors, nerve growth factors, immunotherapy, and/or a pancreatic transplant.

Potential Complications of Diabetes Mellitus

The most common complications of diabetes mellitus are diabetic ketoacidosis, dermopathy, and neuropathy (all discussed on other cards). In addition, diabetics are prone to infections for a variety of reasons that include decreased sensations and immune responses. They are at risk for development of acute coronary syndrome (ACS), in which impaired coronary blood flow leads to myocardial damage and infarction. People with diabetes can develop atherosclerosis, cerebrovascular accidents (strokes), and nephropathies. The latter includes diabetic nephropathy, in particular, which occurs in up to 30% of diabetic patients. It is characterized by systemic vascular changes in the kidney, scarring of the glomeruli, peripheral edema, diminished kidney function, low urine output, and/or microalbuminuria, all potentially leading to end-stage renal disease (ESRD). Patients with diabetic nephropathy should receive some combination of strict glycemic control, protein restriction, fluids, diuretics, nutritional support, antihypertensives, dialysis, and/or pancreas-kidney transplantation.

> **Review Video: End Stage Renal Disease**
> Visit mometrix.com/academy and enter code: 869617

General Physical Therapy Considerations in Patients with Diabetes Mellitus

Diabetic patients need to ingest extra carbohydrates before and during exercise to offset the hypoglycemia that otherwise occurs. The therapist should be aware of the individual's blood glucose levels (often notated as BS levels) before, during, and after the session as they can fluctuate daily, especially in response to any process that can alter glucose metabolism (for example, infections or exercise). These fluctuations can be great in patients with poor glycemic control. Patients should receive insulin injections during exercise in order to moderate lipolysis and hepatic glucose production; otherwise, they can develop hyperglycemia and ketogenesis. It is better to inject the insulin into the abdomen, rather than the exercising limb, in order to avert hypoglycemia. When dealing with patients on CSII pump insulin therapy, care should be taken not to disrupt the catheter. Therapy may need to be postponed in patients newly receiving IV insulin for stabilization.

> **Review Video: Diabetes Education: Health Belief Model**
> Visit mometrix.com/academy and enter code: 954833
>
> **Review Video: Diabetes Type I**
> Visit mometrix.com/academy and enter code: 501396

Hypoglycemia

Hypoglycemia, or hyperinsulinism, is a condition in which there is a low blood glucose level, less than 50 mg/dl, due to too much serum insulin. Fasting hypoglycemia transpires before eating and can be caused by a variety of factors that include beta-cell and other tumors, liver failure, and growth hormone deficiency. Postprandial hypoglycemia after meals can be due to inappropriate insulin release, diabetes, or hurried gastric emptying. Hyperinsulinism can be induced by administration of insulin or oral hypoglycemic agents. Individuals in a state of hypoglycemia may experience hypertension, rapid heartbeats, hunger, tremors, dizziness, vision problems, seizure, paralysis, or even loss of consciousness. They may be given glucose, in the form of fruit juice or honey, and glucagon or other drugs. Those prone to hypoglycemia should be strictly monitored when receiving insulin and oral hypoglycemics, and they should make dietary changes to keep up glucose levels. Extreme solutions include surgical interventions, such as subtotal pancreatectomy.

Parathyroid Gland and Functional Tests

The parathyroid gland, located in the neck area, secretes parathyroid hormone (PTH). PTH targets three sites, each contributing to increasing blood calcium levels: the bones, where PTH mobilizes stored calcium; the kidneys, where it aids calcium reabsorption; and the small intestine, where it increases its absorption. Parathyroid hormone can be measured directly using various radioimmunoassays or urinalysis, with normal levels between 10 and 60 pg/ml. Serum calcium levels are often measured because they are directly related to PTH levels (and function). Normal adults should have a serum calcium level of 8.5 to 11.0 mg/dl. Urinary calcium levels can also be measured, with reference values of 50 to 300 mg/dl. Gastrointestinal and renal function tests are also reflective of parathyroid function.

Hyperparathyroidism

Hyperparathyroidism refers to a condition in which overactive parathyroid gland(s) produce high levels of parathyroid hormone (PTH) and blood calcium, along with decreased bone mineralization and renal function. The underlying cause can be primary (parathyroid gland hyperplasia or adenoma), secondary (renal failure, other tumors), or tertiary (unrelated to serum calcium levels). Patients with hyperparathyroidism present with excessive calcium in their urine and blood (hypercalciuria and hypercalcemia, respectively). The hypercalcemia causes them to have bone demineralization and resorption, kidney stones, joint and bone pain, gastrointestinal issues, hypertension and arrhythmias, and neurological problems. Hyperparathyroidism is treated with modalities, such as partial or total parathyroidectomy, fluid replacement, diets low in calcium but high in vitamin D, and pharmacologic agents. The latter fall into two categories: calcimimetic drugs like cinacalcet (Sensipar) that bind to receptors on the parathyroid gland and suppress PTH secretion; and vitamin D and its analogs (calcitriol, doxercalciferol, etc.), which are multifunctional, ultimately resulting in the establishment of more normal calcium and other levels.

Hypoparathyroidism

Hypoparathyroidism is a condition in which there are low levels of parathyroid hormone (PTH) due to underactivity of the parathyroid gland. The underlying cause is usually damage to the parathyroid or thyroid gland(s), for example, radiation damage or metastases. Patients have low calcium levels (hypocalcemia), spasms and convulsions, dysrhythmias, tingling in their digits, thinning hair, dry skin and nails, and cataracts. They are generally put on a high-calcium, low-phosphate diet. Pharmacologic interventions include administration of PTH, supplemental vitamin D, and calcium-containing nutritional supplements.

Osteoporosis

Osteoporosis is a metabolic bone disorder in which there is diminished bone density, organization, and strength, putting the individual at risk for fracture. The condition can be primary, most often in postmenopausal women, or secondary to the use of certain drugs or presence of other metabolic conditions. Osteoporosis is diagnosed according to the person's bone mineral density as measured by Dual Energy X-ray Absorptiometry (DEXA) since it is the most prognostic factor. Clinical presentations of osteoporosis include back pain that is alleviated by rest, curvature or anterior wedging of the spine, and the existence of vertebral, compression, hip, or pelvic fractures. Treatments include daily supplemental calcium and vitamin D, estrogen or estrogen/progesterone replacement therapy, the use of bisphosphonate supplements like alendronate to reduce bone resorption, use of raloxifene (a selective estrogen receptor modulator or SERM), calcitonin supplements, and administration of parathyroid hormone. Other management strategies include fracture care and physical therapy for exercise prescription.

Osteoporosis and Physical Therapy

The physical therapist must be aware of any weight-bearing restrictions and the existence of fractures and complications, if present, that can impact exercise strategies. If patients have stable vertebral compression fracture(s), they should wear an abdominal corset. If they have postural issues and/or back pain, they should use a walker that is adjusted such that they can walk as upright as possible; exercises that strengthen the chest extensors are suggested. Every effort should be made to prevent trauma or fracture to the patient's bones, particularly during resistive exercises.

Osteomalacia and Paget's Disease

Osteomalacia and Paget's disease are two metabolic bone disorders. Osteomalacia is the presence of low serum calcium, vitamin D, or phosphate, resulting in decreased bone mineralization, diminished calcium absorption in the gut, and hyperparathyroidism. It occurs mainly in women or in the form of rickets in children. Patients have soft bones, bone pain, central myopathies, and a characteristic shuffling walk. Children with osteomalacia have a soft cranial vault and swollen joints, while adults with this disorder are at risk for femoral neck fractures. Patients are given calcium and vitamin D supplements, and if possible, the underlying cause is addressed.

Paget's disease occurs in older individuals and is chiefly characterized by the presence of thick, malleable, brittle bones, usually in the axial skeleton or femur. The etiology is probably viral or inflammatory. Individuals may or may not have symptoms, such as bone pain that cannot be alleviated, bone malformations, warm skin over the involved bones, headaches, and/or hearing loss. Management includes administration of calcitonin and bisphosphonates like alendronate or etidronate.

Gastrointestinal System

Physical Examination for Gastrointestinal Problems

The physical examination for evaluation of gastrointestinal problems can be performed by the physical therapist, physician, or nurse. The history portion should include questioning about signs and symptoms associated with gastrointestinal pathology, namely the presence of diarrhea, constipation, nausea, jaundice, abdominal pain, heartburn, and coughing up of blood. Stool and urine characteristics, such as color changes in either or the presence of bloody or black stools should be noted. History of hernia, hepatitis, drug or alcohol misuse, and intolerance for fatty foods should also be documented. The four abdominal quadrants (right upper and lower, left upper and lower, in total encompassing all the primary GI and accessory digestive organs) should be inspected for asymmetries, scars, incisions, tubes, and the like. The clinician should use light and deep palpation to examine for abdominal tenderness, including upon quick release (rebound) and muscular resistance, both of which suggest underlying pathologies. He should also palpate superficial organs and masses. In addition, the clinician should use a scope to auscultate the abdomen for bowel sounds and bruits, to mediate percussion to approximate the size of the liver and spleen, and to identify ascites, masses, or trapped air.

Diagnostic Laboratory Tests

Evaluation of the Gastrointestinal System for Presence of Tumors

Several laboratory tests are used to diagnose the presence of gastrointestinal tumors. These include the CEA, 5-HIAA, occult blood, serotonin, and *Helicobacter pylori* tests:

- CEA or carcinoembryonic antigen, which should be less than 2.5 ng/ml in an adult nonsmoker (higher in a smoker), is a tumor marker found in venous blood that is useful for monitoring recurrence (not definitive diagnosis) of colorectal cancer.

- 5-HIAA, or 5-hyroxyindoleacetic acid, is a urinary metabolite of serotonin that is diagnostic for carcinoid tumors; normally 1 to 9 mg should be present over a 24-hour period. Blood levels of serotonin itself can also be used to indicate carcinoid tumor when elevated above the normal levels of 50 to 200 ng/ml.
- The occult blood test is used to screen for bowel cancer; it involves looking at three stool specimens for the presence of occult (imperceptible) fecal blood.
- *Helicobacter pylori* tests are used to diagnose this infection, which causes the majority of peptic ulcers and gastric carcinoma. There are three types of *H. pylori* tests, serological, for IgG class antibodies specific for the microorganism; the urea breath test, which identifies its presence in the stomach; and a tissue biopsy.

Evaluation of the Gastrointestinal System for Abnormalities Other Than Tumors

Laboratory tests used to evaluate the gastrointestinal system for abnormalities other than tumors include the gastric stimulation test, measurement of blood gastrin, a jejunal/duodenal biopsy, and the lactose tolerance test:

- In the gastric stimulation test, stomach acids are aspirated via a nasogastric tube at rest and after stimulation with pentagastrin. The test assesses the stomach's ability to produce acid secretions by measuring gastric pH (which should be pH 1.5 to 3.5) and acid output at baseline and peak (which should go up in terms of mEq/hr).
- Gastrin is the hormone responsible for hydrochloric acid release in the stomach; elevated values relative to the reference 25 to 90 pg/ml are diagnostic for Zollinger-Ellison syndrome.
- Jejunal/duodenal biopsies are taken from small bowel areas and examined histologically for indications of irritable bowel syndrome, Celiac disease, and malabsorption.
- In the lactose tolerance test, the patient is given oral lactose after fasting, and sequential blood glucose (reference value > 30 mg/dl) and urine lactose (reference value 12 to 40 mg/dl per 24 hours) levels are measured. If these do not rise, the test is indicative of lactose intolerance-lactase deficiency, which often causes abdominal cramping and diarrhea.

Non-Imaging Diagnostic Procedures

Non-imaging diagnostic procedures to evaluate the gastrointestinal system include esophageal pH, esophageal manometry, the acid perfusion test, GI cytological studies, and an abdominal paracentesis or tap:

- The esophageal pH test uses an implanted capsule to look at pH changes in the esophagus.
- The esophageal manometry measures lower esophageal sphincter (LES) pressure using an endoscope.
- The acid perfusion, or Bernstein test, is used to differentiate between esophageal- and cardiac-derived heartburn by injecting hydrochloric acid into the esophagus via a tube or endoscope.
- GI cytological studies involve analyzing tissue specimens obtained endosmotically for the presence of benign or malignant cells.
- For an abdominal paracentesis or tap, peritoneal fluid is obtained via a needle or trocar and stylet; normal fluid should be clear, odorless, and pale yellow.

Imaging Diagnostic Procedures

Screening tools include colonoscopy and sigmoidoscopy:

- A colonoscopy screens for presence of colon polyps and tumors using an endoscope inserted into the rectum (and excision, if found).
- Sigmoidoscopy uses a fiber optic tube inserted rectally to examine up to the level of the sigmoid colon.

Diagnostic imaging tools include KUB X-ray, barium enema, barium (or Gastrografin) swallow, computed tomography scan, gallium scan, gastric emptying scan, GI scintigraphy, and esophagogastroduodenoscopy:

- A KUB X-ray is an x-ray image of kidneys, ureters, and bladder.
- In a barium enema, the colon is evacuated of feces and the contrast medium barium is instilled rectally; structural abnormalities are visualized via fluoroscopy or x-ray.
- In a barium (or Gastrografin) swallow, the contrast agents are taken orally instead. Upper GI and small bowel series are targeted in barium swallow studies.
- Computed tomography (CT), with or without IV or oral contrast medium, can be used to detect many abnormalities.
- In a gallium scan, radioactive gallium 67 is injected and images taken at various times depending on the suspected issue.
- For a gastric emptying scan, images are taken periodically after ingestion of a food/radionuclide mix.
- GI scintigraphy uses radionuclide-labeled RBCs to look for GI bleeding. Esophagogastroduodenoscopy is endoscopic examination of the upper GI tract.

Laboratory Tests for Enzymes Associated with Injury to the Hepatic, Biliary, and/or Systems

High levels of a number of enzymes indicate injury to the hepatic, biliary, and/or pancreatic systems:

- Alanine aminotransferase (ALT) is very specific for liver damage during acute hepatitis.
- Alkaline phosphatase (ALP) can be elevated not only in liver disease but also in bone disease and hyperparathyroidism; its isoenzymes (I-ALP) can be used to differentiate between these sources of damage.
- Another enzyme indicative of liver inflammation, damage, or necrosis is aspartate aminotransferase (AST).
- Amylase is measured in serum and also in urine (if serum values are normal) to confirm diagnosis of acute pancreatitis.
- Lipase levels are also a means of diagnosing pancreatitis or pancreatic disease.
- Gamma-glutamyltransferase (GT, GGT, and other forms) is an overall system marker for hepatobiliary disease.
- Elevated levels of the catalyzing enzyme 5'-nucleotidase (5' or 5'-NT) are indicative of biliary obstruction or liver cancer.
- ALP, AST, and 5'-NT are indicative of cholestasis, impaired bile flow from the liver to the duodenum.

Laboratory Tests Other Than Enzyme Levels That Are Associated with Hepatic, Biliary, and/or Pancreatic System Changes

Two tumor markers are often quantified: alpha 1-fetoprotein (AFP1), elevated in hepatocellular carcinoma (and pregnant women); and carbohydrate antigen 19-9 (CA 19-9), whose levels can be correlated to pancreatic cancer stage. Bilirubin levels are indicative of liver function and presence of jaundice. Bilirubin is measured as direct (conjugated) and indirect (unconjugated), which, if elevated, indicate hepatic and prehepatic jaundice, respectively. Normal values should be: total, 0.3 to 1.2 mg/dl; direct, 0 to 0.2 mg/dl; and indirect, less than 1.1 mg/dl. Viral hepatitis screening and diagnostic tests quantify antibodies against hepatitis virus antigens (HAV, HAB, HCV, HDV, HEV, and HGV) and HBV's important surface antigen, HBsAg. Hepatic protein tests include protein electrophoresis, which separates out proteins; and serum proteins, both of which are mainly quantify albumin; albumin is normally in the range of 3.5 to 5.0 g/dl and depressed in hepatic diseases. Other possible laboratory tests include ammonia (NH_3) for monitoring of liver failure, high ceruloplasmin levels for liver diseases, elevated fecal fat, elevated prothrombin time (PT), a sweat test for diagnosis of cystic fibrosis, and urine urobilinogen to screen for hemolytic anemia or liver damage.

Diagnostic Procedures for the Hepatic, Biliary, Pancreatic, and/or Splenic Systems

Most diagnostic procedures for evaluation of the hepatic, biliary, pancreatic, and/or splenic systems are imaging techniques. The primary diagnostic tool is ultrasound of the liver, biliary tract, pancreas, and spleen, which identifies gallstones, neoplasms, hematomas, cysts, and abscesses well. Computed tomography (CT) of the same area, with or without contrast medium, is also used. Several specific types of tests use injection of radionuclides. These include the hepatoiminodiacetic acid scan (HIDA) for examination of the gallbladder and biliary ducts; the liver biliary scan, which is a general diagnostic test for biliary tract disorders; and the liver-spleen scan, which images those areas to primarily look for enlargement. There are also two methods of cholangiopancreatography (CP) utilized: magnetic resonance CP (MRCP), which is good for visualization of ducts, the gallbladder, and obstructions; and endoscopic retrograde CP with pancreatic cytology (ECRP), which looks for stones, pancreatitis, and cancer. Regular MRI and PET (positron emission tomography) are other imaging techniques. A non-imaging procedure is the percutaneous liver biliary biopsy, which is used to identify pathological changes and disease progression in the liver.

Laparoscopy

A laparoscopy is a procedure in which a fiber optic tube called a laparoscope is introduced through an incision near the umbilicus into the abdominal cavity for visualization of the region. It has both diagnostic and therapeutic applications. Diagnostic applications include extraction of a tissue biopsy, fluid aspiration, location of the source of ascites, location of an intraabdominal hemorrhage after blunt trauma, staging of various diseases (hepatic, lymphoma, metastases, tuberculosis), and assessment of patients who have fever of unknown origin or abdominal pain. Laparoscopy also has therapeutic utility. It is used for a number of surgical procedures, including appendectomy, hernia repair, gastrectomy, colectomy, vagotomy, tying of fallopian tubes, and gastric bypass. Laparoscopy is also used to aspirate cysts and abscesses, break up adhesions, and remove tissue in patients with endometriosis or cancer with adjunct laser use.

Esophageal Disorder Dysphagia

The general term for difficulty swallowing is dysphagia. Dysphagia can be proximal, meaning it occurs in the upper portions of the esophagus; or distal, signifying it occurs lower in the esophagus. It can occur upon ingestion of solids and/or liquids, there can be concomitant heartburn or chest pain, and the patient may regurgitate or cough. Dysphagia has four classifications—neurologic, obstructive, inflammatory or infectious, and congenital:

- Neurologic dysphagia occurs as part of some type of neurologic or neuromuscular disease, such as stroke, myasthenia gravis, or multiple sclerosis, and is usually responsible for proximal dysphagia.

- Obstructive dysphagia is due to neoplasms, bony growths, or anatomic abnormalities that change the shape of the esophagus. In proximal dysphagia, these abnormalities are usually diverticula or webs, while in distal dysphagia the anomalies are usually rings at the gastroesophageal junction.
- Inflammatory or infectious dysphagia is caused by inflammatory diseases, such as tonsillitis or GERD (discussed elsewhere), candida or herpes infections, or occurs when a patient is immunocompromised.
- Congenital disorders causing dysphagia include tracheoesophageal fistula and atypical arteries resulting in compression of the esophagus.

GASTROESOPHAGEAL REFLUX DISEASE

Gastroesophageal reflux disease, or GERD, is the backflow of gastric acid into the esophagus, causing heartburn, choking, nausea, or hoarseness. The backflow occurs because the lower esophageal sphincter (LES) does not relax properly. The etiology of GERD is unclear, with factors like fat or alcohol consumption and gastric or esophageal motility disorders mentioned as possibilities. Frequent GERD is associated with development of Barrett's esophagus, in which columnar epithelium is substituted for normal mucosa in distal portions of the esophagus, and, later, esophageal adenocarcinoma. It is managed with through strategies that can include consumption of many small meals, upright dining, use of antacids, or surgery.

Review Video: What is GERD?
Visit mometrix.com/academy and enter code: 294757

ESOPHAGEAL MOTILITY DISORDERS

Inadequate esophageal motility results from smooth spasms or atypical contraction patterns. There are other esophageal disorders that may cause this symptom in addition to GERD. These generally present as anterior chest pain. One esophageal motility disorder is achalasia, where again the LES does not relax and causes pressure, esophageal dilation and hypertrophy, obstruction, chest pain, and regurgitation. Another disorder is diffuse esophageal spasm in which there is normal peristalsis in the top portion of the esophagus but erratic contractions in the bottom portion, giving the patient chest pains.

PEPTIC ULCER DISEASE AND GASTRITIS

Peptic ulcers are defined as areas of loss of internal mucosa at least 5 millimeters diameter in size and located in the esophagus, stomach, or duodenum; they penetrate into the muscularis mucosa. Both gastric and duodenal ulcers can be caused by *Helicobacter pylori* infections, NSAID use, and other factors. Individuals with gastric or stomach ulcers ostensibly have normal gastric acid secretion but cannot deal with its effects. The pain associated with gastric and duodenal ulcers is different, occurring during or after eating, possibly with nausea for gastric ulcers, and feels sharper or gnawing but is relieved with food or antacids for duodenal ulcers. Peptic ulcers in general are treated with antacids, drugs for *H. pylori* (metronidazole, clarithromycin, amoxicillin), and removal of causative agents. Recurrent peptic ulcerations in association with gastric acid hypersecretion and pancreatic gastrinoma are termed Zollinger-Ellison syndrome.

Gastritis is an all-purpose term for lesions in the mucosal layer of the stomach that cause burning or pain. It can occur acutely or chronically, the latter being either nonerosive, due to *H. pylori*, or erosive, due to NSAID overuse or alcohol abuse.

Review Video: Peptic Ulcers and GERD
Visit mometrix.com/academy and enter code: 184332

Gastrointestinal Hemorrhage

Gastrointestinal hemorrhage, or GI bleeding, is generally divided into two types depending on location. An upper gastrointestinal bleed (UGIB) is due to duodenal or gastric ulcers, gastric erosion, esophageal varices (dilated blood vessels), and/or use of nonsteroidal anti-inflammatory drugs (NSAIDs). A lower gastrointestinal bleed (LGIB) is caused by diverticulitis or other inflammatory bowel diseases, neoplasms, and/or rectal and anal lesions. The clinical signs of GI bleeding are dark brown vomit and bloody or black, tarry stools. If hemodynamic instability from GI hemorrhage is severe enough, it can cause shock. Therefore, customary interventions are intravenous fluids, blood transfusions, and nasogastric tubes. Common diagnostic tools include endoscopy, sigmoidoscopy, and colonoscopy.

Gastric Emptying Disorders

Gastric retention, or gastroparesis, is reduced gastric emptying. It can occur subsequent to a variety of conditions, including constriction of the pylorus, ketoacidosis, hyperglycemia, electrolyte imbalances, neuropathies, post-surgical stasis, and pernicious anemia. Gastric retention is treated with drugs that encourage gastric mobility.

Dumping syndrome, or increased gastric emptying of liquids and possibly solids, occurs when stomach ulcers or surgical procedures disrupt the usual digestive sequence. A sign of dumping syndrome is hypoglycemia and its associated symptoms, such as sweating, dizziness, and palpitations. The condition is managed with dietary modification and drugs.

Hernias

A hernia is the abnormal protrusion of an organ through the walls of its cavity.

- Abdominal hernia is a distension of the bowel, causing muscle weakening. Risk factors include obesity, surgical procedures, presence of ascites, and heredity. Patients have abdominal bulging visible upon changing position, coughing, or laughing; pain; nausea and vomiting; fever; rapid heartbeat; and possibly abdominal rigidity. The herniation is treated by wearing a corset or with surgery.
- Hiatal hernia is unusual stomach outcropping that extends upward through the diaphragm. Potential causes are similar to abdominal hernia. Patients experience epigastria pain after meals and while lying down. They are treated with dietary modifications, acid-reducing drugs, and surgery. During bronchopulmonary hygiene or mobility exercises, pain may be aggravated.

Diverticulitis or diverticular disease is a form of herniation where the mucosa of the large colon protrudes through muscle layers of the intestinal wall. Symptomatic diverticulitis is characterized by left lower quadrant and referred low back pain, frequent urination, protruding abdomen, fever, constipation, bloody stools, and other GI problems. It is managed by adding increased dietary fiber, nasogastric tube insertion, IV fluids, pain and anti-infective drugs, and surgery.

Inflammatory Intestinal Disorders

Inflammatory intestinal disorders include:

- Appendicitis: inflammation of the appendix of the large intestine; can be simple (intact appendix), gangrenous (focal necrotic areas), or perforated (wall largely destroyed); caused by obstruction and infection; manifests as right lower quadrant or other abdominal pain, GI problems, low-grade fever; treated with anti-infectives or appendectomy

- Peritonitis: inflammation in peritoneal cavity; caused by bacterial infections, chemicals, or perforation of the GI tract; signs include fever, abdominal tenderness and protrusion, pain when breathing deeply, GI issues, low urinary output, cardiac problems; treatments include antibiotics, electrolytes, colloids, pain drugs, nasogastric suctioning, pressure monitoring, and laparoscopy (possibly with surgery)
- Crohn's disease: chronic inflammation in any portion of GI tract; etiology unknown; may be due to hereditary factors, immunological mechanisms, infections, etc.; characterized by constant abdominal cramping, right lower quadrant mass, low-grade fever, diarrhea; treated with corticosteroids, cytokines, antibiotics, fluids, suctioning, and/or resection
- Ulcerative colitis: chronic inflammation of the mucosal layer of colon and rectum; etiology unclear; symptoms include lower abdominal cramping, rectal bleeding, diarrheic stools, fever, dehydration, tachycardia; managed with corticosteroids, suppositories, surgical resection, antidiarrheal agents, and supplemental blood or iron

Intestinal Obstructions

Blockage of the bowel portion of the intestine generally causes the intestinal contents to fail to move forward. Intestinal obstructions can be mechanical, such as herniation, tumors, or impacted feces. Paralytic ileus, on the other hand, is a functional inhibition of the propulsive movement as a result of some traumatic event, such as surgery, spinal fracture, peritonitis, or narcotic use (including for post-surgical pain). Patients with intestinal obstructions have abdominal distension and pain, vomiting, severe constipation, bloody stools, high-pitched or absent bowel sounds, tachycardia, and hypotension. In particular, the abdominal distension can impact other functions, so the physical therapist should try and mobilize patients after surgery to prevent this difficulty. Interventions include supportive management, nasogastric tube introduction, surgical resection of mechanical obstructions, and colostomy (creation of an artificial anus) in severe cases.

Intestinal Ischemia

Intestinal ischemia, or lack of blood within the intestinal tract, can be caused by a number of cardiac complications (emboli to the superior mesenteric artery, chronic vascular insufficiency, hypotension, etc.), intestinal strangulation, or use of various drugs, particularly those with vasoconstrictive features. Symptoms include diverse degrees of abdominal pain, gastrointestinal problems, abdominal distention and tenderness, tachycardia, and hypotension. If the ischemia is severe, there can be abdominal rigidity and fever due to necrosis or gangrene; these symptoms, if present, are potentially life-threatening. The ischemia is treated with revascularization procedures, such as angioplasty, anticoagulation therapy, and use of vasodilators or, in some cases, vasopressors to enhance blood perfusion. Other management tools include resection and reanastomosis, anti-infective drugs, intravenous fluids, analgesics, and nasogastric tube insertion. Another name for this disorder is ischemic colitis.

Irritable Bowel Syndrome

Irritable bowel syndrome (IBS), or spastic colon, is basically erratic motility of the large bowel. This inconsistency can be due to ingestion of milk products, emotional responses, hormones, toxins, neurotransmitters, or colon distention. There is increasing evidence that one important cause is bacteria in the small intestine. Signs of IBS include disseminated abdominal pain, constipation or diarrhea, tender sigmoid colon, and onset of symptoms after eating or stress. Pharmacologic interventions include antibiotics, laxatives or antidiarrheal agents, and antispasmodic drugs. Other management tools are dietary changes and a food diary to find causative agents, counseling, and, occasionally, surgery.

Malabsorption Syndromes

A malabsorption syndrome is any condition in which the small or large intestine cannot absorb nutrients and electrolytes. There are many situations that can cause malabsorption, including AIDS, pancreatitis and pancreatic carcinoma, Crohn's disease, celiac sprue (sensitivity to gluten), lactase deficiency, amyloidosis, Zollinger-Ellison syndrome, and Whipple's disease. Because patients cannot absorb nutrients and electrolytes, they experience anorexia and weight loss, as well as diarrhea and/or steatorrhea (fatty stools), abdominal distension, and bone pain. Some management tools are antibiotic therapy; dietary changes; and supplemental fluids, electrolytes, vitamins, and minerals.

Gastrointestinal Polyps

Gastrointestinal (GI) polyps are typically benign adenomas in the colon or rectum. Patients with GI polyps may or may not have rectal bleeding, constipation or diarrhea, or cramping pain in the lower abdominal area. Because these benign polyps can eventually develop into carcinomas, it is important to screen for their detection with techniques such as colonoscopy, proctosigmoidoscopy, endoscopy, barium enema, and/or tissue biopsy. If found, a polypectomy with electrocautery or, in some cases, surgical resection is performed. Patients should reduce risks for colorectal cancer, which include obesity, alcohol overconsumption, and smoking.

Intestinal Tumors and Anorectal Disorders

In addition to these colon adenomatous polyps, other tumors that may be found in the intestine include other adenomas, lipomas (benign fatty tissue tumors), leiomyomas, and lymphoid hyperplasia. Tumors can not only be cancerous, but they may also impede motility and absorption. Anorectal disorders generally manifest clinically as pain upon defecation and blood stools; they include hemorrhoids, fistulas, fissures, rectal prolapse, and an imperforate anus.

Morbid Obesity and Surgical Treatments

Obesity is delineated as chronic excess body fat with a body mass index (BMI) ≥ 30. Morbid obesity is generally defined as having an even higher chronic BMI. Most obese people have other illnesses, in particular conditions such as hypertension, diabetes, renal disease, and obstructive sleep apnea. Dietary changes and behavioral modifications to reduce weight generally do not work for most morbidly obese people and consequently surgical procedures are now prevalent for management. The major choices are:

- Roux-en-Y gastric bypass: the formation of a small gastric pouch to limit intake to 20 to 30 ml using stapling, bypassing the distal stomach and proximal small bowel; can be done laparoscopically or open.
- Vertical banded gastroplasty: the creation of a small gastric pouch with permanent stapling and a band at the pouch's outlet that slows emptying to the small intestine.
- Adjustable gastric banding: the creation of a small pouch in the upper stomach with an adjustable silicone band, again providing a narrow opening to the small intestine for slow emptying.

The major physical therapy consideration after these types of surgeries is the size of the patient, usually necessitating assistance or some type of bariatric equipment.

Hepatitis

Hepatitis is inflammation and cell death in the liver. Hepatitis is most often viral in origin, with identified hepatitis viruses including hepatitis A, B, C, D, E, and G (HAV, HBV, HCV, HDV, HEV, and HGV, respectively). Hepatitis can also be caused by excess alcohol consumption, exposure to toxins, and several diseases. Most cases are caused by HAV, HBV, or HCV. HAV is spread via the fecal-oral route; HBV and HCV are transmitted by blood or other bodily fluids. Hepatitis from HAV is generally acute, while HBV and HCV can cause both acute and chronic liver damage. Clinically, hepatitis presents as jaundice (yellowing of skin, mucous membranes, and whites of eyes), dark urine, malaise, fever, headache, nausea, and abdominal pain. In terms of management, there are vaccines available to prevent development of HAV and HBV, the latter of which is also protective for HDV as the hepatitis D virus is active only in the presence of HBV. HBV vaccines should be administered to physical therapists and other healthcare workers. Individuals with hepatitis are instructed to get plenty of rest and eliminate causes (if due to alcohol or toxins). They are given fluid and nutritional support, anti-inflammatory agents, and antiviral drugs.

Liver Cirrhosis

Cirrhosis is a chronic, progressive liver disease in which there is cell damage and scarring. It is often complicated by jaundice, presence of ascites, clotting difficulties, and hypertension in the portal vein leading to the liver. Chronic infection with the hepatitis viruses HBV (and potentially HDV) or HCV is one major cause of hepatic cirrhosis. There are many other possible etiologies, including alcohol or drug abuse, biliary obstruction, alpha1-antitrypsin deficiency, cystic fibrosis, cardiac failure, Wilson's disease (copper metabolism defect), and others. Symptoms of cirrhosis include recent weight changes, jaundice, fatigue, bowel changes and GI bleeding, fever, diminished urine output and amber urine, and mental problems. Much of patient management is supportive, such as administration of IV fluids, blood or its products, colloids, vitamins, electrolytes, and/or supplemental oxygen. If possible, the underlying cause and complications are treated medically or surgically. Other possible interventions include paracentesis, dietary and behavioral alterations, and liver transplantation.

Hepatic Ecephalopathy

Hepatic encephalopathy, sometimes called portal systemic encephalopathy (PSE), is a state in which cirrhosis or other liver diseases lead to neuropsychiatric problems. The main cause appears to be ammonia intoxication from defective liver metabolism. The patient exhibits altered states of consciousness, such as stupor or confusion; diminished intellectual functions; changes in personality and behavior; and a variety of neuromuscular anomalies. The latter abnormalities include things like garbled speech, lack of coordination, altered reflexes, and presence of Babinski's sign. Hepatic encephalopathy can evolve into coma if untreated. The core treatment for hepatic encephalopathy is administration of nonabsorbable disaccharides (sugars). Other management tools include restoration of proper fluid, electrolyte, and/or acid-base balance; supplemental O_2, agents for detoxification of the ammonia; anti-infective drugs; gastric cleansing; and elimination of causative agents (including surgically if needed).

Cholecystitis and Gallstones

People who have cholecystitis, or inflammation of the gallbladder, almost always have gallstone formation as well. Gallstone development, or cholelithiasis, is linked to lack of mobility in the gallbladder, excess cholesterol in the bile, and crystals in the bile due to a surplus of insoluble bilirubin. Patients with cholecystitis generally have extreme right upper quadrant (and possibly referred interscapular) abdominal pain, a sensitive and rigid abdomen, jaundice, gastrointestinal problems, and fever. Surgical options for management are laparoscopic removal of the gallbladder (cholecystectomy) or short-term placement of a drain in the gallbladder (cholecystostomy). Other management resources include administration of chenodeoxycholic and ursodeoxycholic acid to dilute the gallstone(s), placement of a nasogastric tube, IV fluids, pain relief, and anti-infective medications.

Pancreatitis

Pancreatitis is inflammation of the pancreas due to excessive release of pancreatic enzymes into the peritoneal cavity and the destruction of pancreatic tissues. Acute pancreatitis is associated most often with the presence of gallstones or drug abuse, but there are many other potential causes, such as hepatitis, peptic ulcers, obstructions, traumatic procedures, and renal failure. Patients with pancreatitis present with a constant, dull abdominal pain in the epigastria, left upper quadrant, or umbilical region, possibly extending further. They might have jaundice, depressed bowel sounds, diminished urine output, GI problems, fever, rapid heart rate or hypotension, pleural effusions, and/or pneumonitis. Their pain is usually controlled through use of narcotics, often via patient-controlled pump analgesia. Patients are generally fed only parenterally, given IV fluids and electrolytes, antacids, and oxygen. They may also need mechanical ventilation and monitoring.

Drug Classifications for Gastrointestinal Problems

The drug classifications that might be used for gastrointestinal problems include:

- Antacids: to suppress acids in cases of mild GERD and heartburn; to neutralize gastric acid, raise pH by preventing pepsin creation, and form viscous protective barrier; depending on form, can cause constipation, diarrhea, heart problems; examples include various hydroxides and carbonates.
- Antidiarrheals: to alleviate diarrhea; to inhibit or lessen GI motility; can cause constipation and CNS depressive effects; examples include diphenoxylate/atropine (Lomotil), loperamide (Imodium).
- Antispasmodics: to manage irritable bowel syndrome; to selectively inhibit gastrointestinal smooth muscle and suppress colonic motor activity; can cause neural side effects, such as dizziness and blurred vision; examples include dicyclomine (Bentyl), hyoscyamine (Hycosin and others).
- Cytoprotective drugs: to protect against stress- or drug-induced GI ulcers; sucralfate complexes with exudates to form a protective coating, misoprostol is a prostaglandin analog; side effects include diarrhea (both), constipation sucralfate), abdominal pain, and fetal maldevelopment (misoprostol).
- Histamine-2 receptor antagonists (H_2RAs): to block receptors and gastric acid secretion; generally, well tolerated; examples include cimetidine, famotidine, etc.
- Proton pump inhibitors (PPIs): to suppress acid in cases of GERD, ulcers, etc.; to inhibit ATPase enzyme systems, thus suppressing gastric acid secretion; well tolerated; examples include esomeprazole, omeprazole, etc.

Laxatives for Treatment of Constipation

Laxatives fall into five categories as follows:

1. Bulk-forming: absorb water in the intestine, creating a thick fluid that encourages peristalsis and lessons transit time; can cause impaction and bloating and should be accompanied by drinking water; examples include psyllium, methylcellulose, polycarbophil
2. Osmolar agents: absorbed in the colon, creating distention and subsequent peristalsis; can cause nausea, distention, irritation; examples include glycerin suppositories, magnesium citrate or sulfate (contraindicated in patients with renal problems as they cause toxicity), polyethylene glycol
3. Emollients: soften stool by reducing the surface tension between water and oils in stool, thus allowing for absorption of water; examples include docusate (Colace), mineral oil (Fleet and others); mineral oil types can suppress absorption of vitamins and some drugs

4. Stimulants: irritate intestinal smooth muscle, stimulating its peristalsis; can cause GI irritation, fluid and electrolyte aberrations; examples include senna (Senokot), bisacodyl (Dulcolax)
5. Chloride channel activator: one example called lubiprostone (Amitiza), a fatty acid that enhances intestinal water secretion; can cause headache, diarrhea, nausea

Colostomy

A colostomy is a surgical procedure done to redirect stool from a damaged part of the colon. There are three types of colostomy performed:

- In an end colostomy, the portion of the bowel that is functioning is diverted onto the surface of the abdomen, folded back onto itself to form a stoma or opening, and sutured onto the skin.
- Double-barrel colostomies are generally temporary and involve creation of two stomas of the abdominal wall: one from the functional proximal portion of the intestinal system to drain stool, and another from the rectum to draw off mucous (a mucous fistula).
- The third type is also usually provisional, the loop colostomy, in which a loop of the bowel is extruded through an incision in the abdominal wall and another incision is made in that bowel portion for stool passage.

All of these procedures drain the stool into an external pouch, which must be securely closed and fastened to the patient before any physical therapy mobility exercises are done. Another procedure with a similar function of diverting stool is an ileostomy, in which the ileum of the small intestine is usually directed to a more distal and operational part of the intestine or to an internal pouch.

Surgical Resection for the Gastrointestinal System

Surgical resection techniques for the gastrointestinal system include:

- Colectomy: the resection of part of the colon via open laparotomy or laparoscopy, often in conjunction with a colostomy or ileostomy.
- Gastrectomy: partial (or complete) removal of the stomach; types of partial resection include Billroth I for the pyloric section and the Billroth II for the distal part of the stomach and the duodenum.
- Resection and reanastomosis: the resection of any nonfunctional part of the gastrointestinal tract followed by reconnection of the operational proximal and distal portions.
- Whipple procedure: excision of the duodenum, some of the stomach, the jejunum, gallbladder, common duct, and regional lymph nodes; followed by a reanastomosis; only indicated for severe cases of pancreatitis or pancreatic cancer; also called pancreaticoduodenectomy.

Patients who have abdominal pain from any of these or other surgical procedures may be more comfortable lying on their side or bending their knees.

Genitourinary System

Patient History for Genitourinary Examination

The history portion of a physical examination evaluating for genitourinary issues should include a description of the pain the patient is experiencing and his voiding patterns, including changes observed. Micturition changes that should be noted and potential causes (in parentheses) include:

- Less forceful urinary flow (obstruction, enlarged prostate)
- Increased urinary frequency (enlarged prostate, inflamed bladder)
- Urinary urgency (infections)
- Incontinence (sphincter and autonomic malfunction)
- Dysuria, or pain upon voiding (infections, etc.)
- Hematuria, or bloody urine (generally indicative of serious pathology, such as cancer)
- Nocturia, or nighttime frequency (congestive heart failure, diabetes)

In addition, small daily urine output should be noted as either oliguria (< 400 ml/day) or anuria (< 100 ml/day), both suggestive of end-stage renal disease (ESRD) or acute shock, renal failure, etc. A large single urine voiding, called polyuria, should also be documented, potentially indicating diabetes, chronic renal failure (CRF), or too much fluid intake.

Physical Examination for Genitourinary Issues

The physical examination when evaluating for genitourinary issues should include questioning and probing specific to the genitourinary system. The history portion is addressed on another card, and basically should include documentation regarding the involved pain and micturition patterns. The clinician should observe the patient for evidence of abdominal or pelvic distention; peripheral edema; incisions, tubes, and other indications of interventions related to genitourinary pathology; and skin changes. He should palpate the kidney region to see whether the patient experiences a sharp or dull pain, indicative of distention or inflammation. He should also use percussion on the kidneys to check for pain and tenderness, which suggests infection or polycystic kidney disease. Finally, the clinician should use auscultation to listen for bruits in the upper abdominal quadrants, which can point to impaired perfusion to the kidneys and renal malfunctions.

Urinalysis and Potential Abnormalities

A urinalysis, in which urine is sterilely collected and analyzed, examines the color, clarity, and odor of urine. Abnormalities are indicated by physical parameters, such as specific gravity, osmolarity (range 300 to 1300 mOsm/kg, i.e. dilute to concentrated), and pH (should be 4.5 to 8.0), as well as the presence of a variety of substances. Several potential abnormalities are usually related to diabetes mellitus, including glycosuria and ketonuria, presence of glucose or ketones, respectively. Bilirubinuria, the presence of bilirubin, is generally indicative of liver and hepatocellular disease. Other possible abnormalities are generally suggestive of genitourinary problems. These include bacteriuria, bacteria in typically cloudy urine, which are indicative of urinary tract infection; proteinuria, the presence of large proteins that have not been filtered out, which may be associated with renal failure but has other causes; hematuria, blood and red blood cells in the urine, found in urinary tract bleeding and a number of kidney diseases; and the presence of crystals, which can appear with urinary tract stones, chronic renal failure, or toxic kidney damage.

Imaging Techniques for Genitourinary Pathologies

Imaging techniques used for the diagnosis of genitourinary pathologies include:

- Radiographic examinations:
  - Kidneys, ureters, and bladder (KUB) x-ray: identifies tumors, stones, and calcifications with a screening radiograph that looks at these structures
  - Pyelography: uses radiopaque dyes injected intravenously or through a cystoscope (retrograde pyelography) to visualize structures and obstructions
  - Renal arteriography and venography: examines the blood supply to or from the kidneys by injecting radiopaque dye into the renal artery (angiography) or vein (venography) and capturing a radiograph
- Ultrasound: is the preferred imaging test to rule out urinary tract obstructions; visualizes kidneys and a variety of other structures; also used to help place biopsy needles and nephrostomy tubes
- Computed tomography (CT) scan: visualizes many structures; the definitive test for renal stone diagnosis
- Magnetic resonance imaging (MRI): definitive test for identifying thrombi in renal veins; often used to identify genitourinary tumors

Non-Imaging Tests Used for Genitourinary Pathologies

Non-imaging tests used for diagnosis of genitourinary pathologies include:

- Creatinine tests: two types, both used to assess renal function; plasma Cr (creatinine) is increased above normal (0.5 to 1.5 mg/dl) and Cr clearance is decreased relative to normal range (75 to 135 ml/min) if renal function is decreased
- Blood urea nitrogen (BUN): abnormally high levels (above normal of 5 to 30 mg/dl) indicative of diminished renal function or fluid intake, infection, high protein intake, or increased muscle catabolism
- Cystometrogram: a urodynamic study in which a catheter is put into the bladder, saline is instilled, and pressure measurements of the bladder wall are taken to assess its tone, sensations upon filling, etc.
- Renal biopsy: percutaneous needle extraction of renal tissue for examination
- Bladder, prostate, and urethral biopsies: transrectal or transperineal insertion of a cystoscope, panendoscope, or needle for extraction of these tissues
- Endoscopic examination of the bladder: insertion of a flexible, fiber optic scope through the urethra into the bladder for visualization; two similar techniques known as cystoscopy and panendoscopy

Acute Renal Failure

Acute renal failure (ARF) is abrupt, rapid decline of renal function, leading to diminished urine output. By far the most common type is prerenal ARF, which is triggered by a decrease in renal blood flow subsequent to trauma, shock burns, profuse bleeding, or dehydration. Other types include intrarenal ARF, which is instigated by some sort of primary damage to the kidneys; and postrenal ARF, in which there is an obstruction distal to the kidney. Regardless of type, mortality rates are high and the clinical course is similar. The patient goes through four phases:

1. An asymptomatic phase
2. An oliguric or anuric stage of a week or more, during which urine output greatly diminishes and patients experience GI problems, confusion, and the potential for congestive heart failure
3. A diuretic stage, where these parameters, renal function, and urine output generally improve
4. A recovery phase of up to a year, defined as the point after which BUN levels are normal

During ARF, patients usually have hemodynamic instability, anemia, infections, and acid-base and electrolyte imbalances. Management includes hydration, renal replacement therapies, transfusions, nutritional adjuncts, treatment of the causative agent, and, in some cases, diuretics.

Chronic Renal Failure

Chronic renal failure (CRF) is the irreparable diminution of renal function and decreased urine output due to permanent damage to nephrons in the kidney. The underlying etiologies are certain systemic diseases (primarily diabetes and hypertension) and a number of primary renal diseases, such as glomerulonephritis, pyelonephritis, polycystic kidney disease, and obstructions. CRF is generally asymptomatic until the majority of nephrons have already been obliterated. End-stage renal disease (ESRD) is the evolution of CRF to severely decreased renal function. Clinical manifestations can include reduced bone density, hemodynamic instability, anemia, infections, and acid-base and electrolyte imbalances. Depending on the situation, patients with CRF are treated conservatively with a number of pharmacologic agents addressing their complications (antihypertensive, anti-infectives, antacids, etc.), nutritional adjuncts, and dietary changes; or more aggressively, with renal replacement therapies or renal transplantation. Those who have not been ambulatory are often given anticoagulants; the physical therapist should be aware of patient clotting times.

Pyelonephritis

Pyelonephritis is inflammation in the kidney subsequent to infection. The renal pelvis is most often involved. The condition can be either acute or chronic:

- Acute pyelonephritis is caused by bacterial infections (*Escherichia coli*, Pseudomonas, etc.) that have entered the kidney through urine reflex or other intrusions. It is more common in women. The patient can present with frequent urination, chills and fever, tenderness on palpation, flank or groin discomfort, GI problems, pain on urination, and/or blood or leukocytes in the urine. Acute pyelonephritis is generally treated with antibiotics, particularly ciprofloxacin (Cipro) for a week.
- Chronic pyelonephritis is characterized by persistent kidney inflammation and resultant scarring. Its causes include autoimmune processes related to infection, kidney stones, and acute pyelonephritis. Many of the signs are similar to acute cases with two notable additions: possible presence of hypertension and renal insufficiency. The latter can lead to renal failure. Management includes treatment of the underlying cause, if identified, and a longer course, up to six months, of the ciprofloxacin, ampicillin, ofloxacin, or trimethoprim/sulfamethoxazole.

Glomerulonephritis

Inflammation of the kidney's glomerulus is termed glomerulonephritis. Hematuria, slight proteinuria, hypertension, and dependent edema are hallmarks when acute. Four common types are:

1. Immunoglobulin A nephropathy (Berger's disease): immune dys-function, where IgA antibody complexes in the glomerulus impact filtration; due to cirrhosis, rheumatic diseases, etc.; signs include blood and protein in urine, oliguria; managed with anti-inflammatory drugs, such as glucocorticoids, ACE inhibitors, and cytotoxic drugs
2. Postinfectious glomerulonephritis: acute renal inflammation after infection, usually group α- or β-hemolytic streptococci; characterized by acute onset fluid retention, hypertension, distal edema, pro-teinuria, anemia, and dark, bloody urine with red blood cell casts; managed with antibiotics, antihypertensives, diuretics, fluids and electrolytes, and hemodialysis, if needed
3. Rapidly pro-gressive glomerulonephritis (RPGN): cases that proceed quickly to very low output and renal failure; due to infection, multiple system or auto-immune diseases; treated with anti-inflammatory drugs, antico-agulants, plasmapheresis, hemodialysis, and renal trans-plantation
4. Chronic glomerulonephritis: scarring and destruction of glomeration and vascular sclerosis accumulating over years; causes include hepatitis, diabetes, systemic lupus erythematosus, others mentioned above; patient has uremia, proteinuria, and hyper-tension; managed with steroids, anti-infectives, cytotoxic agents, dialysis, renal transplants, and treatment of the underlying cause

Nephrotic Syndrome

In nephrotic syndrome, the glomerular basement membrane in the kidneys becomes highly permeable, leading to excretion of albumin and other proteins, diminished osmotic pressures, and peripheral edema. Nephrotic syndrome can be caused by a variety of underlying diseases, such as diabetes, systemic lupus erythematosus, IgA nephropathy, vascular diseases, and renal transplant rejection. It can also occur in acute situations, such as preeclampsia and allergic or drug reactions. Patients have low serum albumin and high serum lipid levels, lipiduria, vitamin D deficiency, and widespread peripheral edema. Pharmacologic agents used for management include steroidal anti-inflammatory drugs, diuretics, and anticoagulants. Other management strategies include albumin and protein replacements, dietary changes (low-fat, low-salt diet), and treatment of the fundamental cause.

Nephrolithiasis

Nephrolithiasis is the formation of renal calculi, or kidney stones. These kidney stones are differentiated in terms of their composition, which can be calcium oxalate, uric acid, cystine, or struvite (a combination of magnesium, ammonium, and phosphate). Causes include high amounts of these substances or others that enable crystal formation in the urine; obstruction in the urinary tract; a low-fluid, high-protein diet; infections; metabolic problems; and certain drugs. The prominent sign is great pain in the flank or groin, particularly when the stone is moving. Other possible signs include GI problems, fever, blood in the urine, and variability in urine pH and various serum substances. Kidney stones are diagnosed using a CT scan (without contrast). Patients are either given drugs that enhance stone evacuation (corticosteroids, calcium channel blockers, alpha-blockers), the stone is extracted with an ureteroscope, or it is shattered with real shock wave lithotripsy. Patients are also given analgesics, taken off any precipitating medications, put on external urinary drainage, and prescribed anti-infectives. Future stone formation is addressed with dietary changes and drugs, such as thiazide diuretics. Stones can also occur in other parts of the urinary tract (urinary calculi or urolithiasis).

Interstitial Nephritis

Interstitial nephritis is the inflammation, damage, and subsequent scarring of interstitial tissues in the kidney. It results in diminished kidney function and potentially chronic renal failure. The causes include infections and obstructions in the urinary tract and reactions to NSAIDs or other medications. The signs of interstitial nephritis are urine abnormalities, namely excessive urination, nighttime frequency, and the presence of pus, blood, or protein in the urine. Treatment of interstitial nephritis includes fluids; dialysis; nutritional adjuncts; anti-infective drugs; surgical removal of obstruction, if appropriate; and renal transplantation.

Renal Vascular Abnormalities

The most common renal vascular abnormality is renal artery stenosis or occlusion, in which the renal artery lumen is either narrowed or blocked, respectively. The causes are vascular in nature (atherosclerosis, emboli, thrombi, bacterial endocarditis) or diabetes mellitus. Renin, a kidney enzyme that breaks down proteins and controls blood pressure, is overproduced, resulting in hypertension. Other signs can include pain in the flank or upper abdomen, presence of bruits, blood in urine, peripheral edema, and ACE inhibitor-induced acute renal failure. Diagnosis is established using renal angiography or other imaging techniques. It is managed with anticoagulants, ACE inhibitor-type antihypertensives, analgesics, dialysis, and surgery (usually angioplasty with or without stent placement). A rarer abnormality is renal vein thrombosis, in which some sort of trauma causes accrual of plaque in the renal vein. This can cause renal infarcts, flank pain, appreciable hematuria, proteinuria, and oliguria. It is addressed with anticoagulants or thrombolytic agents.

Cystitis

Cystitis is inflammation of the bladder wall. Acute infectious cystitis, due to infections, is the most common type, with predisposing factors like sexual activity, diabetes, neurogenic bladder, urinary tract obstructions, or use of an indwelling catheter. Cystitis can also be caused by exposure to chemicals or radiation or as an autoimmune manifestation. People with cystitis urinate often (including at night) and urgently, they have pain upon voiding, and they have suprapubic and/or low back pain. There are a number of drugs to treat cystitis, including ciprofloxacin, cephalexin, nitrofurantoin, trimethoprim-sulfamethoxazole, and others. Patients should also increase their fluid intake. More drastic interventions include hydrodistention of the bladder, followed often by instillation of anti-inflammatory or other agents; and surgical procedures, such as total or partial cystectomy or denervation of the bladder.

Neurogenic Bladder

Neurogenic bladder is paralysis of the bladder due to cortical or spinal cord lesions, resulting in lack of central nervous system control. If the lesion is higher than the sacral level of the spinal cord, the individual cannot voluntarily control voiding. If the lesion is lower in the spinal cord, the patient loses control of both voluntary and involuntary voiding. A person with neurogenic bladder usually has nocturia and frequent microleakage and is prone to urinary infections. The condition may be alleviated if the underlying neurologic disruption can be addressed. Other management tools include use of anti-infective drugs for associated infections, voiding aids like suprapubic pressure or double voiding, and catheterization.

URINARY INCONTINENCE

There are four types of urinary incontinence: stress, urge, overflow, and functional:

- Stress incontinence is an involuntary loss of urine provoked by circumstances that cause increased intraabdominal pressure, such as coughing or exercising; it occurs in people with some type of muscular weakness in the genitourinary system.
- Urge incontinence is urine leakage upon ostensible bladder fullness; this has multiple causes, including cystitis, stones, obstructions, and neurologic disorders.
- Overflow incontinence is leakage resulting from an overdistended bladder; the causes can be mechanical, such as an obstruction, or the result of urinary retention from a noncontractile or neurogenic bladder.
- Functional incontinence is a situation where a physical, cognitive, or psychological issue prevents voiding; it is most often caused by depression, hostility, dementia, or other neurologic illness.

BENIGN PROSTATIC HYPERPLASIA

Benign prostatic hyperplasia (BPH) is the non-cancerous enlargement of the prostate gland in men. The condition is found in about half of men once they reach their 50s. BPH affects normal voiding patterns because it can result in urinary tract infections and acute urinary retention. Signs of the latter include diminished urinary flow, post-void dribble, difficulty urinating, frequent voiding with only partial emptying, and nocturia. A digital rectal examination will reveal palpable lobes of the gland. BPH is treated with alpha1-adrenergic drugs like tamsulosin (Flomax) or terazosin (Hytrin), which encourage voiding by relaxing the smooth muscle in the area. Another drug category used is the 5-alpha-reductase enzyme inhibitor finasteride (Proscar), which suppresses male hormones and gradually shrinks the prostate gland. Other interventions include occasional self-catheterization; anti-infectives, if there is infection; several types of prostatectomy (prostate removal); and other surgical techniques.

PROSTATITIS

Inflammation of the prostate gland is referred to as prostatitis. Prostatitis can be due to acute or chronic presence of bacteria, principally *E. coli, Pseudomonas aeruginosa,* or *Enterococcus*. Most cases, however, are considered nonbacterial or prostatodynia, meaning there are symptoms but no bacterial precipitant, with or without physical findings, respectively. Symptoms of prostatitis are urinary frequency including at night, urinary urgency, pain on urination, difficulty starting a flow, sexual problems, and bladder irritability. If the origin is acute bacterial, there is also fever with rectal, perineal, or low back pain. Management includes dietary changes to reduce symptoms (removal of alcohol, spicy foods), use of antipyretics, anti-infective drugs (if bacterial), alpha1-adrenergic blocking agents (if prostatodynia), and resection of the prostate.

ENDOMETRIOSIS

Endometriosis is the presence of endometrial tissue external to the uterus, particularly in other parts of the pelvis and the ovaries. The origin of endometriosis is unclear, but most believe it is due to backward menstrual flow from the uterus into the pelvic cavity. A laparoscopic assessment is usually done to differentiate endometriosis from pelvic inflammatory disease or presence of neoplasms in the ovaries, uterus, or bowel. The hallmark sign of endometriosis is dysmenorrhea, severe pain during menstruation. Other symptoms include pelvic pain related to the menstrual cycle, pain upon intercourse, and pain in the lower back and lower extremities. Women with endometriosis are given hormonal therapies targeted at reducing the aberrant endometrial tissue growth, including contraceptives, nasal nafarelin, Danazol, and medroxyprogesterone acetate. Surgical options include laparoscopic excision of the tissue and the uterine nerve, and, if childbearing is not an issue, total hysterectomy (removal of the womb) with bilateral salpingo-oophorectomy.

Renal Replacement Therapy

Renal replacement therapy is a process that reestablishes relatively normal concentrations of electrolytes and other solutes, optimal fluid volumes, and filtered urine in patients with acute renal failure (ARF) or chronic renal failure (CRF). There are several ways of accomplishing this, but each utilizes three principles:

1. The first is the principle of diffusion, which means that solutes (dissolved substances, such as electrolytes) move from high concentration zones to those of lower concentration.
2. The second is osmosis, the principle that fluids tend to move from a region of lesser solute concentration to one of greater solute concentration.
3. The third principle utilized is ultrafiltration, or removal of water and fluids by the establishment of pressure gradients between arterial blood and a membrane or compartment used to accomplish the dialysis.

There are three common techniques for renal replacement therapy: peritoneal dialysis, intermittent hemodialysis, and continuous renal replacement therapy (CRRT). All are discussed in detail on other cards.

Peritoneal Dialysis

Peritoneal dialysis (PD) is one type of renal replacement therapy for patients with acute or chronic renal failure. A dialysate fluid is infused into the peritoneal cavity using an indwelling catheter positioned surgically or non-surgically. The water and solutes in the dialysate use diffusion and osmosis to pass across the semipermeable peritoneal membrane and establish equilibrium with blood vessels in the abdominal cavity. Excess fluid and solutes in the peritoneal cavity are then drawn out of the peritoneal cavity. PD can be done using an automated system, which automatically cycles the entire exchange process of instillation, equilibrium, and drainage. An alternate method is continuous ambulatory PD, in which gravity is used for the instillation and drainage processes, with each exchange cycle done about four times daily. Peritoneal dialysis is appropriate for patients who do not require rapid reestablishment of fluid and electrolyte balance, patients in shock, cardiac patients after surgery or with critical disease, and those in which hemodialysis is impossible (poor vascular access, transfusion refusal). It should not be used in individuals with abdominal area issues (peritonitis, adhesions, hernias, abdominal surgery) or coexisting pulmonary complications.

Intermittent Hemodialysis

In intermittent hemodialysis, the patient's arterial blood is removed via an internal arteriovenous fistula, a looped graft, or an external cannula or shunt (generally temporary). Using an external pumping system, the patient's arterial blood is circulated through a dialyzer that acts as an artificial kidney and eventually returned to the individual's venous circulation. In the dialyzer, there is dialysate fluid with normal plasma electrolyte concentrations. As the patient's blood passes through the semipermeable tubing in the dialyzer, normal fluid volumes, electrolyte balance, and acid-base balance are established through diffusion and osmosis; nitrogenous wastes are also removed. The blood returned to the patient is cleaner and more balanced. Long-term intermittent hemodialysis is usually done three or four times weekly in three- to four-hour sessions. Intermittent hemodialysis is used for patients with both chronic and acute renal failure (hypotension as potential side effect), as well as individuals with severe edema, metabolic acidosis, large area burns, transfusion reactions, poisoning, postpartum renal insufficiency, and crush syndrome. It should not be used in patients with bleeding tendencies or other major chronic diseases.

Continuous Renal Replacement Therapy

Continuous renal replacement therapy (CRRT) is the slow removal of fluid, electrolytes, and solutes, similar to normal kidney function. CRRT can be done for over a month with external hemofilter changes daily or every two days. It can be done with intermittent hemodialysis in chronic renal failure but is more likely to be used in situations, such as acute renal failure with other organ failure, acute cardiovascular issues, sepsis, or uremia. It is contraindicated for patients with congestive heart failure, poisoning, shock, atherosclerosis, hypercatabolism, high potassium levels, and low arterial or colloid oncotic pressure. There are five types:

1. Continuous arteriovenous hem filtration (CAVH): uses femoral artery and vein for access; driven by pressure gradients; heparin introduced before filter, filtrate-controlled infusion fluid after prior to return
2. Continuous venovenous hem filtration (CVVH): internal jugular or subclavian veins used for access; utilizes mechanical pump and external exchange filter
3. Continuous venovenous hemodialysis (CVVHD): akin to CVVH, except dialysate solution is utilized to help remove waste products by diffusion
4. Continuous venovenous hemodiafiltration (CVVHDF): employs convection, diffusion, and ultrafiltration for clearance
5. Slow continuous ultrafiltration (SCUF): uses only filtration to extract fluid without reestablishing other parameters

Surgical Interventions for Genitourinary Disorders

Possible surgical interventions for genitourinary disorders include:

- Nephrectomy: surgical removal of the kidney; performed open or laparoscopically; types include radical nephrectomy (all of kidney plus ureter, adrenal gland, and adjacent fatty tissue), simple nephrectomy (entire kidney plus part of ureter), and partial nephrectomy (only the infected or diseased part of kidney)
- Transurethral resection (TURP and others): urethral insertion of rectoscope to resect implicated tissues for TURP (indicated for benign prostatic hyperplasia)
- Open prostatectomy: surgical excision of prostate gland and possibly its capsule in men with prostate cancer
- Percutaneous nephroscopic stone removal: removal of urinary tract stones using percutaneous nephrostomy tube to break them up and remove them in a basket or via flushing
- Bladder neck suspension: suturing of urethra to pubic bones in women with stress incontinence to re-establish continence
- Open urologic surgery: varied types include cystectomy (bladder removal), nephrolithotomy (use of incision to remove kidney stone), pyelolithotomy (kidney stone extraction from kidney's pelvis), ureterolithotomy (removal of urinary stone from ureter), etc.
- Urinary diversion: redirection of obstructed urinary flow (discussed on another card)

Surgical Procedures for Urinary Diversion

There are several possible surgical procedures for diversion of obstructed urinary flow:

- In a supravesical diversion, a nephrostomy is done, which involves insertion of a nephrostomy tube into the renal pelvis and drainage into an external collection appliance.
- In an incontinent urinary diversion, the urine stream is diverted through a stoma, or surgical opening, into an external collection device. The ureters are often implanted into a section of the ileum of the small intestine as well.
- Continent urinary diversions use portions of the ileum, ileocecal segment, or colon to create an internal reservoir. This internal reservoir is attached to an abdominal stoma that the patient must from time to time drain by self-catheterization.
- Another procedure is the restructuring of the distal ileum into what is called an orthotopic neobladder and its attachment to the ureters and urethra.

Fluids and Electrolytes

Fluid and Electrolyte Imbalance

Homeostasis is the internal regulation of an environment or system to maintain stability and constancy. In the human body, cellular functions are impaired when homeostasis is out of balance. Correct homeostasis is dependent on the relative concentration of intracellular and extracellular fluids, the types and concentrations of electrolytes, the permeability of cellular membranes, and operational kidney function. Fluid imbalance can be either hypovolemia, a fluid volume deficit, or hypervolemia, a fluid volume excess or overload. Electrolytes are substances containing free ions in solution (for example, plasma), such as acids, bases, salts, and arterial blood gases. There are established normal levels for these electrolytes in serum that should be maintained for normal cellular function. Fluid volumes and electrolyte levels are interrelated. The electrolyte levels of most interest are sodium and potassium. A sodium deficit is termed hyponatremia (< 135 mEq/L); an excess is hypernatremia (> 145 mEq/L). A potassium deficit is hypokalemia (< 3.5 mEq/L); an excess is hyperkalemia (> 5 mEq/L).

Contributing Factors and Major Diagnostic Findings for Fluid Imbalances

Hypovolemia is caused by diarrhea, vomiting, hemorrhage, burns, diabetic complications, or fluid shifts into interstitial spaces. Signs of hypovolemia include a weak rapid pulse, low blood pressure, dehydration, confusion, and muscle cramps. Patients have high BUN, blood urea nitrogen, and serum sodium levels. Their hematocrit can be high if plasma fluid has shifted from intravascular to interstitial spaces and low if they have experienced blood loss.

Hypervolemia results from water shifting from the vascular system into intracellular space, too much sodium or fluid intake or retention, blood transfusions, and congestive heart or renal failure. Patients present with dyspnea, high blood pressure, a bounding pulse, dependent edema, and heart CHF S3 heart sound and cough. Characteristic laboratory findings include low hematocrit, low BUN, and decreased serum potassium levels.

Contributing Factors and Major Diagnostic Findings for Electrolyte Imbalances

Hyponatremia is due to diuresis with SIADH, renal disease, hyperglycemia, or renal disease, or it can occur as a drug side effect. Patients may be nauseous and confused or have muscle problems like twitching and cramps. Laboratory findings include low serum and urine sodium levels, high plasma protein concentrations, and elevated hematocrit.

Hypernatremia is seen in patients with a water deficit, diarrhea, diabetes insipidus, hyperventilation, or large intake of sodium bicarbonate, sodium chloride, or corticosteroids.

Patients can exhibit evidence of dehydration, high body temperature, neuromuscular and cardiac problems, pulmonary edema, and oliguria. Sodium concentrations are high in serum and low in urine.

Hypokalemia is caused by low potassium intake or its loss through renal disease, polyuria, or diarrhea. Symptoms include fatigue, leg cramps, weak pulse, low blood pressure, constipation, and/or ventricular fibrillation. Patient ECGs show ST depression or prolonged PR interval, arterial pH and bicarbonate are high, and patients are slightly hyperglycemic.

Hyperkalemia causes include high potassium intake, renal failure, diuretics, ACE inhibitors, NSAIDs, or heparin therapy. Most symptoms are cardiac- or muscular-like dysrhythmias, paralysis, etc. ECG findings show ST depression and other abnormalities, and patients have low arterial pH.

Multi-System

Pelvic Floor Dysfunction

Possible pelvic floor dysfunctions include prolapse, incontinence (urinary or fecal), pain, and hypertonus (extreme tenseness). Prolapse is the slippage of pelvic organs out of their normal alignment. Causes include increased abdominal pressure and weakness in muscles, fascia, or ligaments. Prolapse usually occurs as a result of pregnancy, gets progressively worse, and is provoked by constipation or straining upon elimination. The pressure exerted and heaviness of prolapse causes low back and abdominal pain and makes voiding difficult. Urinary and/or fecal incontinence, or content leakage, often transpires concurrently with prolapse, although neurological and muscular problems can cause it as well. Pelvic pain and hypertonus are other types of pelvic floor dysfunction. Origins of these are varied, including trauma during delivery, other gynecologic problems, scar tissue adhesions, etc. The major precipitant of pelvic floor dysfunctions is childbirth, but women who have never had a child can also have them due to factors like straining with constipation, cigarette use, hysterectomy, obesity, and chronic cough. High caffeine consumption is a risk factor for urge incontinence.

Diastasis Recti

Diastasis recti is the severance of the rectus abdominis muscles along the midline of the linea alba, which also disturbs abdominal muscles internal to them. It occurs most often in pregnant women, particularly as the pregnancy proceeds, or during delivery, but it can be found in other women and even men. Effects of diastasis recti include low back pain and functional limitations, such as difficulty changing from supine to sitting positions. Severe separations can result in diminished fetal protection or herniation of abdominal organs (the latter indicating needed surgery). All pregnant women should be tested for diastasis recti before performing abdominal exercises. In the diastasis recti test, the woman lies in hook position with bent knees, slowly lifts her head and shoulders off the floor, and stretches her hands toward her knees until the spines of the scapulae are lifted. The therapist uses the fingers of his hands to feel the abdominal midline at the umbilicus, which will descend into the gap if there is a separation. The number of fingers that can fit into the gap is noted. The test is also done at spots above and below the umbilicus as the diastasis can occur there as well.

Corrective Exercise for Diastasis Recti

If a diastasis recti test indicates that the separation of the rectus abdominis muscles is greater than 2 cm, only corrective abdominal exercise must be done until it shrinks to 2 cm or less. These corrective exercises are limited to the head lift or the head lift with pelvic tilt. In the head lift, the patient is in a hook-lying position (supine with bent knees) with hands crisscrossed over the midline at the diastasis. She should exhale and raise her head until there is a bulge, while mimicking normal abdominal action with her hands (i.e. pulling toward midline). She then releases her head back and relaxes. A sheet wrapped around the separation area may be needed to provide additional support. The head lift with pelvic tilt is similar except that a posterior pelvic tilt is held during the exercise, which means the pelvis is actively lifted posteriorly.

Pregnancy

Postural Back and Sacroiliac/Pelvic Girdle Pain During Pregnancy

The majority of pregnant women have postural low back pain at some juncture. It transpires because of pregnancy-related postural changes and diminished function of abdominal muscles and ligaments. Suggested interventions for relief of the pain are rest, position changes, low back exercises, attention to proper body mechanics and posture, and application of superficial pain relievers. Sacroiliac pain originates from the L5/S1 area and is characterized by stabbing pain in the posterior pelvis (buttocks), possibly radiating to the back thigh or knee. The pain occurs in many positions and is not relieved by rest. Pelvic girdle or pubic symphysis dysfunction may occur concurrently or alone. This pain includes tenderness at the symphysis, which radiates to the groin and mid-thigh and is aggravated by weight bearing. Patients with these types of pain should modify their activities to avoid asymmetrical trunk, pelvis, or leg use. They should not perform exercises that involve weight bearing on one leg, full-range hip abduction, or too much hyperextension, and they should be taught how to stabilize their pelvis during transitions and/or use stabilizing belts or corsets.

Varicose Veins, Joint Laxity, and Compression Syndromes During Pregnancy

During pregnancy, the increased weight of the uterus, along with venous stasis and distension, combine to put the woman at risk for varicosities, including swollen leg veins, termed varicose veins. Varicosities can also occur in the rectum and vulva. If the woman has varicose veins and pain, she should wear elastic support stockings, elevate her legs whenever possible, perform lower-extremity exercises, and avoid other exercises that require dependent positioning of the legs.

During pregnancy, ligaments lose tensile quality, making their joints more lax and prone to injury. These changes can continue into early postpartum. Therefore, pregnant women should do types of exercise that will not place excessive stress on their joints, for example, swimming, walking, etc.

Pregnant women are more prone to various nerve compression syndromes, for example, carpal tunnel syndrome (CTS) or thoracic outlet syndrome (TOS), because of factors like postural modifications, retention of fluids, and hormonal differences. Possible interventions include splints for CTS, postural correction exercises, and other corrective measures.

Guidelines for Management of the Pregnant Woman

Prior to beginning an exercise program with a pregnant woman, the therapist should assess the patient's posture, musculoskeletal problems, and fitness level. S9he) should educate the patient about dealing with physiological responses associated with pregnancy that can impact the program. For example, supine exercises after the first trimester should be short and done with support under the right hip to circumvent vena cava compression of the uterus. Patients should transition from supine to standing or sitting positions slowly to avoid orthostatic hypotension. They should not hold their breath because this places stress on the uterus, pelvic floor, and cardiovascular system. Pregnant women should limit activities that put weight on only one leg as they aggravate sacroiliac and pelvic girdle pain. They should maintain hydration while exercising. Exercise types should include rhythmic warm-up activities, gentle selective stretching (nothing asymmetric), mild aerobics for cardiovascular effects, postural and strengthening exercises, and, after cool-down, pelvic floor exercises, relaxation methods, and labor and delivery techniques. If the woman has any persistent pain, leakage, contractions, bleeding, cardiac problems, or the like, the exercise should be stopped and a physician consulted.

High-Risk Pregnancy

Any condition, preexisting or pregnancy-related, that could potentially cause death or illness constitutes a high-risk pregnancy. These conditions include:

- Diabetes: a condition characterized by high glucose levels and excessive urine; preexisting types 1 or 2 or pregnancy-related (called gestational diabetes)
- Pre-eclampsia: pregnancy-related hypertension, edema, and pertinacious urine, usually occurring during third trimester; if severe, termed eclampsia, which can lead to convulsions, coma, or death
- Multiple gestation: development of more than one fetus
- Placenta previa: low attachment of placenta close to cervix
- Incompetent cervix: dilation of cervix as early as 16 weeks gestation
- Preterm rupture of membranes: breakage of amniotic sac and fluid loss
- Premature onset of labor: labor before mature fetal development, anywhere before 37 weeks gestation

Multiple gestation, placenta previa, incompetent cervix, and preterm rupture of membranes can all result in premature labor and delivery and endanger the fetus.

Management Guidelines for a High-Risk Pregnancy

A woman with a high-risk pregnancy is generally restricted to bedrest. The optimal positioning for her is lying on her left side with pillows between her knees and under her abdomen, which averts compression of the vena cava. Other possibilities include short-term supine positioning, with a wedge under the right hip; or modified prone, defined as lying on the side, leaning toward prone and pillow supported. The patient should do range-of-motion (ROM) exercises on all joints. ROM exercises done side-lying or supine, with a wedge under the right hip, are suggested. Stretching, strengthening, and movement exercises should be done within the limits imposed by a doctor. Ambulation is usually not allowed in a high-risk pregnancy, but if it is (for example, to go to the lavatory), posture and perhaps a few other techniques can be taught. It is important, however, to avoid the Valsalva maneuver. Relaxation techniques, bed-mobility exercises, transfer techniques, and preparatory exercises for labor should all be done.

Tumors

The terms "tumor" and "neoplasm" are often used interchangeably to mean a new growth or a tissue mass of abnormal size. Tumors can be benign, slow-growing masses, largely resembling nearby tissues, or malignant (cancer), meaning they are expanding uncontrollably, usually with cellular changes. Tumors are classified beyond these definitions in terms of their cell and tissue type of origin, anatomical location, amount of dysphasia (change from normal cell type), and degree of spread. Tumors are designated with a prefix reflective of the organ involved and a suffix that indicates cellular type. Benign tumors end in "-oma," while most malignant tumors are carcinomas or sarcomas, depending on whether they derive from epithelial or mesenchymal tissues, respectively. Mesenchymal tissues include connective tissues, muscles, and lymphoid tissues. There are also bone marrow-derived tumors (leukemias etc.), nerve tissue, and other cancer types. Neoplasms are also defined in terms of grade from I to IV, which reflects the degree of differentiation from normal cell type, and stage, which defines the extent of tumor and its spread (both discussed further elsewhere).

TMN System for Tumor Staging

Tumors are generally staged by the TMN system, which defines three parameters: the extent of the primary tumor (T); the amount of regional lymph node involvement (N); and the presence of distant metastasis, or spread to other parts of the body (M). An "X" after one of these notations indicates the parameter cannot be assessed, a "0" (zero) means none is observed, and a number indicates the size or degree of presence. For the primary tumor, there is an additional choice, Tis, which means carcinoma, or tumor in situ (site of origin). Choices for each parameter include:

- Primary tumor: TX, T0, Tis, T1, T2, T3, T4
- Regional lymph node involvement: NX, N0, N1, N2, N3
- Distant metastasis: MX, M0, M1 (any presence)

Thus, a tumor might be staged by this system as T1 N1 M0, which for many tumors would be a stage II in other systems. Specific types of tumors are generally assigned a stage from 0 to IV based on their TMN combination. These stages differ somewhat, depending on the organ of origin.

Neoplasms Grading

Grading of neoplasms reflects the degree of dysplasia, or differentiation of the cells involved from their initial cell type. Grading is useful because a higher level of differentiation from normal indicates the tumor is more aggressive and potentially lethal. The grades are:

- Grade I: tumor cells look much like the original tissues
- Grades II and III: tumor cells are somewhat differentiated and have a changed but relatively intermediate appearance
- Grade IV: tumor cells are so modified that they have lost their original distinctive features (anaplastic), and it is hard or impossible to establish their initial cell of origin

Risk Factors for Neoplasms

The etiologies of neoplasms, or cancer, are caused either by genetics or exposure to external, environmental factors. The latter include viruses, a variety of chemical agents, physical agents, certain chemotherapeutic drugs, and the hormone estrogen. Many of the chemical agents are related to tobacco use or workplace exposure (benzene, tar, soot, etc.). Physical agents include ionizing radiation, ultraviolet light, and asbestos exposure. Lung and oral cancers are highly linked to history of smoking. Other cancers, such as breast, ovarian, prostate, stomach, and skin, have proven or suggested genetic components. Aging puts people more at risk for certain cancers, such as colorectal. Dietary factors contribute to stomach and breast cancer.

Symptomatic and Diagnostic Evaluation for Malignancy

As malignancies grow, depending on the location, they tend to produce symptoms of changing bowel or bladder habits, a sore that will not heal, unusual bleeding or discharge, thickening or a lump in the breast or in other places, indigestion or dysphasia, obvious transformation in a wart or mole, and/or a nagging cough or hoarseness (American Cancer Society's acronym CAUTION). Other symptoms include inexplicable weight loss or pain, fever, tiredness, anorexia, anemia, and seemingly peripheral syndromes related to hormone release by the tumor. Diagnostic tests are usually specific to the type of suspected cancer.

For example, colon cancer testing might include carcinoembryonic antigen (CEA) and CA19-9 blood tests, stool guaiac, sigmoidoscopy, and/or colonoscopy. Potential breast cancer can be diagnosed using mammography. Biopsy, in which some of the tissue is removed and analyzed for presence and characteristics of tumor cells, is a common diagnostic tool. Imaging tools include positron emission tomography (PET) scanning, CT scanning, radiography, MRI, computerized axial tomography, and bone scans.

Surgical Interventions for Cancer

Surgical removal of a tumor is just one type of therapeutic intervention. Other possible interventions include radiation therapy, chemotherapy, various biotherapies, physical therapy, and supportive measures. Types of surgery include:

- Surgical removal of portions of the tumor for purposes of staging is termed exploratory surgery.
- Excisional surgery is the cutting out of the suspected cancerous cells and some of the adjacent normal tissue; it is followed by a pathological determination of cancer cell type and extent of removal. A variation is Mohs' surgery, where tumor layers are removed and inspected microscopically until all abnormal cells have been eliminated.
- Patients considered terminal might undergo debunking, partial resection to decrease tumor size and make them more comfortable.
- A lymph node dissection or resection of regional lymph nodes is often done to restrain cancer spread.
- Following other procedures, two additional types of surgery might be performed: skin grafting and/or reconstructive surgery. Skin grafting can impact therapy as the patient usually remains on prolonged bedrest.

Radiation Therapy

Radiation therapy can be used as a standalone modality to treat cancer; in conjunction with surgical resection or chemotherapy; prophylactically, for limitation of cancer growth; and/or as a palliative measure in incurable patients. Most radiation therapy performed is some variation of external bean radiation therapy (EBRT), where the radiation is delivered externally. Another type is brachytherapy, in which a radioactive source is placed into a body cavity or other internal space. Intraoperative radiation therapy (IORT) is the conveyance of a large amount of radiation directly to the tumor site during surgery. Radioimmunotherapy, in which radiation is transported to a site via specific antibodies, is a burgeoning option. Patients receiving radiation therapy typically have a variety of immediate or later-onset side effects, including swelling of limbs, neuropathies, bone marrow suppression, fibrosis, gastrointestinal problems, etc. Radiation therapy precludes the therapist from delivering massage or heat therapies in that area. Physical therapy is contraindicated when there are implanted radioactive seeds. Range-of-motion exercises are good, however, to prevent contracture.

Chemotherapy

Chemotherapy is the pre- or post-operative use of certain drugs to shrink the size of the tumor or prevent metastasis. Methods of delivery include systemically through IV or central lines and direct site injection via a catheter. The most effective chemotherapeutic agents act by damaging DNA in rapidly dividing cells like tumor cells; they are also usually very toxic. There are quite a few classes of chemotherapeutic drugs utilized (summarized on another card). Some of the typical side effects of use are gastrointestinal problems, hair loss, pain, and loss of other fast-growing cells (i.e. blood components). The latter makes patients prone to infections and sepsis as they are often neutropenic, deficient in the white blood cells called neutrophils that help fight infection. White blood cell, red blood cell, and platelet counts should all be monitored, in addition to vital signs. One of the biggest considerations is the patient's possibly severe nausea and vomiting, which may delay therapy. Chemotherapeutic drugs also tend to suppress appetite and absorption of nutrients, and therapy is dependent on nutritional status.

Antiemetic Drugs

Antiemetic drugs are given to cancer patients to prevent or treat nausea and vomiting related to chemotherapy, radiation therapy, and/or surgery. There are four classes of antiemetic drugs:

1. 5-HT3-receptor antagonists: act by blocking serotonin; the best tolerated of all classes but can cause headache, constipation, and dizziness; examples include dolasetron (Anzemet), ondansetron (Zofran), and others
2. Benzamides: block dopamine receptors and, at high dosages, serotonin receptors; have many neurologic side effects, such as dystonia, Parkinsonian-like symptoms, uncontrollable limb movements; also cause fatigue, diarrhea; examples include metoclopramide (Reglan)
3. Butyrophenones: block dopamine stimulation; cause QT prolongation on ECG, putting patients at risk for torsades and requiring monitoring; can alter central temperature regulation, and make patient either restless or drowsy; examples include droperidol (Inapsine), haloperidol (Haldol)
4. Cannabinoids: mechanism unclear; can cause palpitations, vasodilation, and neurologic changes; examples include dronabinol (Marinol)

Chemotherapeutic Agents

Chemotherapeutic Agents that Affect Nucleic Acids

Classes of chemotherapeutic agents affecting nucleic acids include:

- Alkylating agents: act by cross-linking DNA and inhibiting its replication; patients must be monitored for pulmonary toxicity and renal function; potential adverse effects are somewhat agent-specific, i.e. hemorrhagic cyclophosphamide and ifosfamide (also encephalopathy), pulmonary fibrosis for carmustine
- Antimetabolites: inhibit nucleic acid synthesis by replacement; potential adverse effects include swelling of palms and soles, diarrhea, bruising, bleeding, hepatotoxicity, etc.; examples include cytarabine, fluorouracil, methotrexate, and others
- Antitumor antibiotics: block DNA and/or RNA synthesis; several types, the most common being anthracyclines, which can cause cardiotoxicity and have lifetime limits; other adverse effects include nausea and vomiting, hair loss, etc.; anthracyclines include Adriamycin, daunorubicin; others include bleomycin, dactinomycin
- Plant alkaloids: inhibit replication through a number of mechanisms; can cause peripheral neuropathy, low blood pressure, edema, diarrhea, headache, SAIDH, etc., depending on type; includes camptothecins, epipodophyllotoxins, taxanes, and vinca alkaloids
- Platinum compounds: inhibit DNA synthesis through alkylation; may cause severe nausea and vomiting, nephrotoxicity, peripheral neurotoxicity, and hearing and balance problems; examples include carboplatin, cisplatin

Chemotherapeutic Agents That Act by Mechanisms Other Than Directly Affecting Replication

These chemotherapeutic agents include:

- Biological response modifiers: work by triggering immune-mediated host defense mechanisms; can cause hypo- or hypertension, fever, organ toxicity, pain, nausea, etc.; examples include interferon-alpha 2b, levamisole, aldesleukin

- Monoclonal antibodies (mAbs): combine with specific antigens on tumor cells, causing apoptosis (cell death), toxicity, or lysis; similar possible adverse effects as biological response modifiers as well as mAb-specific reactions for some; examples include Bevacucizumab (potential rash), cetuximab (potential interstitial lung disease), trastuzumab, etc.
- Hormones and their antagonists: effective only in hormone-dependent tumors; work by inhibiting or diminishing production of said hormone; can cause vaginal bleeding, thromboembolisms, menstrual problems, edema, bone loss, impotence, etc., depending on type; types include androgens and antiandrogens, estrogens and antiestrogens, progestins, aromatase inhibitors, gonadotropin-releasing hormone (GNRH) inhibitors, and luteinizing hormone-releasing hormone (LHRH) agonists
- Tyrosine kinase inhibitors: can cause hepatotoxicity, fluid retention, neutropenia, etc.; examples include gefitinib, imatinib

Biotherapy for Treatment of Malignancies

Several types of modalities are considered biotherapy, including hormonal therapy, immunotherapy, use of monoclonal antibodies, and bone marrow transplantation:

- In hormonal therapy, sources like the ovaries or adrenal glands, which influence hormonal levels, are removed surgically or obliterated pharmacologically. Hormonal therapy is most often used to deal with breast or prostate cancer.
- In immunotherapy, agents that boost immune responses against the cancer or the immune system, in general, are administered. Monoclonal antibodies are specific to tumor cell antigens, which they target when administered; a radioactive tag may be included for added radiation effects.
- Bone marrow transplantation may be indicated for treatment of certain cancers as other therapies may have depleted bone marrow cells.

Pulmonary Cancers

The vast majority of lung cancers are of the type called non-small cell lung cancer (NSCLC), all of which are carcinomas and include squamous cell carcinoma, adenocarcinoma, or large cell undifferentiated carcinoma. NSCLC is staged as stage 0 (tumor in situ); stage IA or IB (≤ or > 3 cm in size with no peripheral lymph node or metastatic involvement); stages IIA or IIB with some combination of peripheral lymph node involvement or larger size; stages IIIA or IIIB, where there is also lymph node involvement but the main distinction is the location of tumor and lymph node invasion; or stage IV, which indicates distant metastases. Patients have chronic cough, shortness of breath, adventitious breath sounds, and coughing up of blood. Those with stage IA, IB, IIA, or IIB NSCLC are generally managed surgically with lung pneumonectomy, lobotomy, or a wedge resection; tracheal repair; sleeve resection of the bronchus; a rib resection; and/or a pleurectomy. Post-operative complications can be averted with deep-breathing exercises, mucus-clearance, incisional splinting, and upper-extremity range of motion. More advanced NSCLC is basically untreatable surgically. About 15% of lung cancer patients have another type called small-cell lung cancer (SCLC).

Musculoskeletal Cancers

Musculoskeletal, or bone, cancers are often metastases originating in other primary tumor sites. The major symptoms are site pain and often fracture. There are quite a few types of possible benign and malignant primary tumors in bones as well. Malignant varieties include myeloma, malignant lymphoma, several types of chondrosarcoma that affect the cartilage, fibrosarcoma in the fibrous tissues, osteosarcoma of the bone itself, and others. Surgical options consist of insertion of rods, plates, or prosthetic devices to shore up the affected bones. It is important for the physical therapist to clarify the patient's weight-bearing condition and obtain physician approval before initiating mobility exercises; measures should be taken to prevent falls.

Breast Cancer Staging

Breast carcinoma is staged from stage 0 to stage 4:

- Stage 0 is carcinoma in situ, either lobular or ductal.
- Stage I is invasive breast cancer that is ≤ 2 cm in diameter with no or extremely minimal lymph node involvement.
- In stage II breast cancer, either the primary site is ≤ 5 cm with up to three axillary lymph nodes affected or it is larger with no lymph node involvement.
- There are several scenarios that are classified as stage III: more axillary node involvement, larger size in association with axillary spread, involvement of the ipsilateral internal mammary lymph nodes, or some skin or chest wall association.
- Distant metastases are the distinguishing feature for stage IV breast carcinoma; typical metastatic sites include the lungs, bones, brain, liver, or adrenal glands.

Surgical Options for Breast Cancer

There are several types of mastectomy (breast removal) or less invasive procedures performed for breast cancer:

- A radical mastectomy is the most invasive, involving removal of the breast tissue, skin, pectoralis major and minor, ribs, and associated lymph nodes.
- A modified radical mastectomy only removes the breast, skin, and a sampling of the axillary lymph nodes.
- In a simple or total mastectomy, the breast removal and lymph node sampling are done at different times.
- In a partial mastectomy, only the tumor itself and a wedge of adjacent tissue are cut out.
- The least invasive surgical technique is a lumpectomy, also known as a local wide excision, in which the malignancy itself is excised and the axillary lymph nodes are resected separately.
- In addition, most breast cancer patients later undergo reconstructive surgery to make a more natural-appearing breast. These procedures include surgical insertion of saline implants and muscle flap transfer reconstruction, which uses muscle and skin from the stomach or back.

Surgical Interventions for Gastrointestinal Cancers

Colorectal cancer is the most prevalent of gastrointestinal malignancies. Others consist of esophageal, stomach, liver, and pancreatic cancer. Surgical interventions for colorectal cancer include abdominal perineal resection, in which the lower two-thirds of the rectum are removed; anterior or low-anterior resection, which excises the upper third of the rectum; hemicolectomy, which cuts out part of the colon; and gastroduodenostomy and gastrojejunostomy, which remove a portion of the stomach plus the duodenum or jejunum, respectively. GI surgeries, in which some or part of the stomach is removed, are termed gastrectomies. Surgical interventions involving the hepatobiliary system include the Whipple procedure for pancreatic cancer, in which the duodenum and proximal pancreas are excised; and liver resection for liver cancer, with options including segmental resection or subsegmental (partial) resection. Hepatic cancers are often metastases from other areas, not primary. Pancreatic tumors are generally aggressive and are also often treated with adjunct chemotherapy and radiation.

Surgical Interventions for Genitourinary System Cancers

Genitourinary system cancers are those affecting the reproductive and ancillary organs. They are usually managed by excision of the entire, or sometimes part, of the affected organ:

- Cancer of the uterus is addressed with a hysterectomy, which involves removal of the uterus through the abdominal wall or vagina. In a total abdominal hysterectomy, the body of the uterus and the cervix are excised, whereas a subtotal abdominal hysterectomy leaves the cervix intact.
- There are several surgical options for ovarian cancer, including oophorectomy, or excision of one ovary; and bilateral salpingo-oophorectomy, in which both ovaries and the oviducts are removed.
- Prostate cancer surgery is generally radical prostatectomy, the excision of the entire prostate.
- Testicular cancer is addressed with orchiectomy, removal of one or both testes.
- Colorectal cancer is generally considered a gastrointestinal cancer.
- Anal cancer is rare.

Leukemia

Leukemia is one category of hematologic cancers in which the malignant cells are white blood cells (WBCs). These WBCs displace normal cells in the bone marrow and eventually enter the bloodstream, potentially leading to anemia, thrombocytopenia, leukopenia, infections, bruising, and weakness. Leukemias are defined in terms of the maturity of the malignant cell and the WBC type involved:

- Acute leukemias involve relatively immature WBCs, evolve rapidly, and are generally found at younger ages. Examples include acute lymphocytic leukemia, affecting lymphocytes and generally occurring between ages 3 and 7; and acute nonlymphocytic leukemia, involving precursor stem cells, which usually manifests later between ages 15 and 40.
- Chronic leukemias involve more mature WBCs, evolve more slowly, and generally occur later in life. Examples include chronic myelogenous leukemia, in which granulocytes are implicated, and chronic lymphocytic leukemia; the general age ranges for these two types are 25 to 60 years old and over 50 years of age, respectively.

Leukemias are managed with radiation, chemotherapy, hormone therapy, and/or bone marrow transplantation.

Review Video: Leukemia
Visit mometrix.com/academy and enter code: 940024

Lymphoma

Lymphoma is a hematologic cancer in which malignant lymphocytic cells dwell in lymph tissue, either lymph nodes or the spleen. This causes the lymph nodes to enlarge. Blood vessels and organs eventually are permeated with these malignant cells, potentially causing a variety of undesirable and possibly lethal effects, such as blood vessel occlusion, infarction, a variety of nerve disorders, joint hemorrhage and rheumatism, and infection. The most widespread lymphoma is Hodgkin's lymphoma, which is typically confined to a single node and spreads in a methodical fashion. Non-Hodgkin's lymphoma generally involves more than one nodal region, often with extranodal involvement and erratic proliferation. Lymphomas are staged a bit differently than most other cancers, with stage I being single nodal or organ involvement; stage II involving two or more lymph node sites on the same side of the diaphragm or some bordering extralymphatic organ;

stage III, where nodal areas on both sides of the diaphragm and/or some contiguous extralymphatic organs are affected; and stage IV, in which there is dispersed organ involvement. Treatments for lymphoma include radiation and/or chemotherapy.

Review Video: Lymphoma
Visit mometrix.com/academy and enter code: 513277

Multiple Myeloma

Multiple myeloma is a type of hematologic cancer in which malignant plasma cells manufacture only monospecific antibodies, making the blood very viscous. Multiple myeloma is considered a bone marrow cancer because plasma cells are B-cell-derived lymphocytes that produce antibodies and the abnormality initially occurs in the bone marrow, spreading to other organs in due course. Findings include depressed numbers of all normal hematologic cells, bone pain, and, in later stages, often fractures, renal stones, renal failure, and/or amyloidosis. There is a unique staging system based primarily on serum beta-2-microglobulin levels, which become higher as the disease progresses and median survival time decreases:

- Stage I is defined as serum beta-2-microglobulin < 3.5 mg/L, plus serum albumin ≥ 3.5 g/dl.
- Stage II is either a similar beta-2-microglobulin concentration with serum albumin < 3.5 g/dl or a serum beta-2-microglobulin in the range of 3.5 to less than 5.5 mg/L.
- Stage III is defined as serum beta-2-microglobulin ≥ 5.5 mg/L. By stage III, the median survival time is only 29 months.

Multiple myeloma cannot be cured, but it is managed with radiation, chemotherapy, biotherapy, and/or bone marrow transplantation. The therapist should consult the doctor before doing mobilization exercises.

Skin Cancer

Skin cancer is suspected when a person has skin lesions that are irregularly shaped, variably colored, nodular or ulcerative, bleeding or crusting, and/or have undergone changes in size, thickness, or color. Skin cancers are designated in terms of cell type involved. The most dangerous is malignant melanoma, which originates in the pigment-producing melanocytes and can spread to lymph nodes, the brain, bones, and other areas. It is defined similar to the above by the ABCD rule (A = asymmetry, B = irregular border, C = varied color, D = diameter > 6 mm). The most widespread skin cancer is basal cell carcinoma. generally found in sun-exposed areas. Lesions that are bleeding or crusting, elevated with central indentation, nodular, or have poorly defined borders can all be basal cell carcinoma. It is diagnosed with laboratory examination of a biopsy and is usually excised without further problems. Squamous cell cancer is also usually found in radiation-exposed areas. Here, lesions are generally elevated and crusty or keratotic, and metastasis is possible. Kaposi's sarcoma, a connective tissue cancer with reddish-purple skin patches, is also considered a skin cancer. Physical therapy considerations include proper positioning and use of range-of-motion exercises to avoid contractures.

Brain and Other Neurologic Cancers

Brain tumors can be primary or secondary as a result of metastases. Brain tumors are classified as glioma (from connective glial tissue), neuronal (from nerve cells), meningioma (affecting the protective meninges), or poorly differentiated neoplasms. Central nervous system tumors, including brain tumors, compress nerve tissues and can cause neurologic changes regardless of whether they are benign or malignant. These changes often continue even after tumor removal if nerve tissue has been damaged. Potential effects include cognitive losses, inability to control bladder and bowel functions, sexual problems, skin changes, hemiplegia, and lack of muscle control. Patients often require assistive devices, skin care, splinting, positioning, help performing daily activities, and training to improve cognition, gait, and balance.

Interventions/ Equipment & Devices; Therapeutic Modalities

Cardiac, Vascular, and Pulmonary Systems

Surgical Thoracic Procedures

Respiratory abnormalities are often addressed with one of the following surgical thoracic procedures:

- Pneumonectomy: removal of a whole lung with or without resection of mediastinal lymph nodes
- Lobotomy: resection of one or more lung lobes
- Segmentectomy: excision of a section of a lung
- Wedge resection: excision of a small wedge-shaped section of lung tissue regardless of segment divisions
- Bronchoplasty (sleeve resection): partial surgical removal and reanastomosis (reconnection) of a bronchus
- Laryngectomy: partial or complete excision of one or more vocal cords
- Tracheostomy: surgical procedure in the trachea to create a stoma or surgical opening for a tracheostomy tube
- Tracheal resection and reconstruction: partial surgical removal and reanastomosis of the trachea and/or main stem bronchi
- Lung volume resection: removal of portions of emphysematous lung tissue
- Rib resection: removal of part of one or more ribs

Non-Surgical Thoracic Procedures

Respiratory abnormalities are often addressed with one of the following non-surgical thoracic procedures:

- Laryngoscopy: the use of a fiberoptic scope to visualize the larynx
- Mediastinoscopy: the use of an endoscope to visualize the mediastinum
- Pleurodesis: the obliteration of the pleural space by introduction of a chemical agent into it using a thoracoscope (endoscope) or a thoracostomy (incision and chest tube)
- Thoracentesis: the removal of pleural fluid using percutaneous needle aspiration
- Thoracoscopy: video-assisted examination of the pleura or lung tissue through the chest wall with an endoscope called a thoracoscope

Cardiac Catheterization

Cardiac catheterization is an invasive process in which a flexible radiopaque catheter is delivered into the heart for visualization of the anatomy. The procedure is used in conjunction with angiography, percutaneous transluminal coronary angioplasty (PTCA), cardiac muscles biopsies, and electrophysiologic studies (EPSs). During angiography, a radiopaque contrast substance is injected via catheter to look at blood vessels or chambers. Various types include aortography of the aorta and its valve, coronary arteriography of the coronary arteries, ventriculography of either ventricle and the AV valves, and pulmonary angiography. EPSs involve insertion of an electrode catheter via the femoral vein into the right ventricle to look at electrical conduction in the heart.

Cardiac catheters can be right-sided or left-sided and are typically inserted into the subclavian vein or femoral artery, respectively. The side for insertion is selected depending on the suspected cardiac issues on that side. A common use of right-sided catheterization is to monitor cardiac pressures in patients with heart failure. Patients that have undergone cardiac catheterization must remain on bed rest from four to six hours with the selected extremity immobilized.

Thrombolytic Therapy

Thrombolytic therapy is the intravenous use of thrombolytic agents during an acute myocardial infarction (MI). The basis of this therapy is that most individuals experiencing a MI have coronary artery thrombosis or blood clots. The therapy should be given within six hours (some say 24 hours), unless the patient is at risk for excessive bleeding. The therapeutic agents administered fall into two classes. Fibrin-selective agents like tissue plasminogen activator (t-PA) quickly lyse clots, while non-selective ones like streptokinase and anisoylated plasminogen streptokinase activator complex act more slowly but are retained systemically longer.

Percutaneous Revascularization

There are several types of percutaneous revascularization procedures, all of which are designed to reestablish blood flow in occluded coronary arteries. The procedures include:

- Percutaneous transluminal coronary angioplasty (PTCA): involves insertion of a balloon system at the lesion site in the coronary artery via a catheter guided within a sheath inserted into the femoral, radial, or brachial artery; the balloon is inflated to reduce the lesion; often used in conjunction with endoluminal stents
- Endoluminal stents: tubes placed within the coronary artery to increase the intraluminal diameter
- Directional coronary atherectomy: insertion of a catheter featuring a cutter (or laser) and balloon on either end; the balloon is inflated so that it presses the cutter or laser against the atheroma (plaque), which is cut out through rotational ablation (cutter) or removed via laser
- Coronary laser angioplasty: use of laser energy to remove plaques

Coronary Artery Bypass Grafts

Coronary artery bypass grafts and transmyocardial revascularization are two methods of revascularization of the myocardium in patients with cardiac disease. A coronary artery bypass graft (CABG) is indicated when there is complete blockage of the coronary artery or if percutaneous revascularization procedures are ineffective. The incisions are either minimally invasive or performed through a median sternotomy, and the blood vessels commonly used for the vascular graft are the saphenous vein or the left internal mammary artery (LIMA). Patients who have had a CABG with median sternotomy should keep upper-extremity use to a minimum for about two months afterwards.

Transmyocardial Revascularization

The other technique, transmyocardial revascularization, is indicated for patients who cannot endure CABG or angioplasty. It employs a catheter with a laser tip to construct channels from unblocked coronary arteries into a region of the myocardium where there is blockage.

Myocardial Revascularization

The types of secondary procedures typically performed after myocardial revascularization include:

- Ablation procedures: the use of a catheter to reach and remove ectopic foci using low-power, high-frequency alternating current, possibly in conjunction with surgical ablation (the latter mostly for atrial fibrillation)
- Implantation of a cardiac pacemaker or automatic implantable cardiac defibrillator: the implantation on the myocardium of a unipolar or bipolar electrode to generate an action potential that controls arrhythmias (discussed further on another card)
- Valve replacement: replacement in patients with valvular disease of the defective valve with a mechanical (more durable and long-lasting but often thrombogenic) or biologic one (from a cadaver or animal tissue); typically involves median sternotomy for access
- Cardiac transplantation: a procedure generally performed only on patients with end-stage cardiac disease
- Cardiac medications: the use of drugs that fall into a number of categories, such as antiarrhythmic agents, anticoagulants, antihypertensives, fibrinolytics, and others

Cardiac Pacemaker or Automatic Implantable Cardiac Defibrillator

Both cardiac pacemakers and automatic implantable cardiac defibrillators (AICDs) are used to manage arrhythmias. Pacemakers use unipolar or bipolar electrodes on the myocardium to generate an action potential. They are utilized in patients with sinus node disorders, atrioventricular disorders, tachyarrhythmias, or when improved atrioventricular and/or biventricular synchrony is needed. Pacemakers are classified according to whether or not certain chambers are paced, sensed and triggered, or inhibited if sensed; whether or not there is rate modulation; and the location of multisite pacing.

Rate modulation, the capacity to modulate heart rate based on activity levels or physiologic needs, is an important concept for physical therapists. If there is no rate modulation, only low-level activity with small incremental changes should be performed; if there is rate modulation, then blood pressure must be watched when the patient's heart rate is near the upper limit of rate modulation.

An AICD is indicated for management of critical, uncontrollable ventricular arrhythmias, such as tachycardia or fibrillation. AICDs work by discerning the heart rhythm and then defibrillating the myocardium to establish normal rhythm.

Cardiac Catheterization

Cardiac catheterization is an invasive process in which a flexible radiopaque catheter is delivered into the heart for visualization of the anatomy. The procedure is used in conjunction with angiography, percutaneous transluminal coronary angioplasty (PTCA), cardiac muscles biopsies, and electrophysiologic studies (EPSs). During angiography, a radiopaque contrast substance is injected via catheter to look at blood vessels or chambers. Various types include aortography of the aorta and its valve, coronary arteriography of the coronary arteries, ventriculography of either ventricle and the AV valves, and pulmonary angiography. EPSs involve insertion of an electrode catheter via the femoral vein into the right ventricle to look at electrical conduction in the heart. Cardiac catheters can be right-sided or left-sided and are typically inserted into the subclavian vein or femoral artery, respectively. The side for insertion is selected depending on the suspected cardiac issues on that side. A common use of right-sided catheterization is to monitor cardiac pressures in patients with heart failure. Patients that have undergone cardiac catheterization must remain on bed rest from four to six hours with the selected extremity immobilized.

Respiratory Dysfunction

If, upon inspection, the clinician finds a patient has dyspnea, tachypnea, an asymmetric respiratory pattern, or posture issues, a number of physical therapy interventions are suggested. These include repositioning of the patient, postural exercises, relaxation techniques, energy-conservation maneuvers, trunk and shoulder stretching, incentive spirometry, and supplemental oxygen. Findings on palpation of asymmetric respiration or palpable fremitus due to pulmonary secretions suggest a range of possible interventions, including coughing maneuvers, upper-extremity and diaphragmatic exercises, postural drainage, manual techniques, functional activity, incentive spirometry, and perhaps a flutter valve. The same type of measures are indicated if there is increased dullness on percussion or decreased or unusually-positioned breath sounds on auscultation, both of which indicate retained pulmonary secretions. If the patient has an ineffective cough, possible interventions include repositioning, huffing, and coughing techniques; functional activity; a tracheal tickle (external stimulation); suctioning; bronchodilator use; and possibly incisional splinting.

Vascular Surgery

Incisions made during vascular surgery should be examined before initiating physical therapy as they can drain or weep during activity, necessitating compression and/or stabilization by the nurse. As pulmonary infections are common in patients with abdominal and other painful incisions, the therapist should use techniques to prevent these infections, such as assisted coughing and manual procedures. Vital signs must be monitored prior to, during, and after activity as post-operative systolic blood pressures generally need to be maintained within a range that does not reduce perfusion (BP too low) or damage the graft (BP too high). Diminished distal peripheral pulses are problematic and should be reported to the nurse and doctor. The physical therapist should take direction from the physician in terms of the extent of weight bearing allowed on the affected extremity. Grafting done in the hip joint area may restrict hip flexion.

Vascular and Hematologic Disorders

The physical therapist's role is optimization of functional mobility and activity tolerance within the context of the patient's disease-related limitations. Patients with peripheral vascular disease usually have other issues, such as coronary artery disease, diabetes, chronic obstructive lung disease, impaired sensation, renal insufficiency or failure, heart failure, venous insufficiency, liver disease, aortic dissection, and others. The therapist must be familiar with each of these conditions and how they might impact therapy. At rest and during interventions, vital signs (blood pressure, heart rate, oxygen saturation, respiratory rate) must be constantly monitored, and blood work, particularly CBCs and coagulation profiles, should be performed daily. The laboratory data should be taken into account as physical therapy may need to be deferred or modified. If values indicate risk of bleeding (low platelets, high INR) in a patient with a hematologic disorder, allowable activity levels are related to fall and hemorrhage prevention. Similarly, for patients with vascular diseases, edema management (for example, through compression) and measures to deter thrombus formation are the most important considerations.

Musculoskeletal System

Range-of-Motion Exercises

Range of motion (ROM) is the amount of allowable angular motion at a joint between two bones acting as levers. It is correlated to the functional excursion, the distance the attached muscle can shorten to after maximal stretching. ROM exercises are used therapeutically to maintain joint and soft-tissue mobility. There are three basic types of ROM exercises.

- Passive ROM (PROM) is movement produced entirely by an external force, such as the therapist, with no voluntary muscle contraction involved. PROM is appropriate in areas where there is acute inflammation or in patients that should not move parts of their body, such as those on bed rest, paralyzed, or in a coma.
- Active ROM (AROM) is movement produced by active contraction of the muscles crossing the indicated joint. AROM exercises are indicated for patients able to contract the needed muscles, for aerobic conditioning, and in areas distal to an area immobilized by fracture, etc.
- Active-assisted ROM (A-AROM) is a variation of AROM in which the involved muscles are aided by an additional manual or mechanical outside force. A-AROM is useful in patients with weak musculature.

Other types of ROM exercise are self-assisted ROM and continuous passive motion (CPM), the continuous use of a mechanical device.

Contracture

A contracture is adaptive shortening or hypomobility of the skin, fascia, muscle, or joint capsule, resulting in decreased mobility or flexibility of the structure. Contractures are usually described in terms of the affected shortened muscle, for example, shortening of the elbow flexor, which would be an elbow flexion contracture. They are also often identified in terms of the pathology, as either myostatic (no specific muscle pathology), pseudomyostatic (due to spasticity or rigidity associated with nervous system disorders), arthrogenic (intraarticular pathology), periarticular (involving associated connective tissues), fibrotic (due to fibrotic changes in connective tissue), and irreversible (usually stemming from fibrotic types).

Stretching

Stretching is any type of therapeutic exercise that elongates pathologically shortened soft-tissue structures. The goal is to increase range of motion (ROM). Stretching is indicated anytime ROM is limited due to contractures, adhesions, or scar tissues; in patients with muscle weakness and shortening of opposing tissue; in cases where restricted motion can result in deformities; as part of a fitness program; and before and after exercise to lessen soreness. Stretching is contraindicated with recent fractures, tissue trauma, joint hypermobility, etc. Modes of stretching include:

- Passive: stretching of soft tissue with force applied opposite to direction of muscle shortening
- Cyclic: repeated passive stretch, generally using a mechanical device
- Self-stretching: passive stretching of a joint or soft tissue utilizing another body part to apply force
- Selective: stretching of only certain muscle groups, allowing others to adaptively shorten for functional improvement
- Static: elongation of soft tissues just past the point of resistance and holding
- Ballistic: high-speed and high-intensity intermittent stretch
- Manual: force applied by someone else just past resistance
- Mechanical: use of equipment to produce stretch
- Active: part of functional movements
- Proprioceptive neuromuscular facilitation techniques: discussed elsewhere

Effective Stretching Intervention Terms

Effective stretching interventions incorporate appropriate use of:

- Alignment: the positioning of a limb or the body in a way that allows the stretch force to target the appropriate muscle group
- Stabilization: securing of one site of attachment of the muscle while force is applied to the other bony attachment
- Intensity of stretch: magnitude of stretch force applied
- Duration of stretch: period of time the stretch force is applied during the cycle
- Speed of stretch: how fast the initial stretch force is applied
- Frequency of stretch: number of stretching periods in a day or week
- Mode of stretch: the manner in which the force is applied, the amount of patient involvement, or the source of the stretch

Joint Mobilization

Joint mobilization is the use of manual techniques to control pain and treat joint dysfunctions that reduce range of motion. It addresses specific joint configurations. Joint-play techniques are utilized to reduce pain, muscle guarding, and spasm; reverse joint hypomobility; correct malpositioning or subluxation; treat progressive diseases; and prevent the potential effects of immobility. Prior to use of passive joint mobilization, the patient is examined and evaluated for quality of pain, capsular restriction, and the presence of subluxation or dislocation. There are two possible schemes for grading dosages: graded oscillation techniques and sustained translatory joint-play techniques (detailed elsewhere). The treatment force is applied close to the opposing joint surface either parallel or perpendicular to the treatment plane, such that the entire bone moves and one joint surface glides over the other.

Passive Joint Mobilization Grading

There are two possible grading systems applied in passive joint mobilization techniques:

- Graded oscillation techniques:
  - Grade I: small rhythmic oscillations at the low end of the available joint play range
  - Grade II: large rhythmic oscillations in the available joint play range, not reaching the limit
  - Grade III: large rhythmic oscillations performed up to the limit of available joint play and then past it into tissue resistance
  - Grade IV: small rhythmic oscillations near the limit of available motion stressed into the tissue resistance range
  - Grade V: small-amplitude, high-velocity thrusting method at limit of available motion
- Sustained translatory joint play techniques:
  - Grade I (loosening): small amplitude distraction not involving capsular stress
  - Grade II (tightening): application of sufficient distraction or glide to tighten surrounding tissues, involves entire range of available joint play
  - Grade III (stretching): larger distraction or glide past tissue resistance, placing stretch on joint capsule and adjacent structures

Resistance Exercise

The types of resistance exercise are defined in terms of the form of resistance. Broadly speaking, all resistance exercises can be categorized as either manual, meaning the resistance is applied by another person or the individual, or mechanical, involving use of some type of equipment.

Resistance exercises can also be differentiated as static, dynamic, isokinetic, or open- or closed-chain. Isometric exercise, in which muscles are under tension and contract but do not change length (such as pushing against a resistance), is a static form of exercise. Dynamic forms of resistance exercise include concentric, in which the muscle shortens while overcoming a load (such as lifting a hand weight), and eccentric, in which less force is used and the muscle fibers lengthen (such as lowering the weight). Isokinetic exercise is also dynamic exercise in which the velocity of limb movement is held constant with a dynamometer but the force is varied. Open- versus closed-chain exercise refers, respectively, to whether the movement is unrestricted or the peripheral segment is restricted with a fixed external resistance.

Aquatic Exercise

Aquatic exercise is performance of exercises while immersed in a pool or tank of water. Water has buoyancy (an upward force, causing flotation), hydrostatic pressure exerted on immersed objects, viscosity (friction between water molecules), and surface tension. All of these properties make it ideal for performing activities in an environment that is relatively weightless and relaxing, does not put much pressure on joints, acts as a resistance, and keeps certain cardiac parameters in check. Aquatic exercises are means of doing range-of-motion, resistance, weight-bearing, cardiovascular, and functional activity replication exercises. One of the basic principles of aquatic exercise is that fluid in motion adheres to hydromechanics, meaning that slow movement produces parallel or laminar flow, faster movement produces turbulent or non-parallel flow, and turbulence and viscosity together produce drag and increased resistance. Another consideration is thermodynamics, the conversion between forms of energy and the effects of parameters, such as temperature, pressure, and work; for example, with immersion, individuals dissipate less heat. Moreover, the person is governed by a center of buoyancy (at the sternum when vertical) instead of a center of gravity.

Acetabular Fracture

Appropriate physical therapy for stable fractures is touch-down or partial weight bearing, gentle range of motion (ROM), positioning, breathing exercises, and uninvolved breathing exercises if on bed rest. For unstable fractures, partial or as tolerated weight bearing and gentle hip ROM are indicated.

Hip Dislocation

For patients with hip displacements without fracture, appropriate physical therapy interventions are partial or as tolerated weight-bearing mobility and, depending on the doctor's instructions, positioning and certain exercises.

Intracapsular Femoral Head and Neck Fractures

Suggested physical therapy for type I is partial (PWB) or non-weight bearing mobility, active/active-assisted ROM, and lower extremity; similar interventions are used for types II, III, and IV, except for mobility, which should be PWB or as tolerated (for type IV).

Extracapsular Femoral Head and Neck Fractures

The appropriate physical therapy interventions for intertochanteric Evans type I and subtrochanteric Russell-Taylor types IA, IB, or IIA are all similar. They include partial weight bearing for functional mobility, gentle hip range-of-motion (ROM) exercises, and distal lower-extremity strengthening exercises. Comparable ROM and distal lower-extremity exercises can be used for the other types of extracapsular fractures, but weight bearing needs to be more restricted. Touch-down weight bearing (TDWB) is suggested for intertochanteric Evans type II fractures, and non-weight bearing or TDWB exercises for functional mobility are the only ones that should be used for patients with subtrochanteric Russell-Taylor type IIB fractures.

For simple or nondisplaced closed fractures, the suggested physical therapy approach is non-, touch-down, or as tolerated weight bearing for functional mobility, and gentle range-of-motion (ROM) exercises. For the other two types, physical therapy should be limited to non- or touch-down weight bearing, and other interventions should include lower-extremity ROM exercises as directed by the physician, and positioning, breathing exercises, and unaffected-extremity exercises if on bed rest. Single crutches are often used for transfer.

Distal Femoral Fractures

For supracondylar distal femur fractions that are simple or nondisplaced, the appropriate physical therapy interventions are non-weight bearing mobility and distal and proximal active/active-assisted range-of-motion (A/AAROM) exercises. If the supracondylar fracture is displaced or comminuted, the management is different (as described elsewhere) and the patient is often on bed rest. This means positioning, breathing exercises, and unaffected-extremity exercises are indicated, as well as distal and proximal A/AAROM; the type of functional mobility should be partial weight bearing. For nondisplaced unicondylar fractures, physical therapy should include non- or touch-down weight bearing and distal and proximal A/AAROM. Patients with unicondylar fractures with displacement should do touch-down weight bearing, gentle ROM exercise, and continuous passive motion as medically directed. Appropriate physical therapy for patients with intercondylar fractures is touch-down or light partial weight bearing, anything that will maintain functional ROM in the hip and ankle and, eventually, gentle ROM and exercises for the quadriceps.

Patellar Fractures

Appropriate physical therapy interventions for both are partial or as tolerated weight bearing, making sure the fracture is not stressed and, for the displaced type, eventual active-assisted range of motion exercises as directed. Comminuted patellar fractures are managed with ORIF, a partial or total patellectomy with quadriceps tendon repair, or immobilization using a long leg cast or brace or a posterior splint with the knee in full extension or minimal flexion. Functional mobility should be limited to non-, partial, or as tolerated weight bearing, and strong quadriceps contractions should be avoided.

Tibial Plateau Fractures

For a non-displaced fracture suggested physical therapy includes touch-down or partial weight bearing and active-assisted range-of-motion (ROM) and/or continuous passive motion. For displaced fractures involving a single condyle or split compression, physical therapy is the same as for nondisplaced fractures described above. For displaced fractures that are impacted or significantly comminuted involving both condyles, only non-, touch-down, or partial weight bearing should be done along with positioning, breathing and uninvolved-extremity exercises (if on bed rest), and, eventually, knee A/AAROM.

Tibial Shaft and Fibula Fractures

Appropriate physical therapy interventions for minimally displaced closed fractures are touch-down, partial, or as tolerated weight bearing, quadriceps strengthening, and edema control. With moderate displacement, only non- or touch-down weight bearing should be done, along with knee range-of-motion (ROM) exercises, quadriceps strengthening, and edema management. Severely displaced or comminuted closed or open fractures should be addressed with ankle and possibly knee ROM exercises, quadriceps strengthening, and edema control.

Distal Tibial Fractures

The appropriate physical therapy interventions for patients with minimally or moderately displaced distal tibial fractures are non-weight bearing functional mobility, knee range of motion (ROM) exercises, strengthening of the proximal joint, and edema control. For those with severely displaced closed fractures, lower-extremity isometrics and neutral ankle positioning should be done instead of knee ROM. For open fractures, ankle ROM exercises and neutral ankle positioning are substituted.

Ankle Fractures

For closed, nondisplaced fractures appropriate physical therapy is non- or partial weight bearing functional mobility, exercises to strengthen the proximal lower extremity, and edema management.

For closed fractures that are displaced, or open ankle fractures, the suggested physical therapy regimen is non-weight bearing mobility; proximal lower-extremity strengthening; foot and ankle exercises, as prescribed by the physician; and edema control.

Calcaneal Fractures

The suggested physical therapy regimen for patients with any of these calcaneal fractures is non-weight bearing functional mobility; strengthening and range of motion exercises for the proximal lower extremity; ankle and forefoot exercises, as prescribed by the doctor; and edema management.

Forefoot Fractures

The suggested physical therapy interventions are the same for any of these types, namely proximal lower-extremity strengthening and range of motion, edema management, and, depending on the location and severity of the fracture, non-, partial, or as tolerated weight bearing mobility.

Cervical Spine Fractures

Patients with stable vertebral body fractures, or isolated spinous process (laminal) fractures, require only functional mobility, posture training, and body mechanics. Those with Hangman's (bilateral pedicle) fractures or odontoid process cervical spine fractures, which are more serious, should be approached differently. For these patients, the appropriate physical therapy interventions include posture and body mechanics training; therapeutic and active assisted/passive range-of-motion exercises, tailored to the neurologic injury; balance and scapular exercises, if they wear a halo vest; and functional mobility with logroll precautions. Logroll precautions mean turning the patient in bed so that the head and torso are a unit.

Thoracolumbar Spine Fractures

Regardless of type, the appropriate physical therapy interventions are functional mobility with logroll precautions, postural and body mechanic training, and therapeutic exercise and active-assisted passive range of motion as indicated by the neurologic injury.

Proximal Humeral Fractures

Suggested physical therapy for any of these types of fractures is non-weight bearing functional mobility, pendulum exercises and passive range of motion (ROM) as prescribed, edema control, and ROM exercises for the elbow, wrist, and hand.

Humeral Shaft Fractures

Regardless of type, the appropriate physical therapy interventions include non-weight bearing functional mobility, isometric scapulothoracic exercises, wrist and hand exercises, edema control, and shoulder and elbow active/active-assisted range of motion drills as prescribed by the doctor based on the type of immobilization.

Distal Humeral & Olecranon Fractures

The appropriate physical therapy regimen for any olecranon fracture is non-weight bearing functional mobility, distal and proximal joint active ROM, edema management, and elbow active-assisted ROM that is not painful, per physician order.

Radial Head Fractures

The appropriate physical therapy regimen for any radial head fracture is non-weight bearing functional mobility, distal and proximal joint active ROM, edema management, and elbow active-assisted ROM that is not painful, per physician order.

Forearm Fractures

Suggested physical therapy for all of these forearm fractures includes non-weight bearing functional mobility, distal and proximal range-of-motion exercises, and edema control. In addition, intraarticular radius fractures (including comminuted ones) indicate use of active and passive movements if the patient has external fixation.

Hip Arthroplasty

The main concern of the therapist is to help the patient attain safe functional mobility in areas such as bed mobility, transfers, and walking with assistive devices. The patient should lie flat part of the time to stretch the anterior hip muscles. To facilitate transfers, the bed height may need to be raised and elevated and seating surfaces, such hip and commode chairs, may need to be used. The patient will probably need to wear a shoe on the uninvolved side at first to accommodate for a phenomenon known as "apparent leg length discrepancy" resulting from the inserted hardware. Physical therapy should include passive and active-assisted range of motion, which may require an overhead frame with sling. In order to restore control of the quadriceps and peroneal muscles, reduce muscle spasms, and protect the associated femoral and sciatic nerves, a knee immobilizer and/or ankle-foot orthosis may be needed and isometric exercises for these muscles should be instituted after surgery. Eventually, active-assisted exercises for these muscles are indicated as tolerated. Another area of concern is prevention of DVT and edema, which should be addressed with ankle-pumping exercises, compression stockings or devices, and repetitive sets of quadriceps and gluteus exercises.

Joint Resurfacing

The physical therapy regimen for patients with joint resurfacing is in many respects similar to that for THA, namely emphasis on bed mobility, transfers, hip range of motion (ROM), quadriceps strengthening, and gait training. These patients can only tolerate partial weight bearing for the first four to six weeks. They should avoid bending beyond 90 degrees at the hip, crossing legs, twisting during exercise, or doing anything else restricted by the doctor. Many patients who have joint resurfacing eventually need a THA.

Knee Arthroplasty

Immediately post-operatively, physical therapy should be initiated in patients who have undergone knee arthroplasty. The therapy regimen should emphasize bed mobility, positioning, edema control, transfer techniques, gait training with appropriate assistive devices, strengthening of the quadriceps with active-assisted exercises, passive or active-assisted range of motion (ROM), and antiembolic exercises. Antiembolic exercises to promote venous circulation and isometric strengthening should be done in sets of up to 15 repetitions hourly; they should consist of quadriceps and gluteus sets and ankle pumps. The involved limb should be elevated with pillows, towel rolls, or, if possible, without them to encourage knee flexion. A pillow or towel roll should also be put under the knee during isometric exercises. A towel roll or blanket placed along the lateral aspect of the femur is useful for maintaining a neutral position. Active-assisted ROM exercises are best done using hold-and-relax techniques to minimize muscle guarding. Ice is generally applied after exercises to reduce edema.

MIS Hip and Knee Arthroplasties

Physical therapy for MIS arthroplasties should emphasize maximal functional mobility and is fairly similar to that for those treated by less conservative techniques. Weight bearing as tolerated is usually possible directly after surgery. The key to rapid recovery after MIS or any total joint arthroplasty is early introduction of ambulation (as soon as three hours post-operatively) and other exercises, often in conjunction with short-acting spinal analgesics.

Shoulder Arthroplasty

The physical therapy interventions for patients who have undergone shoulder arthroplasty are fairly similar regardless of procedure (total shoulder arthroscopy, humeral hemiarthroplasty, shoulder surface replacement arthroplasty, or reverse total arthroplasty). The patient should be instructed not to put weight on the surgically altered extremity, including rolling onto it or lifting anything heavier than a coffee cup. While lying down, the arm should be kept neutral (using a pillow or towel) and not permitted to extend past midline. If they wear an abduction brace for stability, they should be instructed as to how to take it on and off for exercise or dressing. Sling use should only be temporary. The types of physical therapy exercises to include are pendulum exercises in all four planes of motion; gentle passive or active-assisted range of motion (ROM); forward elevation in the scapular plane as tolerated; limited external rotation; active abduction and flexion per physician order; and hand, wrist, and elbow ROM to control edema. The latter ROM exercises should be done with elevation and ice packs. Patients who have had reverse total arthroscopy should be immobilized in slight abduction and neutral rotation.

Total Elbow Arthroplasty

Appropriate physical therapy includes functional mobility and activities of daily life training; edema management; ROM exercises, as prescribed; and if accessible, continuous passive motion to the elbow.

Total Ankle Arhtroplasty

Appropriate physical therapy is non-weight bearing functional mobility; edema management; and ankle range of motion and hip and knee strengthening, as ordered.

Resection Arthroplasty

Resection arthroplasty and two-stage reimplantation are procedures commonly performed after a joint arthroplasty region has become infected. During the healing period, physical therapy should primarily address functional mobility, safety, use of assistive devices, retention of muscle strength and endurance, positioning to reduce muscle spasms, and edema control with ice and elevation. Patients who originally had a total hip or knee arthroplasty are usually less restricted during the period of prosthesis removal and can do most isometric, active, and active-assisted exercises. For knee resection patients before reimplantation, range-of-motion exercises should be kept to a minimum to preserve integrity of bone surfaces. As these patients are non-weight bearing, gait can be assisted by wearing a shoe on the uninvolved side and a slipper sock on the involved side, unless there is leg-length discrepancy in a hip patient, in which case the foot coverings are reversed.

Total Femur Replacement

Suggested physical therapy includes toe touch or non-weight bearing, bed mobility, gait and balance instruction, crutch or walker training, and strength and endurance exercise, including upper extremities, which will need to be used. For the first two months, therapy exclusions are active and passive abduction and adduction, external and internal hip rotation, straight leg raises, and hip extension beyond neutral. Adduction can be avoided by moving via log-roll technique with a pillow between the legs.

Hip Disarticulation and Hemipelyectomy

Physical therapy should emphasize bed mobility, including learning to sit up; transfer training; gait and balance instruction; crutch or walker training; and functional strength and endurance, including upper extremities, which will need to be used. A good method of transfer is a reclining wheelchair. Patients who have undergone an internal hemipelvectomy can be started on limited weight bearing mobility and joint motion.

Tibial and Trochanteric Osteotomies

For tibial osteotomy, typical post-operative physical therapy includes bed mobility, transfer training, balance and gait instruction, toe-touch weight bearing, active knee range of motion (ROM), and involved extremity strengthening exercises (ankle pumps, quad and gluteus sets). Eventually, the patient should progress to partial weight bearing, then full weight bearing, and additional extremity strengthening exercises, such as active-assisted straight leg raises, hip abduction/adduction, and heel slides.

For trochanteric osteotomy, appropriate physical therapy includes toe-touch weight bearing; gait and transfer training, including use of the assistive device; ROM and modest strengthening of the involved hip; bed mobility; antiembolic exercises (ankle pumps, etc. as above); and global strengthening and endurance, particularly with upper extremities, which will be used.

Spinal Surgery

The main goal of physical therapy for patients who have undergone spinal surgery is ambulation. This means the therapy is generally limited to functional mobilization, gait and body mechanics training, proper use of assistive devices, and relaxation and breathing exercises to manage pain. Precautions for spinal surgery patients who have undergone a decompression procedure alone (such as microdiscectomy) can generally lift up to 10 pounds, but those who have also had a spinal fusion or instrumentation inserted should follow doctor's orders for lifting restrictions and should avoid bending and twisting. Log rolling out of bed is recommended for all. Use of rolling walkers is suggested for correct gait, and most patients wear braces out of bed. Special considerations related to specific procedures include use of a splinting pillow and corset in patients whose surgery was done anteriorly; use of ice at the site of iliac crest bone grafting to minimize swelling; and chair sitting as tolerated, if interbody fusion cages were inserted. Cigarette smoking is contraindicated for spinal fusion patients. Patients who have had minimally invasive spine surgeries should be treated similarly.

Vertebroplasty and Kyphoplasty

The main goals of post-surgical physical therapy for each are functional mobility and ambulation. The patient should also be taught good body mechanics, how to log roll for bed transfers, and, if indicated, extremity active range-of-motion and light strengthening exercises.

Knee Soft-Tissue and Reconstruction Repairs

The suggested physical therapy for meniscal repair, or meniscectomy, is edema control, proximal and distal range-of-motion (ROM) exercises, functional training per prescribed weight-bearing precautions, and quadriceps and hamstring strengthening, if prescribed. Patients who have had meniscal repair may be instructed to wear a brace or have ROM and weight-bearing restrictions. Physical therapy indications for patients who have had a lateral retinacular release are edema management; gentle ROM and functional training, as prescribed; isometric exercises; and straight-leg raises for quadriceps strengthening. Patients who have had reconstructive surgery on their anterior or posterior cruciate ligaments (ACL or PCL, respectively) should receive edema control, active and passive knee ROM, isometric exercises for the quadriceps and hamstrings, straight leg raises for quadriceps strengthening, and functional training per weight-bearing restrictions. They should also be taught brace use. For those who have undergone a quadricepsplasty, therapy recommendations are limited knee flexion using a hinged brace, ROM and continuous passive motion to maximum of 90 degrees, passive knee extension, active/active-assisted exercises for quads and hamstrings, and functional training per weight-bearing precautions.

Shoulder Soft Tissue Repair and Reconstruction

For both of these types of repairs, the suggested physical therapy is use of a sling, edema control, pendulum exercises, active and active-assisted shoulder range of motion (ROM), and ROM for the hand, wrist, and elbow. Depending on the scope of repair, patients who have had rotator cuff repairs may be prescribed self-assisted ROM exercises. The other common shoulder surgery is an anterior reconstruction, also called Bankart repair, which is indicated for persistent anterior instability. It consists of a shift of the anterior capsule and/or repair of the labrum (fibrocartilage). Indicated physical therapy includes sling use, if needed; edema control; limited passive ROM; and ROM for the hand, wrist, and elbow.

Leg or Hip Casts

Casts are rigid dressings that immobilize joints on either side of a fracture to promote bone healing. Casts for immobilizing portions of the leg include a short leg cast (SLC), a long leg cast (LLC), and a patellar tendon-bearing cast:

- A SLC is used for distal tibia or fibular leg fractures and foot and ankle fractures. It covers from the metatarsal heads to the tibial tubercle and immobilizes the foot and ankle at neutral or in minimal dorsiflexion.
- A LLC is used for proximal tibia and distal femur fractures. It extends from the metatarsal heads to either the proximal/mid-femur or greater trochanter, depending on whether the fracture is in the tibia or distal femur; it immobilizes the knee in full extension or at 5-degree flexion. A variation of an LLC is a cylinder cast, which does not include the foot.
- A patellar tendon-bearing cast is used to promote weight bearing. It extends from the metatarsal heads to the mid- or suprapatellar area and uses a patellar tendon bar to transfer loading forces to the cast. The knee is kept at 90-degree flexion, and the ankle is generally neutral.
- A hip spica cast is used for proximal femur and hip joint fractures or dislocation. It starts at the involved-side lower trunk or pelvis and may extend to the thigh, the involved lower extremity, or even the uninvolved thigh.

Upper Body Casts

Common types of upper body casts follow:

- A short arm cast (SAC) is utilized for radius or ulna fractures and covers from the metacarpophalangeal (MCP) joint to the proximal forearm with the wrist immobilized. A SAC permits elbow, finger, and thumb movements.
- A long arm cast (LAC) is used for distal humerus, elbow, or forearm fractures and extends from the MCP joint into the proximal upper arm or into the axilla or shoulder, if limitation of abduction and rotation is desired. The elbow is generally immobilized in 90-degree flexion.
- A thumb spica is employed for fractures of the distal radius, wrist, or thumb. It covers from the tip of the thumb up to some portion of the forearm, immobilizing the wrist in or close to neutral and keeping the thumb under the adjacent two fingers.
- A shoulder spica is used for complex humerus fractures or shoulder dislocation. It is a combination of a LAC and a modified body cast, attached by stabilizing bars but leaving the shoulder area open. This immobilizes the shoulder in the ideal position for reduction.
- A body cast is usually employed for stable spine injuries. It immobilizes the thoracic and lumbar spine and covers from above the nipple line down to the pubis.

Complications from Use of Casts

The major complications associated with cast use are neurologic issues and skin breakdown. Potential neurologic issues include peripheral nerve compression and, sometimes, damage over bony prominences, as well as development of compartment syndrome, which is the compression of nerves, blood vessels, and muscles inside a closed space and which leads to poor oxygenation and tissue death. Signs of compartment syndrome are unmitigated pain, pallor, weakness, diminished peripheral pulses, and thick tissues. There are many causes of skin breakdown, such as pressure, blister formation from moisture within the cast, and/or skin lesions. The therapist needs to watch for and contact the physician or nurse if any of the following types of symptoms develop: anything listed above indicative of compartment syndrome, nerve damage, or skin breakdown; drainage, odor, burning, tingling, or numbness from within the cast; excessive edema; or a discolored or cool hand or foot. Unless the patient has congestive heart failure, elevation of all distal extremities several inches above the heart is suggested for gravity-assisted venous return. The patient should avoid weight bearing as prescribed, keep the cast dry, and do exercises to keep proximal and distal joints functional.

Functional Bracing

Cervical Regions

Common functional bracing for the cervical regions includes cervical collars, halo vests, and the sterno-occipito-mandibular immobilizer (SOMI). Spine/trunk soft cervical collars are foam cylinders used for injuries that do not require rigid fixation, such as whiplash. A reinforced cervical collar is made of padding, with a semirigid plastic frame that encloses the neck and supports the chin and back of the head, and a front opening that can accommodate a tracheotomy tube; it is indicated when neck movement needs to be more restricted. A halo vest is a vest fastened by vertical rods to a circumferential frame and connected to the forehead by percutaneous pins, immobilizing the cervical or high thoracic spine even more. A SOMI consists of a T-shaped yoke worn over the shoulders and secured at midtrunk, a mandibular support attached to it, and an occipital support connected to that with a metal rod. It is used for instability at or above C4 and thoroughly restricts flexion.

Thoracic or Lumbar Regions

Common functional bracing for the thoracic or lumbar regions includes abdominal binders, the Jewitt brace, and molded thoracolumbosacral orthoses (TLSO):

- Abdominal binders are wide elastic bands fastened with Velcro around the abdomen and/or pelvis, providing external abdominal support.
- The Jewitt brace consists of an anterolateral aluminum frame with padding at the sternum and other areas; it is used to restrict flexion and promote hyperextension in patients with compression fractures.
- A TLSO is a customized thermoplastic shell worn to restrict trunk movement in all directions; it is indicated for deformities or fractures of the thoracic or upper lumbar spine.

Lower Extremities

Common functional bracing for the lower extremities includes lower-extremity post-op shoes, ankle stirrups, short leg walking boots, and solid ankle-foot orthoses (AFO):

- A lower-extremity post-op shoe is a type of sandal open at the toe and dorsum of the foot and secured with Velcro; it is useful for patients with edema, bulky dressings, or foot pain.
- An ankle stirrup (Air-cast) is a molded, air-filled shoe insert used for moderate to severe ankle sprains; its main purpose is limitation of inversion or eversion.
- A short-leg walking boot is a manufactured foam-filled plastic shell encircling the foot and lower leg below the knee; it is used for situations like stable leg fractures or a bruised calcareous, where the patient can bear weight but needs intermittent stabilization or cushioning.
- An AFO is a thermoplastic shell worn posteriorly from below the knee to the plantar aspect of the foot and worn inside the shoe; it provides ankle stability, prevents foot drop, and restrains knee hyperextension and flexion.

Knee or Hip

Common functional bracing for the knee includes knee immobilizers and the Bledsoe brace, and for the hip, a hip abduction orthosis:

- A knee immobilizer is a foam cylinder extending from the calf to upper thigh, which is used to encourage knee extension in patients with ligament injuries.
- A drop-lock or Bledsoe brace is used for more severe knee injuries requiring occasional rigid immobilization, such as cruciate ligament repairs or patellar fractures. The brace consists of metal struts at the thigh and lower leg, which are attached to a hinge device at the knee and can be adjusted to a particular degree of extension or flexion.
- A hip abduction orthosis is utilized in patients with conditions where hip flexion and extension must be limited, such as hip revision or dislocation or trauma to the pelvis or spine. It consists of a padded pelvic band, with lateral extensions attached to a thigh cuff that extends across the knee joint, and an adjustable hip joint.

Shoulder or Upper Extremities

Common functional bracing for the shoulder or upper extremities includes simple arm slings, the Rowe sling, and resting hand splints:

- A simple arm sling is a fabric sling with attached neck strap, which is worn with the elbow internally rotated and in about 90-degree flexion; simple arm slings are used for modest support of shoulder or upper-extremity fractures.

- The Rowe sling is similar except that it has an additional strap around the trunk, which restricts shoulder abduction and external rotation, making it more suitable for situations where greater immobilization is sometimes needed, such as after open rotator cuff repair.
- Resting hand splints are utilized to protect or maintain positioning of the wrist and hand, usually in patients with neuromuscular disorders; they are thermoplastic splints positioned on the dorsal side of the hand, wrist, and forearm.

External Fixators

External fixators are external, percutaneously attached metal (aluminum or titanium) devices used to align fracture fragments and promote reduction during healing. They are commonly used for dealing with severely comminuted or open fractures or fracturing with simultaneous tissue damage or infection. Types include pin or ring fixators, in which the frame is rod-shaped or circular. They are used on extremities, as well as the pelvis. Potential complications include infections at the site, compartment syndrome, union deficits, refracture, loss of reduction, and damage to surrounding nerves, blood vessels, or soft tissues. It is important to avoid contact of the external fixator with other objects. Exercises to maintain full range of motion of the proximal and distal joints are essential.

Traction

Traction is the use of some type of device to distract forces on an extremity in order to diminish fracture and muscle spasm or immobilize a joint. There are basically two types of traction: direct, or skeletal traction, in which pins or wires are driven through the bones; and indirect, or skin traction, in which slings, boots, or belts are attached to the skin. Potential complications include hypomobility of the affected joint in conjunction with hypermobility of the joint near the skeletal pin site, muscle atrophy in the extremity, compartment syndrome, infections at pin sites, bone inflammation, skin breakdown or ulcers, and cardiovascular system deficits. Suggested physical therapy for patients in traction is isometric or active exercises with both involved and uninvolved limbs to avert loss of strength, joint stiffness, and agitation. The therapist should check for skin integrity, pain, and positioning. Generally, he should keep anything involved with the traction apparatus or patient positioning intact.

Neuromuscular and Nervous Systems

Parkinson's Disease

Early physical therapy interventions in patients with Parkinson's disease (PD) are imperative to maximize function. The approach is somewhat dependent on the predominant manifestation exhibited: bradykinesia, tremor, rigidity, postural instability, or the combined gait difficulty. Possible gait interventions include use of aids or cues to enhance attention; breaking down tasks into parts; working toward measurable goals, such as increasing stride length; and practicing different walking patterns. Some patients may need to use a walker or cane. Postural interventions include strengthening exercises for postural extensors, stretching of pectorals and heel cords, rotational exercises to increase range of motion of the neck and trunk (done while supine or side-lying), and relaxation exercises, including deep breathing. Aerobic conditioning is also suggested to combat fatigue.

Multiple Sclerosis

Most physical therapy interventions for patients with multiple sclerosis (MS) speak to the three major neurologic symptoms of weakness, spasticity, and ataxia. Exercises to address weakness should be performed at submaximal levels with interspersed rest periods to avoid fatigue.

Strengthening is an important component, and should focus on high reps of low to moderate intensity. Low-level aerobics should be included. Patients should do exercises in a cool environment. In order to decrease the possibility of spasticity during exercise, slow static stretching exercises should be performed first. Examples include stretching of the heel cord and hamstrings, using a towel or assisted by the therapist; sitting and wall stretches for the hamstrings; stretching the legs against a wall to stretch hamstrings and hip adductors; rotating the lower trunk, using a therapy ball; and transiting from four-point to side sitting for trunk rotation. Interventions for ataxia should focus on postural exercises, functional movement transitions, static and dynamic balance training, and Frenkel exercises for coordination (discussed elsewhere). Assistive devices or orthoses are often used.

Frenkel Exercises

Frenkel exercises are a set of movements done in supine, sitting, or standing position. They are designed to be done slowly and evenly to improve coordination. Typically, there are eight supine movements in the set, involving different combinations of lower-extremity flexions, extensions, abductions, adductions, and/or heel sliding. There are four sitting-position Frenkel exercises, which address issues like sitting steadily, rising and sitting down, etc. There are four more exercises done standing, three of which involve walking along a winding strip, between two parallel lines, or along a floor tracing. Frenkel exercises are good interventions for patients with ataxia, such as those with multiple sclerosis.

Proprioceptive Neuromuscular Facilitation

Proprioceptive Neuromuscular Facilitation

Proprioceptive neuromuscular facilitation (PNF) is a physical therapy intervention strategy that focuses on improving functional performance through increasing strength, flexibility, and range of motion. The goals of PNF are to help the patient develop head and trunk control, begin and sustain movement, manage shifts in center of gravity, and control the trunk and pelvis at midline while moving extremities.

PNF expounds that there are 10 components to this improved motor learning:

1. Manual contacts: application of hands to the skin over the target muscle groups in the direction of preferred movement
2. Mirroring: therapist mimicking of the patient's body position and mechanics
3. Use of stretch: facilitation of muscle activity
4. Manual resistance: minimization of internal resistance and application of external resistance
5. Irradiation: the concept that muscle activity spreads out or overflows from the point of resistance
6. Facilitation of joints through traction and approximation
7. Timing or sequencing of movement
8. Use of diagonal patterns of movement
9. Use of visual cues
10. Concise verbal input in three phases: preparation, action, and correction

Upper-Extremity Patterns

One basic tenet of proprioceptive neuromuscular facilitation (PNF) is the use of diagonal combinations of joint movements, called patterns. The therapist aids the patient through manual contact and other principles of PNF. Extremity patterns are designated in terms of the direction of movement at the proximal joint, the resultant movement, and directions for flexion and extension.

Upper-extremity (UE) patterns are either diagonal 1 (D1) or 2 (D2), depending on whether the pattern moves counterclockwise or clockwise, respectively. The flexion or extension designation describes the starting position for the joint in question. The pattern starts in flexion or extension, goes through some sequence of internal or external rotation, plus adduction or abduction.

A UE-D1 Flexion pattern is shoulder Flexion/Adduction/External Rotation and a UE-D1 Extension pattern is the opposite, Extension/Abduction/Internal Rotation.

A UE-D2 Flexion pattern is Flexion/Abduction/External Rotation, and UE-D2 Extension pattern is Extension/Adduction/Internal Rotation. Flexion patterns always involve shoulder external rotation, forearm supination, and radial wrist deviation, while extension patterns involve shoulder internal rotation, forearm pronation, and ulnar wrist deviation.

UE patterns are combined in the lifting and reverse lifting and chopping patterns.

Scapular and Pelvic Patterns

Proprioceptive neuromuscular facilitation (PNF) uses therapist-assisted diagonal patterns to achieve its goals. Scapular patterns are somewhat unique because they take into account scapulohumeral biomechanics. They begin in elevation or depression and end in the opposite. Elevation, a type of flexion, is when the scapula, or shoulder, is pulled up or shrugged, and depression is a type of extension in which it is depressed and retracted downward. Both can be done to the anterior or posterior side with the patient side-lying.

Pelvic patterns are analogous in that there is a limited range of motion in the pelvis, the patterns are similarly named, and side-lying positions (with flexed legs) are generally used. Here, the most germane patterns are the Anterior Elevation and Posterior Depression Pelvic patterns, which involve pulling the pelvis up and forward or back into the therapist's, respectively.

Lower-Extremity Patterns

Lower-extremity (LE) patterns for proprioceptive neuromuscular facilitation (PNF) are named similarly to upper-extremity patterns, for example, LE-D1 Flexion and so on, with D1 patterns moving counterclockwise and D2 ones moving clockwise. Here, hip internal rotation is always paired with abduction and hip external rotation with adduction. In addition, the patient also goes through a posterior or anterior pelvic tilt during the pattern. The main patterns are:

- LE-D1 Flexion: hip Flexion/Adduction/External Rotation, basically plantar flexion of the foot and pulling the leg across
- LE-D1 Extension: hip Extension/Abduction/Internal Rotation
- LE-D2 Flexion: hip Flexion/Abduction/Internal Rotation
- LE-D2 Extension: hip Extension/Adduction/External Rotation

Common Techniques That Address Mobility and Stability

Proprioceptive neuromuscular facilitation (PNF) techniques that address mobility and stability include:

- Rhythmic initiation: focuses on enhancing mobility by sequentially introducing passive, active-assisted, and, eventually, active or slightly resisted movements
- Rhythmic rotation: applies passive movements in a rotational fashion to encourage relaxation, reduce tone and lessen spasticity, and, ultimately, improve joint mobility

- Hold relax active movement: consists of sequences of resisted isometric contraction, followed by relaxation and incremental lengthening of position; goal is to increase range of motion
- Hold relax: is essentially the same as hold relax active movement, except usually includes verbal cues; patient-controlled movement is ideal
- Contract relax: uses resisted isotonic or isometric contraction of a short muscle to available range of motion (ROM), followed by verbal instruction to move it further, hold for a least five seconds, and then relax; used to increase ROM
- Alternating isometrics: therapist uses manual contact or resistance alternately, against opposing muscle groups, to enhance stability, strength, and endurance in them; also involves verbal cues to maintain stability
- Rhythmic stabilization: primarily promotes stability by simultaneous contraction of muscles around the target joint, while applying a rotary force

Common Techniques That Address Controlled Mobility or Skill Development

Proprioceptive neuromuscular facilitation (PNF) techniques that address controlled mobility or skill development include:

- Slow reversal: uses concentric contraction of muscles and reversal of manual contacts at end of range of motion to other direction to develop smooth transitions
- Slow reversal hold: variation of slow reversal, in which a resisted isometric contraction is held before reversing direction; useful for moving from emphasis on stability to mobility, as well as controlled mobility and skill
- Agonistic reversals: involves concentric contraction of muscle, an isometric hold against resistance, eccentric contraction through resistance during return to baseline position, and holding at the end; primarily promotes functional stability in a controlled manner; bridging exercise is a good example
- Resisted progression: application of resistance during perfection of a skill, such as creeping or walking

Cerebrovascular Accident

Physical Therapy Considerations

An important consideration with cerebrovascular accident patients is positioning, which should rotate between supine, with support on the involved side under the patient's scapula, pelvis, and knee; side-lying on the uninvolved side, with involved leg and arm crossed over and supported by pillows; and side-lying on the involved side, with involved affected shoulder forward and protracted, forearm in supination, and, again, support. The patient should be assisted with bridging, pushing the hips upward, and bridging with approximation or compression applied through the knee. Early types of bedside interventions include hip extension over the edge of the bed or other surface, straight leg raises with the uninvolved extremity, lower trunk rotation in hook lying position, hip and knee flexion while supine, separation and pushing against the patient's toes to inhibit toe clawing and promote ankle dorsiflexion, scapular mobilization (all of which involve manual contact by the physical therapist or assistant), and double arm elevation by the patient alone. Use of facilitation techniques is, for the most part, controversial or unproven. Inhibition techniques, such as slow, rhythmic rotation and weight bearing, are useful. Air splints are often used to help with positioning, reduction of tone sensory awareness, or early gait training.

Physical Therapy Interventions Related to Performance of Functional Activities

Functional movements should be taught as early as possible to a cerebrovascular accident patient. One of the first functional activities is rolling, both to the involved and uninvolved sides. Since the roll is initiated from the opposite side, rolling to the involved side is actually easier, but rolling to the uninvolved side can be aided by having the patient assume the hook lying position and grasp hands together before rolling. The patient should learn to scoot in the supine position. Transfers should be taught, particularly supine-to-sit and wheelchair-to-bed/mat transfers. Supine-to-sit transfers should be learned on both the uninvolved and involved sides. Techniques include rolling onto the uninvolved side, followed by moving lower extremities off the bed; and a diagonal pattern, where he scoots to the edge through bridging, brings the lower extremities off the surface, and, while tucking the chin, reaches forward with the unaffected arm. The main wheelchair-to-bed/mat technique used is the stand-pivot transfer (described elsewhere).

Physical Therapy Interventions Related to Functional Positioning

Once the cerebrovascular accident patient can accomplish short-sitting, sitting on the side of the bed or other surface with flexed knees and hips and feet planted on the floor, functional positioning can be addressed. The first interventions should concentrate on the patient's sitting posture, starting with guiding the pelvis through an anterior pelvic tilt, eventually into neutral, followed by positioning the trunk such that the shoulders are aligned over the hips, and positioning of the head upright. Adjunct sitting interventions include weight bearing on the involved hand, weight-shifting with arms resting in lap or bearing weight, sitting balance or isometric activities, reaching activities, and bilateral proprioceptive neuromuscular facilitation patterns performed seated. When possible, sit-to-stand transitions should be taught; these include techniques like standing in front of the patient with hands on the paraspinals to help him shift forward from sitting, guarding the patient from the involved side as he gets up, and use of the uninvolved arm for independent transfers. Early standing activities should include weight-shifting with assistance in all four directions, while observing for posture, joint control, and balance.

Ambulation Progression and Common Gait Deviations

The clinician helps the cerebrovascular accident patient through various stages to achieve ambulation. The initial stage, once the patient can stand, is to practice weight shifting in all four directions. The second is to have them learn to advance the uninvolved lower extremity both forward and backward with weight bearing, while blocking the involved leg to prevent knee buckling. After that the patient should be taught how to advance the involved leg forward; this may require tactile cues at the hip or the foot behind the patient's by the PT or PTA. Extremity advancement steps are sometimes done with the patient seated. The next progression is stepping backward with the affected lower extremity, and the last step is putting several steps together, engaging both extremities. Advancing the involved leg during the swing phase and weight shifts during the stance phase of gait should be stressed. The patient normally uses a cane on the involved side, while the clinician provides support on the unaffected side. Common gait deviations to look for include hip retraction, hiking, circumduction, or inadequate flexion; knee instability, hyperextension, or undue flexion during stance or too little flexion during swing; and ankle inversion, eversion, footdrop, or toe clawing.

Advanced Physical Therapy Interventions

A natural progression in physical therapy interventions for cerebrovascular accident, or stroke, patients is performance of prone activities; transitioning from prone on the elbows into the four-point or quadruped position; four-point activities, such as creeping; changing from the four-point into the tall-kneeling position; tall-kneeling activities, such as lifting; moving from tall-kneeling to half-kneeling; half-kneeling activities; and finally, the modified plant grade position. The latter is a standing position with weight bearing on all four extremities (for example, arms on a table); from this position, many types of exercises can be done, such as alternating isometrics, squats, or functional activities. During mid- to late recovery, physical therapy approaches include negotiation of stairs, both climbing and descending, with clinician assistance and wearing a safety belt; exercises to develop fine motor skills, coordination, and balance; and advanced exercises for ambulation-involved joints, especially the ankle. Useful equipment for balance exercises includes tilt boards and the Swiss ball.

Traumatic Brain Injuries

In the acute period after medical stabilization, one of the most important considerations for patients with traumatic brain injuries (TBIs) is positioning. The best positioning for the TBI patient is not supine, but rather side-lying, semiprone, or even prone, to reduce tonic labyrinthine reflexes. The prone position with various props is preferred for a TBI patient using mechanical ventilation or a tracheostomy tube. Sensory stimulation and activities to increase patient awareness are indicated early. After the patient is transferred to an inpatient rehabilitation setting, the previously mentioned positioning should be continued along with some time spent in a wheelchair (regular or tilt-in-space type). Range-of-motion exercises should be begun, particularly stretching, as well as functional mobility training as TBI patients typically lack postural and motor control. Assisted sitting and standing activities and transfers should be incorporated. Activities addressing some of the associated cognitive deficits should be included when possible. Eventually, interventions can incorporate a variety of balance exercises using moving surfaces.

Spinal Cord Injuries

Acute Care for Spinal Cord Injuries

A good deal of physical therapy for spinal cord injury (SCI) patients in the acute setting should focus on improvement of respiratory function. This includes breathing exercises and diaphragmatic breathing in patients with C4 to T1 injuries, glossopharyngeal breathing for those with C1 to C3 damage, lateral expansion or basilar breathing in those with T1 to T12 injuries, incentive spirometry, manual chest stretching, postural drainage techniques, and assisted cough techniques. Acute care management should also focus on prevention of joint contractures, improvement of muscle function, prevention of other complications, and acclimation of the patient to the upright position (usually with a tilt table). Range-of-motion (ROM) exercises are essential, concentrating on stretching in upper regions and passive ROM in the lower paralyzed extremities. Strengthening exercises, usually employing manual resistance, should be performed.

Inpatient Rehabilitation Phase

Some of the earliest interventions for spinal cord injury patients should be mat activities. Mat activities include learning how to roll (flex and rotate head, extend arms above head, turn with momentum), exercises in prone position (scapular strengthening, for example), transitions to prone on elbows, exercises in prone on elbows position (for example, alternating isometrics), shifts from there to supine, transitions to supine on elbows (assisted or independent, utilizing neck shift forward and side weight shift to come onto other elbow), and movement from there into long-sitting (extension of both lower extremities). Another emphasis should be on how to perform transfers (discussed elsewhere). Eventually patients with C7 tetraplegia should be taught how to self-stretch their hamstrings (in long-sitting or supine position), gluteus maximus, hip rotators, and ankle plantar flexors. Patients with paraplegia can move on to advanced mat activities, such as the sitting swing-through, hip swayer, trunk twisting and raising, prone push-ups, creeping, and tall-kneeling exercises with or without crutches. Other potential components include cardiopulmonary training, wheelchair use, circuit training, aquatic therapy, and for some, eventually, ambulation training.

Genetic Disorders Involving the Neurologic System in Children

Some important genetic disorders involving the neurologic system are: Down Syndrome: presence of extra 21st chromosome in bodily cells, resulting in intellectual disability, developmental delays, musculoskeletal deficits (such as instability at the atlanto-axial joint involving the two upper cervical vertebra), hypotonicity, flat facial features, a variety of neurological deficits, etc.

Arthropyosis multiplex congenital: a nonprogressive neuromuscular syndrome inherited on chromosome 9 (or 5 in neurogenic form); characterized by multiple contractures

Osteogenesis imperfecta: autonomic dominant disorder affecting collagen synthesis and bone metabolism, making individual prone to bone fractures

Spinal muscle atrophy (SMA): autonomic recessive, progressive neurologic disorder destroying anterior horn cells and lower motor neurons

- Type I acute infantile SMA occurs shortly after birth and is characterized by respiratory and other oral issues and a frog-leg posture
- Type II chronic SMA starts at approximately 2 to 18 months of age characterized by muscle weakness and scoliosis
- later-onset Kugelberg-Welander SMA is similar

Duchenne muscular dystrophy (DMD): X-linked recessive trait in which muscle protein dystrophin is absent; symptomatic only in boys, presenting as progressive weakness (including cardiac and respiratory muscles), diminished range of motion, and contractures

Fragile X syndrome: presence of fragile site on X chromosome; signified by intellectual disability and other neurologic defects

Integumentary System

Burn Care

Physical Therapy Examination Related to Burn Care

Physical therapy for a burn patient may be initiated within a few days of admission. The history should include questions about the burn itself, as well as underlying conditions and secondary injuries that might impact recovery. Specifically, the therapist should ask about the circumstances under which the burn occurred, whether the patient fell or was thrown, where he endured the inhalation injury or carbon monoxide poisoning, the classification and location of the burn, and the possibility of self-infliction or suicidal tendencies. The therapist should inspect the burn site, including proximity of joints and the presence of interventions, such as dressings, tubes, etc. S9he) should also observe the patient's posture and positioning, level of consciousness, swelling, and pain. Pain levels should be assessed at the burn and donor sites at rest; during various types of range-of-motion (ROM) exercises; and before, during, and after physical therapy. Heart rate, blood pressure, respiratory rate, and oxygen saturation levels should be quantified. The therapist should attempt to grossly assess ROM, strength, and functional mobility, although these assessments may be difficult due to bulky dressings, pain, tendon exposure, etc.

Physical Therapy Interventions in Burn Patients

The physical therapist needs to be fully engaged as a member of the burn team by attending rounds. Burn patients generally have multi-organ involvement and tend to have increased metabolic functions. The fluids and pain medications they are receiving affect their vital signs, which can in turn impact appropriate levels of therapy. The status and needs of burn patients change rapidly. Physical therapy interventions may be contraindicated for several days after skin grafting to preclude shearing of the graft. Positioning of the joints in danger of contracture or tightening is crucial. The therapy plan is dependent on a number of factors, such as surface area of the burns, prior functional status, area covered, and patient's age. The goal is to increase functionality, whether through conventional exercises or other means.

Physical Therapy Considerations Regarding Burn Patients

Burn patients generally develop a decreased range of motion quickly due to edema, pain, and immobilization of the nearby joint, which may extend somewhat to other joints if there is generalized edema. This can be addressed with positioning devices, such as splints, pillows, boards, and stretching gadgets like pulleys. Patients tend to have less strength that should, if possible, be tackled with use of active exercise. The patient generally needs protracted bed rest, which can decrease endurance and functional mobility. If he has orthostatic hypotension or deficient lower-extremity mobility, a tilt table may be needed to move the patient, and assistive devices may need to be modified. Cardiovascular active exercises with secondary improvements in range of motion (ROM) and strength are suggested. Burn patients are at risk for scarring, which can be lessened with the use of pressure garments, massage, and ROM exercises. Compliance after discharge can be heightened with expert patient and family education about the process and interventions.

Wound Care

Physical Therapy Goals for Patients with Acute Wounds

The physical therapist performs as part of an interdisciplinary team to treat patients with acute wounds. The therapist's role may vary depending on what is allowed in a particular facility. In general, one major goal is the promotion of wound healing, possibly including assessment, dressing application, and/or cleaning and debridement of the wound. Other goals include minimization of the patient's pain, maximization of mobility and function without jeopardizing wound healing, and education for the patient and his family about wound care and deterrence of complications. In addition, the physical therapist gives recommendations for interdisciplinary acute care and aftercare.

Physical Therapy Interventions for Wound Care

The physical therapist aids the patient with pain management. Sessions should be scheduled to coincide with pain premedication. Some specific interventions are positioning, relaxation methods, deep breathing, and exercise. The therapist should implement practices that increase the patient's range of motion (ROM), strength, and functional mobility. Adequate ROM enables the patient to be positioned for prevention of pressure ulcers, and sufficient strength is important for weight transfer, functional mobility, and adherence to weight-bearing precautions. During exercises, the therapist should be careful not to disturb dressings. Edema management is also important, with a variety of interventions possible, including lymphatic drainage techniques, elevation of the limb, compression, and certain exercises. Lastly, the therapist is responsible for prevention of further damage. Prevention interventions include education of the patient about wound etiology and care, regular repositioning of the patient, dressing removal and other skin care, the use of pressure lessening mattresses and cushions, and, if needed, special footwear.

Other Systems

Gastrointestinal System

Physical Therapy for Gastrointestinal Issues

The objectives of physical therapy for patients with GI problems are the establishment of greatest functional mobility, maximization of endurance and activity tolerance, and deterrence of pulmonary complications. The therapist should keep in mind that most of these patients are very fatigued. Their ability to perform activities is quite dependent on their caloric intake and hematologic status. Patient responses to medications are often unpredictable because of metabolic problems.

Another important consideration is positioning. Lying supine can lead to difficulty swallowing, aspiration pneumonia, portal hypertension, and rupture of esophageal blood vessels. Coughing and forced expirations also aggravate these conditions, and huffing is suggested. Patients who normally rely on NSAIDs for pain management will probably have functional limitations because NSAIDs are typically withdrawn. Pulmonary complications often occur in individuals with ascites or who have had large abdominal incisions, so these patients need pain management before receiving physical therapy, position changes during the therapy, and early mobilization.

Genitourinary System

Physical Therapy for Genitourinary Disorders

Patients with genitourinary disorders usually have fluid and electrolyte imbalances and an inability to regulate cellular waste products. These imbalances can cause alterations in mental status, muscular problems, sensory defects, pulmonary and peripheral edema, and other problems. These issues may require the physical therapist to defer or alter interventions, for example, precluding activities that demand concentration, reducing intensity, and changing positioning. These patients also often have blood pressure irregularities, anemia, or referred pain. If they have undergone surgery, it is important to take measures (such as positional changes, incision splinting during deep breathing, and early mobilization) to avoid pulmonary complications because their abdominal incisions make it difficult to breathe deeply or cough. Incontinence can be addressed by modalities, such as use of a bedside commode, pelvic floor retraining, and home exercise regimens.

Pelvic Floor Retraining

Pelvic floor muscle retraining is used to decrease urinary incontinence and improve pelvic floor strength. It is often used in women of childbearing age but is also appropriate for patients with certain genitourinary disorders. Pelvic floor exercises are done with an empty bladder and often assisted by gravity with hips elevated relative to the heart. There are several types of exercises:

- In the contract-relax exercise, the patient does 10 rounds alternating pelvic floor tightening (as if to stop urine flow or gas release) and relaxing, each portion held for three to five seconds. The goal is to isolate use of the pelvic floor and not use other muscles, such as the abdominals.
- Another exercise is performance of up to 20 quick, successive contractions of the pelvic floor muscles without using accessory muscles and at a standard breathing rate.
- During the "elevator exercise," the patient contracts the pelvic floor muscles either more tightly or less with each subsequent contraction to improve strengthening and relaxation of the pelvic floor respectively.

During pelvic floor relaxation exercises, it is important to emphasize slow, deep breathing and concurrent relaxation of the facial muscles.

Biofeedback for Pelvic Floor Impairments

Biofeedback is a method using monitoring devices to help a patient learn to consciously control normally automatic bodily functions. One biofeedback technique used for pelvic floor impairments is surface electromyography (SEMG), which is generally used in conjunction with pelvic floor retraining exercises (discussed elsewhere) and other modalities. One of these techniques is neuromuscular re-education, which uses isolated contractions of the pelvic floor without excessive utilization of accessory muscles, initially followed by their integration with activities of daily life, lumbar stabilization, and other exercises. Additional interventions include use of visual aids, particularly schematic diagrams of the pelvic floor muscles; and manual intravaginal or intrarectal techniques (depending on the cause).

Multi-System

Pregnancy

Appropriate Level and Type of Fitness Exercise for a Pregnant Woman

It is generally suggested that pregnant women do mild to moderate exercise most days for 15 to 30 minutes. The intensity should be in the range of 12 to 14 on the Borg Rating Scale for Perceived Exertion (basically, moderately hard). Non-weight-bearing aerobic exercises are recommended, while contact sports, high-altitude, and scuba diving should be shunned. Anything that might cause the patient to lose balance and fall should also be avoided. After childbirth, she should gradually resume the earlier program. If a pregnant woman also has diastasis recti, gestational diabetes, musculoskeletal issues, anemia, infections, or is far outside normal weight limits, her exercise program should be modified and monitored by a doctor, as well as the therapist. Conditions that preclude exercise are primarily related directly to the pregnancy, such as vaginal bleeding, pre-eclampsia, placenta previa, premature amniotic fluid loss or labor, an incompetent cervix, or multiple fetuses. Other contraindications include maternal heart, thyroid, serious pulmonary diseases, and type 1 diabetes.

Posture Exercises During Pregnancy and Immediately After Delivery

A pregnant woman should perform certain stretching and strengthening exercises for her posture as pregnancy shifts her center of gravity forward and upward. The stretches should be done gently because a pregnant woman's joints are fragile. Suggested exercises are those that stretch the upper neck extensors and scalene, the scapular protractors, levator scapulae, shoulder internal rotators, low back extensors, hip flexors, hip adductors, hamstrings, and plantarflexor of the ankle. It is suggested that posture exercises for strengthening target the upper neck flexors, thoracic extensors, scapular retractors and depressors, shoulder external rotators, hip extensors, knee extensors, ankle dorsiflexors, and the abdominals. In the latter case, the lower abdominals should be stressed.

Abdominal Muscle Exercises

The following abdominal muscle exercises are suggested for pregnant women:

- Pelvic tilt exercise: The woman is on both hands and knees with a straight back while she isometrically tightens and holds the lower abdominals in a posterior tilt, releases, and then does a small anterior tilt. Additional exercises include side bends in that position, and pelvic tilts while lying on her side and/or standing.
- Leg sliding: The patient lies supine with bent knees, assumes a posterior pelvic tilt, and holds it while sliding one leg as far forward as possible without releasing the tilt. She then brings the foot back and repeats with the other leg.
- Trunk curls: The patient does archetypal curl-downs, curl-ups, and diagonal curls but with crossed hands to protect linea alba. Contraindicated if she has diastasis recti.

- Modified bicycle: While lying supine and keeping her back flat, the woman alternates flexing one leg and (somewhat) extending the other.
- Standard stabilization exercises for the lumbar spine and pelvis are also recommended.

Pelvic Motion Training Exercises

Pelvic motion exercises help alleviate postural back pain and increase mobility in the lumbar, pelvic, and hip regions. Suggested exercises include:

- Pelvic clock: Patient lies on back with knees bent. She pictures a clock on her abdomen, with the umbilicus at 12 o'clock and the pubic symphysis at 6 o'clock. She should begin with several regular pelvic tilts (12 to 6) and weight shifts to either side (3 and 9), eventually establishing a clockwise rotation around the clock, from 12 to 3 to 6 to 9 and back to 12.
- Pelvic clock progressions: These are variations on the above. One possibility is to have the patient go through one half of the clock, return, and then repeat on the other side. Others feature counterclockwise rotation and seated positions.

Modified Upper- and Lower-Extremity Strengthening Exercises

The following modifications of extremity strengthening exercises are suggested for pregnant women:

- Standing push-ups: The individual stands arm's length from a wall and places her palms against it at shoulder height. While in pelvic tilt and with firmly planted feet, she brings her upper body forward by bending her elbows and then uses her arms to push back to her initial position.
- Quadruple leg raising: While propped on hands and knees, the patient does a posterior pelvic tilt and then raises and extends one leg, lowers it, and repeats the sequence on the other side. During lifting, the hip should be at pelvis level or lower, and if the patient is unstable, the leg can be slid along the ground instead.
- Modified squatting: The patient stands with her back to the wall in shoulder-width stance and slides her back up and down the wall. Alternatively, she can stand facing some sort of support and squat. These are good preparatory exercises for childbirth. Perineum and adductor flexibility exercises are as well.
- Supine bridging: In hook-lying supine stance, the woman does a posterior pelvic tilt and raises and holds the pelvis (bridge position). She can repeat this or hold it while flexing and extending the arms.
- Scapular retraction: Instead of doing this exercise prone, patient can do it seated or standing.

Relaxation and Breathing Exercises During Labor

During labor, it is important for the mother to relax muscles that are not involved in the birthing process. It is recommended that she focus on a serene image at tense times during pregnancy, as well as during labor. She should ready her muscles for the process. To do this, while lying comfortably, she should contract and relax muscles in each section of the body, moving from the feet upward to the face, eventually adding slow, deep, relaxed diaphragmatic breathing. She should be aware of the difference between muscles that are tensed and those that are not. When the woman reaches the point where uterus contractions are stronger and nearer together, suggestions for relaxation and breathing include finding a comfortable position, gentle movements (like pelvic rocking), slow breathing, visual imagery or distractions (talking, etc.) that relax her, massaging of painful areas, local application of cold or heat (if needed), face dabbing with a wet wash cloth, and use of quick blowing, not pushing, as delivery nears. When the cervix is dilated, the woman can aid the birth by bracing, breathing in, contracting her abdominal wall, and then slowly breathing out. During the actual delivery, she can use pants or groans to relax the pelvic floor.

Physical Therapy Considerations for Cesarean Section

Delivery of a baby via an incision in the abdominal wall and uterus, instead of through the pelvis and vagina, is a cesarean section. The mother is still at risk postpartum for pelvic floor dysfunction, plus she has just undergone surgery with its attendant perils and complications. When feasible during her recovery, she should initiate preventive exercises, including ankle pumping, lower-extremity range of motion, and walking to prevent vascular complications; pelvic floor exercises to prevent dysfunction; and correct deep breathing, coughing, and/or huffing to increase pulmonary function and discourage development of pneumonia. Abdominal exercises should be incorporated slowly and include corrective ones for diastasis recti. She should receive postural training. Several exercises that alleviate intestinal gas pains should be included, such as limited abdominal curl-ups, bridge and twist, and pelvic tilting and/or bridging, the latter often done in conjunction with another helpful technique, abdominal massage or kneading. Other interventions include massage around the incision site to prevent adhesions and enhance circulation, support of the incision to decrease pain, and incisional splinting to prevent injury and low back pain.

Head, Neck or Facial Tumors

Most head, neck, and facial tumors are addressed by some type of radical neck dissection (RND) or laryngectomy, usually followed by reconstructive surgery. In a RND, the affected organ, musculature, jugular veins, and/or lymph nodes are partially or totally removed. Reconstructive surgery generally involves creating a skin flap over the area or using the pectoralis or trapezius muscle to create a muscle flap. Patients who have undergone these procedures have problems with airway obstruction and clearance of oral secretions, which need to be addressed. They may have additional lung disease, particularly oral cancer patients, who are generally heavy tobacco users. They tend to have difficulty communicating, swallowing, and chewing, and other senses are typically diminished. After consulting with the physician, the physical therapist should institute therapy, emphasizing posture and range of motion in the neck, shoulder, temporomandibular joint, and scapulothoracic region.

Cancer Patients

In addition to the general physical therapy goals for all patients, certain areas are of importance when dealing with cancer patients. The therapist should know the site of the primary tumor and metastases, the surgical procedure performed to assess what procedures can be done, the patient's risk for pulmonary or fracture complications or skin breakdown, and the assistive devices or prosthetics that might be needed. Pertinent laboratory values should be monitored, particularly parameters such as platelet counts, which, if low, make the patient prone to bruising or internal bleeding. If exercise is permitted by the physician, a moderate, progressive, mainly aerobic program for use throughout treatment should be developed (no more than 70% maximal heart rate or 13 on the Borg's Rating of Perceived Exertion).

Equipment & Devices; Therapeutic Modalities

Equipment and Devices

Positioning Seating and Side-Lying in Children

The main goal of using adaptive equipment is to bolster appropriate positioning and movement, not just provide support. Prone positioning in children is aided by half-rolls, bolsters, or wedges that promote head lifting, weight bearing on forearms and elbows, and shoulder control. Wedges and half-rolls are also used to hold up the child's head and upper trunk or knees while supine. Adaptive seating devices include posture chairs, bolster chairs, posteriorly inclined wedges, and benches with pelvic support. If the child has poor head and trunk control, the adaptive chairs may also be outfitted with head support and a lap tray for arm placement. A general requirement for any seating device is that it maintains the 90-90-90 rule for sitting alignment, meaning flexion of feet, knees, and hips should all be about 90^0. If the child has trunk muscle paralysis, an orthotic device may also be used. The side-lying position is good for sleeping, where a long body pillow is used for support, but during the daytime another device used is the sidelyer, which straps the child into the side-lying position.

Standing in Children

Adaptive equipment for standing is beneficial because it promotes growth of the child's long leg bones and, depending on the configuration, allows use of upper extremities. There are prone, supine, and vertical standers available, as well as walkers for mobility. A prone stander holds up the child's front chest, hips, and front surface of the legs. A supine stander is basically a tilt table. A vertical stander supports the child's lower extremities in extension. Benefits of this type of stander include thorough weight bearing, ability to use upper extremities, and adjustability. Mobility in children with motor dysfunction can be facilitated with walkers, either a standard one used in front or a reverse posture control walker supported from behind. The latter is generally preferred.

Wheelchairs

Wheelchairs as Assistive Devices for Children

Wheelchairs are often used for children with cerebral palsy. They can be manual, power-operated, or gait trainers. Most wheelchairs support the trunk and lower extremities, but gait trainers provide considerable trunk support while allowing the individual to use the lower extremities to move it. Children with Duchenne muscular dystrophy, who have weak upper extremities, generally use light sports wheelchairs or power wheelchairs, often in conjunction with arm supports that have feeding apparatuses, voice-activated computers, and/or environmental controls. Children with myelomeningocele usually go through a period where they use some type of mobility device before being able to ambulate on their own. These include manual and electric wheelchairs, as well as caster carts, prone scooters, adapted tricycles, and cyclones.

How to Select an Appropriate Wheelchair

A wheelchair should be selected that encourages good posture and prevents injury to the patient. It should have adequate pelvic control to keep the pelvis neutral and support the curvature of the spine. A general rule is that the wheelchair should maintain a 90-degree angle at the hips, knees, and ankles. This translates to a chair that maintains the thighs horizontal to the floor, a seat depth of approximately 2 inches from the popliteal fossa behind the knee, and a footrest that keeps the thighs parallel to the floor. The types of wheelchairs available include manual, power, sport or light for easier mobility, hemi-height or gait trainers where feet are used for propulsion, and reclining or tilt-in-space types. There are folding and rigid nonfolding types, numerous types of added features, and a variety of wheelchair cushions that help diminish pressure and shear and aid in posture control.

Wheelchairs as Assistive Devices for Adults

Patients who have undergone traumatic brain injuries should use wheelchairs after becoming stable because this orients them to an upright position. A standard wheelchair with attached lap tray is sufficient if the person has a fair amount of trunk and head control; the eventual goal is independent propulsion of the wheelchair. Another option is the tilt-in-space wheelchair, which maintains 90-degree angulation at the hips, knees, and ankles, while allowing the patient to recline. Patients with spinal cord injuries generally need power wheelchairs outfitted with a reclining feature and a sip-and-puff mechanism, a chin cup, or other type of facial control for mobilization if their injury is high, down to about C4, or hand controls if at C5. Lower spinal cord injuries can be accommodated by use of a manual wheelchair or orthoses. A power wheelchair with a seat belt is one option for mobility for individuals with ataxia, lack of muscle control.

Six-Pivot Transfer Technique

All spinal cord injury patients are prepared for the six-pivot transfer technique and other transfers by positioning the wheelchair parallel to the mat or bed, locking the brakes, removing the leg rest, and putting a gait belt on. The six-pivot transfer technique is often used for dependent spinal cord injury patients. The helper shifts the patient's weight forward in the wheelchair. The armrest on the side for transfer is then removed. The assistant helps the patient to flex forward in the direction of the assistant's hip while maintaining knee contact. Another helper should be situated behind the mat table or patient for assistance, if needed. The person in front of the patient then moves the patient's weight forward, places the hips and buttocks onto the transfer table and mat, and positions the patient upright, being careful to maintain contact as the patient does not have trunk control and could lose balance or fall.

Stand-Pivot Transfer and Modified Stand-Pivot Transfer Techniques

The stand-pivot transfer is the most common technique used to transition from a wheelchair to a bed or mat for cerebrovascular accident patients. The modified technique is sometimes used for spinal cord injury patients with partial injuries and some intact lower-extremity innervation. For the stand-pivot transfer, the patient moves his weight forward in the wheelchair until feet are firmly planted on the floor. The transfer is made toward the uninvolved side. The assistant holds the involved arm firmly and encourages the patient to shift weight forward and stand up. Once erect, the patient pivots on his feet and slightly moves the inside, uninvolved leg to sit down on the mat or bed. The assistant guards the patient's knee with his own during standing-up and sitting-down processes. In the modified technique, the patient usually holds his arms around the person helping with the transfer for more support.

Wheelchair Transfer Techniques for Spinal Cord Injury Patients

Transfer techniques for high-cervical injuries (C1 to C4) include:

Dependent six-pivot transfer (discussed elsewhere)

A two-person lift: one person lifts patient legs while the other lifts the trunk

Use of hydraulic power lift

Airlift: patient flexes legs, which rest on or between therapist's thighs; patient is rocked out of the wheelchair and lifted onto transfer surface; must have lower-extremity tone

Modified stand-pivot transfer (discussed elsewhere)

Sliding board transfers: the board is placed on the transfer surface at a 45-degree angle to the wheelchair; patient shifts weight to farther side, while lifting buttocks on the transfer side, and the board is positioned underneath; patient slides over the board onto the mat; done with assistance or for C6 tetraplegia independently

Push-pull transfer: patient turns head and trunk away from transfer surface and scoots over onto the bed or mat by bracing bent arms on armrest, while bending forward; appropriate for C6 tetraplegics

Prone on elbows transfer: patient turns trunk toward table, lifts lower extremities onto surface, and rolls onto it

Lateral push-up transfer: with feet on floor and rotated opposite to direction of transfer, patient uses upper extremities and sometimes a board to complete transfer; appropriate for C7 injuries

Wheelchair-to-Floor Transfers and Righting of the Wheelchair

Spinal cord patients need to be taught the correct way to brace themselves if their wheelchair falls, how to right the chair while seated, and how to get into it from tall-kneeling and long-sitting positions. If the chair falls backwards, the patient should tuck the head in and keep arms inside the chair resting one over the knees. The therapist or assistant can teach this by lowering the patient backwards in the chair.

The other techniques are somewhat dependent on the patient's upper body strength. The way to right a tipped wheelchair while seated is to use one arm to push against the floor and the other arm to push against the front of the chair, while employing the head and upper trunk to shift weight. From the floor, a patient can get into a wheelchair by kneeling tall, facing the chair, and using the arms to push up on the front while lifting and rotating hips into a seated position; this can be reversed for getting out of the chair.

Alternatively, the patient can sit with legs stretched along the floor (long-sitting position) with the back against a stool, which is up against the front of the chair; he then uses the upper extremities to lift the buttocks onto the stool and then into the wheelchair.

Methods of Standing from the Wheelchair

The following methods of standing from the wheelchair are for use in spinal cord injury patients who wear additional orthoses (which are locked during transfer), can use crutches, and are ready to become independent:

- Method 1: The patient positions the wheelchair against the wall, locks the brakes, and puts his crutches behind the chair, leaning on the push handles. The individual then uses mini-push-ups to move to the edge of the chair, crosses one leg over the other to pivot to one side, and uses upper extremities to push against the armrests to bring the body up to standing, facing the chair. The patient secures each crutch, bracing the other arm against an armrest for support. After crutch attachment, he moves a few steps backwards and uses the crutches to stand upright.
- Method 2: The patient shifts forward to the edge of the chair and, with crutches ready, places them flat on the floor just behind the front wheels. The individual bends the head forward and pushes down on the crutches to lift out the chair. Once he feels in balance, he can move the crutches forward as well.

To get back into the wheelchair, the patient faces it, puts the crutches behind it, unlocks the knee joint of one orthosis, and turns in that direction to sit down.

Advanced Wheelchair Skills for Spinal Cord Patients

Advanced wheelchair skills are appropriate for patients who have innervation and strength in their finger muscles. They include:

- Wheelies: These are essential for independent navigation of curbs. The patient must find a balance point on the back wheels while leaning back and grasping the hand rims. The position is attained by leaning forward while pulling back on the rims, followed by moving the shoulders back against the chair while pushing forward on the rims.
- Ascending and descending ramps: Ascending the ramp, the patient should face and lean forward in the wheelchair. The length and strength of pushes on the hand rim are directly related to the ramp's length. Descending a ramp can be done either facing forward and leaning back while applying friction to the hand rims and wheels or facing backwards and leaning forward while lightly grasping the hand rims near the brake. Diagonal and zigzag ramp transfers are also possible.
- Ascending and descending curbs: In order to ascend a curb, the patient faces it and does a wheelie to lift the front casters for clearance, then leans forward, pushing on the hand rims to lift the rear wheels. It is safest to descend forward popping a wheelie on approach and then leaning forward once the rear wheels have cleared the curb. Alternatively, the patient can descend backwards while leaning forward and grasping the rims near the brakes.

Orthoses

Orthoses for Children with Myelomeningocele

Myelomeningocele (MMC) is a congenital disorder affecting the nervous, musculoskeletal, and urologic systems. Children with MMC may need orthoses, or some type of external support, to avert deformities. Initially, this is usually a simple abduction splint between the legs that is secured by a strap to keep the legs in a neutral rotation and a total body splint worn at night. When the child is older, other types of orthoses are indicated for standing and ambulation. The device should be selected collaboratively by the physical therapist, orthopedist, and orthotist. By about age 12 to 18 months, the child should get a customized standing frame and a parapodium ambulation orthosis if the lesion level is thoracic, L1, or L2. By age 24 to 36 months, this patient can proceed to use of a reciprocating gait orthosis (RGO), which holds in various parts of the legs and trunk, or a swivel walker. For those with L3 or L4 lesions, a RGO or hip-knee-ankle-foot orthosis (HKAFO) can be used from 12 to 18 months, followed by a knee-ankle-foot orthosis (KAFO) or ankle-foot-orthosis (AFO) at about 24 to 36 months. Ambulation is facilitated for children with L5 using a KAFO then AFO in the same time frames. Children with S1 to S3 lesions only need an AFO or FO (foot orthosis) from about 12 to 18 months.

Orthoses for Children with Cerebral Palsy

Children with cerebral palsy who are ambulatory generally use an ankle-foot orthosis (AFO), which is also used after surgery or casting. Most AFOs are made of molded polypropylene, which covers from the ankle and foot area up to near the head of the fibula. There are two main types of AFOs available: hinged AFOs and ground-reaction AFOs.

An alternative device useful for children who need medial lateral support for their ankles is the supramalleolar orthosis (SMO), which permits dorsiflexion and plantar flexion while preventing mediolateral movement. An added advantage is that SMOs fit inside tennis shoes.

Orthoses for Nervous System Genetic Disorders

Orthoses are often used as described for patients with the following genetic disorders:

- Arthrogryposis multiplex congenita (AMC): AMC is a congenital, nonprogressive neuromuscular syndrome characterized by numerous joint contractures. An early intervention is use of a Velcro band around the thighs to ensure neutral alignment of legs. To learn to stand, the child may use standing frames, parapodiums, supine standers, or prone standers. Orthoses are used for ambulation at joints where muscles are weak, or walkers are outfitted with supports.
- Osteogenesis imperfecta (OI): This is a disorder in which collagen synthesis and, subsequently, bone metabolism is defective, resulting in brittle bones and associated problems. These children need orthoses for standing and ambulation, usually some type of hip-knee-ankle-foot orthosis (HKAFO), used with a standing frame or prone walker to stand or in conjunction with parallel bars, a walker, or crutches for ambulation.
- Duchenne muscular dystrophy (DMD): This is an inherited or acquired x-linked recessive trait in boys, resulting in muscle weakness. The main use of orthoses in DMD is for heel cord lengthening during ambulation (AFOs, KAFOs), but most patients end up using a wheelchair.

Orthoses for Cerebrovascular Accident Patients

Patients who have had cerebrovascular accidents, or strokes, may need orthoses because they can have varying motor capabilities which can diminish ankle dorsiflexion and gait. Ankle-foot orthoses (AFOs) are the most common, and options include:

- Prefabricated AFOs: These are standard-size AFOs made of plastic that can accommodate a shoe over them. They are useful, at first, for training as they permit some heel strike and limit dragging of the toes.
- Customized ankle-foot orthoses: These are made by an orthotist from a cast of the patient's foot in neutrality or slight dorsiflexion. They are expensive.
- Articulated ankle-foot orthoses: These are usually plastic and have articulated ankle joints that can be locked into various stances. Advantages include a lower cost than customized and the ability to change the angle of articulation during the course of recovery. There are also metal upright orthoses that are hooked to a patient's shoe and allow for articulation.
- Other options include posterior leaf splints, plastic orthoses that restrict dorsiflexion and plantar flexion, and knee-ankle-foot orthoses (KAFOs), which extend up to and lock the knee in extension.

Orthoses for Spinal Cord Injuries

Paraplegics who want to ambulate require orthoses. Options include:

- Knee-ankle-foot orthoses (KAFOs): made of metal and plastic with a thigh cuff, calf band, and external lockable joints at the knee and ankle
- Scott-Craig knee-ankle-foot orthoses: have thigh and front pretibial bands, offset knee joints with locks and bail control, ankle joints with pin stops, cushioned heels, and customized steel footplates
- Reciprocating gait orthoses (RGO): consist of a molded pelvic band, thoracic extensions, bilateral hip and knee joints, plastic back thigh protection, ankle-foot orthoses, and connecting cables
- ARGO: comprised of an RGO used in conjunction with a hydraulic lift for transfer

Ankle-Foot Orthoses for Multiple Sclerosis

Patients with multiple sclerosis (MS) have demyelization of the central nervous system, resulting in weakness, spasticity, and ataxia. They frequently use ankle-foot orthoses (AFOs) to reinforce ankle stability, control knee hyperextension, improve their gait pattern and foot and toe clearance, and conserve energy. Choices include standard polypropylene AFOs, polypropylene AFOs with articulating ankle joints, and double upright metal AFOs with articulating ankle joints. Polypropylene AFOs with articulating ankle joints have additional advantages, such as more normal ankle movement and facility for squatting, while the metal upright types may have straps for correction of inward or outward turning of feet and/or room for different limb volumes. Both polypropylene types are contraindicated for MS patients with considerable spasticity, weakness, or foot edema.

Trunk Cervical and Upper-Limb Orthoses

Orthoses to protect the trunk area include sacroiliac corsets, which prevent dislodging of the sacroiliac; lumbosacral corsets that inhibit spinal hyperextension; and other lumbosacral orthoses restricting various types of motion. More comprehensive protection is provided by thoracolumbosacral orthoses (TLSOs), which restrict flexion, extension, lateral flexion, and rotation. Cervical orthoses impede unwanted motion in the cervical, or neck area, and include soft collars, inflexible cervical-post orthoses, and halos, which are generally used for vertebral fractures in that area. There are also a variety of upper-limb orthoses. Many of these are protective, e.g., shoulder slings to prevent dislocation and wrist-hand orthoses generally used for carpel tunnel syndrome. Other upper-extremity orthoses are designed to assist individuals with neuromuscular weakness, enhance range of motion, or aid paralytic patients with grasping.

Prostheses

Prosthetic devices, or prostheses, are artificial limbs designed to replace all or part of a limb after amputation. Amputation is the removal (generally surgically) of all or part of a limb as a result of trauma or irreparable damage to tissues or vessels due to infection, cancer, diabetes, or peripheral vascular disease. Initially, in the operating room, the patient is usually fitted for an immediate post-operative prosthesis (IPOP) pylon, and several days later, for a temporary or preparatory prosthesis, which is adjustable. Both of these prostheses consist of a socket, suspension belt, pylon, and foot. The patient wears the temporary prosthesis for about six months, during which time volume changes usually occur in the remaining part of the limb. After this time, a customized definitive or final prosthesis is made for use, which usually includes a socket, pylon, and foot.

Prosthesis for Transtibial Amputation

A transtibial, or below-knee, amputation involves removal of the leg up to the center of the tibia. The components of the prosthesis include the socket, suspension, pylon, foot, and a prosthetic socket worn between the socket and residual limb:

- The socket is the portion that abuts against the residual limb. Types include total contact sockets, silicone suction liners, supracondylar/suprapatellar sockets, and patellar tendon-bearing sockets.
- The prosthesis is fastened to the residual limb with suspensions. Various possible suspension systems include vacuum-assisted suspension systems (VASSs), locking devices that use pins or lanyards, elastic sleeves, gel liners, and valves.
- The pylon is the portion between the socket and foot, which aids forward motion and absorption of torque.

- The foot, which replicates foot and ankle motion, is designed based on desired absorption and ambulation characteristics. The standard foot is the SACH, or solid-ankle cushioned heel type, which absorbs shock at heel strike. Multiple-axis types permit plantar flexion, dorsiflexion, eversion, and inversion, while single-axis feet restrict plantar flexion and dorsiflexion. Dynamic response types store energy.

Prosthesis for Transfemoral Amputation

A transfemoral, or above-knee, amputation involves removal of the leg up to the femur in the thigh. The components of the prosthesis made include a prosthetic knee, socket, suspension, pylon, and foot:

- The prosthetic knee can be hinged around a single axis or able to change centers of rotation; various methods of friction control and locking during standing are available.
- The socket abuts against the residual limb. Sockets used for transfemoral amputations are either quadrilateral (four-walled), favored for longer residual limbs; or ischial containment sockets, which are wider from front to back but narrower laterally, providing better support of weight and preferred for shorter residual limb amputations or active patients.
- Suspensions fasten the residual limb to the prosthesis, and possibilities include suction types, hypobaric options that use a ring about 2 inches below the ischial tuberosity, and pelvic belts (either soft belts on the uninvolved side or total pelvic belts).
- Possible pylon types and foot and ankle components are discussed under transtibial amputations.

Other more extensive lower-extremity amputations include hip disarticulation and transpelvic amputation to the thigh and parts of the hip respectively.

Prostheses for Partial Foot Amputations

Partial foot amputations are defined in terms of the specific disarticulation (joint separation) occurring or the toes (rays) or bones removed. For example, a transmetatarsal amputation cuts through the metatarsals, a single-ray resection is removal of one toe, and a Lisfranc disarticulation involves separation of the tarsometatarsal joint. These amputations may not necessitate use of a prosthesis; if they do, prosthetic options include a solid ankle-cushioned heel (SACH) foot or other prosthetic foot. Most solutions are really orthoses, such as toe fillers, custom-molded shoes, or neuropathic walkers, which are ankle-foot orthoses with rocker bottoms.

Prosthesis for Upper-Limb Amputation

A patient who has undergone an upper-limb amputation needs a device that will permit maximal functional use. Depending on where the amputation occurred, these prosthetic devices may consist of a terminal device (TD), wrist and elbow components, a transradial socket, and some sort of power control:

- The terminal device is a prosthetic hand or hook that can be opened and closed either actively using a harness structure or passively with the other uninvolved hand.
- The wrist component to which the TD is attached is designed to allow the person to turn the palms up or down.
- The elbow component permits flexion and extension and can be locked into a particular angulation.
- The transradial sockets, which are located around the radius of the forearm, can be self-suspending, silicone-lined, or transhumeral.

- Options for power control include harness systems that fit around the torso and opposite arm, body-powered controls that employ proximal muscle contractions to regulate the prosthesis, and external battery-powered systems.

Common Types of Upper-Limb Amputations

The level of an upper-limb amputation determines the type of prosthesis used. The main purpose of the prosthesis is to enable the patient to perform fine motor skills and functional activities. Options follow:

- Of the common types of upper-extremity amputations, the smallest would be a wrist disarticulation, in which the carpal bones from the radius and ulna are separated.
- A transradial amputation is removal of the forearm below the area around the ulna and radius bones.
- An elbow disarticulation is a separation of the radius and ulna of the forearm from the humerus bone in the upper arm.
- A transhumeral amputation is removal of the arm below some point of the humerus.
- A shoulder disarticulation is the surgical severance of the shoulder at the glenohumeral joint.

Problems Encountered by Patients with Prosthetic Devices Subsequent to Amputation

For patients adjusting to lower-limb prostheses, gait deviations are prevalent. Prostheses that are too long (and other causes) can create an abducted (wide-based) gait, circumfusion (wide lateral swinging motion), and vaulting (pushing up on the toes of the other leg to swing the leg through). A short prosthesis can result in lateral trunk bending. Lateral or medial whip can occur if there is too much internal or external rotation at the knee. Patients also tend to experience pain after amputation, which can be real residual limb pain, phantom limb pain related to the excised limb portion (generally requiring antidepressants, analgesics, etc.), or other phantom limb sensations, such as numbness or itching. Skin integrity, posture, range of motion, and other parameters are usually affected. There is likely to be edema in the remaining limb, necessitating measurements, initial wrapping, and attention to positioning to avoid contractures.

Implants for Joint Replacement Arthroplasty and Arthrodesis

Implants are surgically implanted artificial body parts or prostheses. Joint replacement arthroplasty is the removal of articulating surfaces of a joint and replacement of both surfaces (total joint replacement) or one surface (hemi replacement). Both are mainly used for late-stage arthritis. The prosthetic implants are composed of inert materials, either rigid inert metals, such as cobalt-chrome or titanium alloys or ceramics, or semirigid plastics like polyethylene. Implant designs range from unconstrained resurfacing to fully constrained and articulated, which provides the most stability. The implants may be affixed with acrylic cement; biologic fixation, which allows the bone to grow into a porous surface; screws; or other methods.

Arthrodesis is the surgical union of joint surfaces. It can be used for late-stage arthritis pain or instability of joints that need not be mobile. The two surfaces are fused using internal pins, screws, plates, bone grafts, etc. Internal fractures are often set temporarily using similar implants.

Gravity-Assisted and -Resisted Devices

Gravity-assisted and -resisted devices work, respectively, with or against the forces of gravity to aid patients in performance of functional activities. Gravity-assisted treadmill devices can be used. For example, bodyweight support (BWS) treadmill training or partial weight-bearing gait training utilizes a harness to suspend patients with incomplete spinal cord injuries during treadmill use.

With aquatic therapy or exercises, many of the devices are gravity-resistive as they are used to provide buoyancy, or ability to float.

These include worn collars, rings, belts, and vests, as well as hand-held swim bars and kickboards. There are also devices to provide resistance to water motion, including balls, paddles, fins, and boots. In addition, there are gravity-assisted or -resisted exercise devices like pulley units used for strengthening.

Protective Supportive and Bariatric Devices

Protective and supportive devices are useful for patients prone to wounds. Most are both supportive and protective and are designed to reduce pressure on bony protuberances. Examples include seat cushions and pressure-reducing mattresses made of foam, gel, static or dynamic air, or water. Bariatric devices are specifically designed for morbidly obese patients of about 350 or more pounds. These include special beds that can support this weight and may incorporate special bed scales, exits, or lifts. Other bariatric-specific devices include wheelchairs, commodes, walkers, and mechanical lifts.

Therapeutic Modalities

When Therapeutic Modalities Are Indicated

Therapeutic modalities are generally used to relieve pain and inflammation and promote healing and functional use. Pain messages are transmitted via nerve fibers to the spinal cord and, ultimately, the brainstem, where they are interpreted as pain. The pain can be acute with a defined aggravating factor and characterized by localized swelling and redness, or it can be chronic, which is vaguer, less defined, and longer lasting. Pain is usually assessed with subjective measurement.

Inflammation is an immunological response to tissue injury and is characterized by pain, edema, redness, and high tissue temperature. Most of these signs are due to vasodilation of blood vessels or increased blood flow. Both pain and inflammation can result in functional limitations. Therapeutic modalities include physical agents, such as thermal agents and hydrotherapy; mechanical interventions, such as compression or traction; iontophoresis; and various forms of electrical stimulation. The choice of modality is dependent on many factors, such as suitability of using heat or the presence of certain conditions.

Thermal Agents as Therapeutic Modalities

Thermal agents are modalities that control pain and edema with superficial application. When heat is applied, blood flow is enhanced locally, increasing the metabolic rate, vasodilation, tissue repair and extensibility, and pain relief. The latter is believed to be due to blockage of the ascending pain pathway, known as the gate control theory. When cold is applied, vasodilation briefly occurs, followed by more prolonged vasoconstriction, and eventually more vasodilation (the Hunting response). Cold stimulates nerve endings, raises the pain threshold, decreases local metabolism, averts edema, and reduces pain, probably via the aforementioned gate control. Mechanisms of temperature transfer with thermal agents include conduction or direct transfer with tools, such as hot or cold packs; convection, which uses circulatory motion (example is fluidotherapy); conversion, or changing cellular parameters, such as with ultrasound, evaporation, or conversion from liquid to vapor as in perspiration; and radiation.

Modalities for Applying Superficial Heat

Superficial heat is applied via hydrocollator packs, paraffin baths, hydrotherapy, short-wave diathermy, or fluidotherapy:

- Hydrocollator packs are padded hot packs (initially about 170°F) that are applied to the skin for approximately 15 to 20 minutes for transfer of superficial moist heat. Home heating pads, microwaveable products, and hot-water bottles are variations.
- Paraffin baths are used primarily for the hands and feet. The bath consists of paraffin wax and mineral oil maintained at roughly 126°F. The wax is applied by dipping the body part, followed by wrapping with a plastic bag (dip and wrap); or sequential dipping, followed by soaking the extremity in the bath for 15 to 20 minutes (dip and submerge).
- Hydrotherapy is the utilization of water for therapeutic reasons, which can mean hot or cold water. Here, hydrotherapy generally means submersion in a warm whirlpool for its relaxing and immune stimulation properties; warm water also promotes wound care.
- Short-wave diathermy utilizes electromagnetic energy (frequency 27.12 MHz), which is converted to mechanical energy in bodily tissues.
- Fluidotherapy uses convection (other modalities use conduction) by employing dry heat and an air stream with suspended cellulose against the skin to decrease edema.

Modalities for Superficial Cryotherapy

Cryotherapy is the application of superficial cold to decrease tissue temperature, reduce blood flow, avert edema, and relieve pain. Three of the common modalities use conduction to decrease local temperature: cold packs, ice massage, and ice baths. Cold packs are stored frozen and then locally applied for about 15 minutes, using a towel between the pack and skin to avert frostbite. Ice massage uses direct application of ice in a massage-type manner, generally for shorter periods. An ice bath or whirlpool is a type of hydrotherapy in which the body part is immersed in a swirling bath of cold water and ice. There are also cold compression units that employ compression sleeves with circulating cold water, and vapocoolant sprays, mostly containing fluoromethane, that utilize evaporation as a mechanism.

Therapeutic Ultrasound

Ultrasound is the utilization of sound waves to transfer energy through conversion. Although ultrasound also has nonthermal effects, its deep heating thermal effects are utilized therapeutically. These include increased blood flow, relaxed muscle, augmented tissue extensibility and range of motion, decreased inflammation, and reduced pain. Ultrasound is contraindicated in regions that include the reproductive areas in pregnant women, eyes, genitals, growth plates in children, recent areas of infection or injury, the area above a cardiac pacemaker, etc. In order to use ultrasound therapeutically, one must set the frequency to achieve desired penetration (1 MHz for 2 to 4 cm deep, 3 MHz for 1 to 2 cm), the mode to continuous (as opposed to pulsed for nonthermal effects), and the intensity to between 0.5 and 1.0 watts per square centimeter. The duration is dependent on the size of the area being treated. Ultrasound waves are also used as delivery vehicles for medications, such as dexamethasone or lidocaine, to control inflammation or pain, respectively, in a process called phonophoresis.

Electrotherapy

Electrotherapy is the therapeutic use of electric currents to alleviate pain. Electric current is applied either as direct current (DC), which flows unidirectionally, or alternating current (AC), which changes direction of flow between electrodes. Cathodes are electrodes with positive charges; anodes have negative charges. Each attracts opposite charges and repels like ones. There are a number of specific modalities using electrical stimulation, which all have different mechanisms and settings.

The current theories as to how electrotherapy controls pain include the gate control theory, which advocates the mechanism involves blocking the ascending pain pathway; the endogenous opioid release mechanism, which poses that natural painkillers, such as endorphins and enkephalins, are liberated with electrical stimulation; and the descending inhibition theory, which expounds that strong electrical stimulation ultimately blocks the perception of pain via a descending pathway. The gate control theory is also believed to account for the effectiveness of heat and cold modalities, while the other two theories are believed to explain therapies employing strong electrical stimulation.

Types of Electrotherapy

Generally, electrotherapy requires setting the following parameters:

- Type of waveform: the number of phases of the pulse; options include monophasic (one direction), biphasic (two directions), or polyphasic (more phases)
- Pulse duration: time in microseconds (μs) between the start and end of a complete waveform; inversely related to frequency
- Frequency: number of pulses per second (pps)
- Amplitude: the peak current during one phase of a pulse (expressed in milliamperes); also related to voltage or potential difference between electrodes
- Ramp time: the number of seconds needed to attain maximum amplitude
- Duty cycle: the percentage of time the modality is on relative to total time
- Modulation: changing of parameters during treatment
- Electrode placement: the number of electrodes (two or four) and the area where electrode leads are placed

Electrical Current, the Tissues Involved, and the Sensations of the Patient

Muscles and tendons are less resistant to passage of electric current than skin and fat tissue. Therefore, for example, areas with considerable adipose tissue require stronger current applied. This can be circumvented somewhat by warming, cleansing, and hair removal. At low levels of electrical stimulation, the patient may not experience any sensation because the nerves have not been activated (subsensory response).

As the level of stimulation increases and A-beta nerve fibers are activated, the typical response is a painless tingling sensory sensation. As A-alpha nerve fibers are activated, they have a motor response of greater tingling and muscle contraction. Once A-delta and C nerve fibers are stimulated, the patient becomes quite uncomfortable and has strong muscle contractions (noxious response). The nature of electrotherapy preludes its use during pregnancy; in areas where there is a pacemaker, defibrillator, or metal device (superficial or implanted); in patients with epilepsy or malignancy; in regions of suspected thrombosis, etc.

Transcutaneous Electrical Nerve Stimulation (TENS)

Transcutaneous electrical nerve stimulation (TENS) is one type of electrotherapy. It reduces acute or chronic pain, ostensibly by the gate control mechanism (blockage of the ascending pain pathway), and improves circulation. In TENS, a battery-operated, portable apparatus is employed to deliver the electrical stimulation, making it ideal for use while active. The electrodes are placed directly over the painful area or nerve trunk, innervating it. The stimulation intensity, or amplitude, is set at a strong but comfortable level, and the optimal frequency for motor effects is 40 to 80 pps.

NEUROMUSCULAR ELECTRICAL STIMULATION (NMES)

Neuromuscular electrical stimulation (NMES) is one type of electrotherapy. Unlike other types of electrical stimulation, which target pain reduction, the main goal of NMES is muscle activation and reeducation. NMES is often done in conjunction with strengthening exercises. It is also used to retrain muscles to alleviate urinary incontinence, to prevent muscle spasticity, and as part of functional electrical stimulation (FES), which incorporates foot or hand switches that are used to maintain contractions as needed. In NMES, one or two active electrodes are placed near the applicable motor point with exit electrodes elsewhere. A biphasic, pulsatile, or burst-alternating current is applied for about 10 minutes or until exercise completion. The amplitude and frequency depend on the desired muscular contraction. The duty cycle is set to deliver electrical stimulation 1:5 to 1:3 of the time to prevent fatigue or, if muscle fatigue is the goal (for example, with plasticity), closer to 1:1.

INTERFERENTIAL CURRENT (IFC) AND HIGH-VOLT PULSED CURRENT (HVPC)

The interferential current (IFC) technique is an electrical stimulation modality indicated for acute or chronic pain control, including for Complex Regional Pain Syndrome. It uses four electrodes placed near the area of pain and two channels of medium-frequency current (4000 pps), which first pass through the skin and then mix and interfere with each other, generating lower-frequency current for healing. The amplitude and beat frequency determine the predominant mechanism of action. For strong but comfortable amplitudes and a beat frequency of 50 to 100 pps, the mechanism is gate control, while for an intensity generating muscle contraction and a lower beat frequency of 5 to 30 pps, it is the endogenous opioid mechanism.

High-volt pulsed current (HVPC) is short pulse duration, sensory threshold monophasic stimulation. It activates many types of fibers and can generate a polarized potential over either electrode, thus minimizing edema or aiding wound healing, in addition to controlling pain.

IONTOPHORESIS

Iontophoresis is an electrical stimulation technique in which medications are conveyed through the skin to a painful or injured area via direct current. The modality is indicated for inflammatory syndromes and trigger-point pain. The electrode used for delivery contains the drugs in ionized form, with the same polarity or electric charge as the electrode itself. Thus, the ionized drug is repelled from the electrode into the skin. The most common drugs delivered by iontophoresis are the anesthetic lidocaine, which is positively charged, and the negatively charged anti-inflammatory agents, dexamethasone and salicylates.

SPINAL TRACTION

Spinal traction employs mechanical forces like weights to stretch tissues and separate vertebral joints through longitudinal pull. The most common types are lumbar and cervical traction. In both, the patient lies supine in slight flexion and halters are attached above and below the segment of interest. Lumbar traction is used to widen the disk space and potentially reduce nuclear protrusion in the lower back. Traction time should be short, less than 10 minutes if continual and less than 15 minutes if intermittent. Greater than 50% of body weight is generally needed for adequate separation, and after release, disk pressure may increase. Cervical traction is indicated for widening of the intervertebral foramina in the cervical region. Conditions that cause this space reduction include spondylosis, spinal stenosis, swollen facet joints, and injuries. The traction is generally gentle, typically using manual not mechanical techniques. Stronger traction is indicated for nerve root irritation without acute joint inflammation, as with spondylosis or stenosis. Mechanical traction should not be used in patients with conditions such as osteoporosis, rheumatoid arthritis, meningitis, or malignancies.

COMPRESSION THERAPIES

Compression is the application of force perpendicular to the cross-sectional area of affected tissue facing it. It is primarily used to restrain edema formation, for example, lymphedema with breast cancer or peripheral edema. The use of compression garments worn on the involved limb and stretch bandages is one simple compression technique. Another is intermittent compression, which utilizes compression sleeves worn over the limb, on which pressure is periodically applied or released. The sleeve pressure is 30 to 60 mm Hg for upper limbs and 40 to 80 mm Hg for lower limbs, and the intermittent on-and-off pressure times generally vary from 30 seconds to 5 minutes with total treatment typically lasting up to a half-hour. Intermittent compression may be used in conjunction with cryotherapy.

Safety, Protection, & Professional Roles; Teaching & Learning; Research & Evidence-Based Practice

Safety, Protection, and Professional Roles

Patient Records

Patient records are legal documents that include all pertinent information related to the individual and his care. These records should contain a patient registration form that documents all important demographic information, such as patient name, address, phone numbers, employer, spousal information, similar data about the responsible party accountable for payment, insurance information and insurance card, and chief reason for the visit. The patient's record should also include a comprehensive medical history, including points that address issues pertinent to care (drugs taken, allergies, etc.). Conditions that could potentially affect care should be tagged with visible colored medical alert stickers. All forms should be signed and dated by the patient. If the patient has any conditions that require consultation with the physician, he must sign a release of information form. The patient should be informed in writing of the right to privacy under the Health Insurance Portability and Accountability Act (HIPAA) and sign a form addressing this. The patient record should also contain pertinent laboratory reports, including tests for infectious diseases (e.g., hepatitis, HIV) and information obtained during the patient visit.

Americans with Disabilities Act

In 1990, the Americans with Disabilities Act (ADA) was federally passed. It mandates that people with disabilities cannot be discriminated against in terms of employment and access to public services, accommodations, and goods. It also makes provisions for more sophisticated telecommunication services to facilitate the hearing and speech impaired. Technically, this act applies to facilities with more than 15 employees, but all physical therapy offices should comply because of the nature of the specialty. Essentially, this means the office should have ramps, entryways, waiting rooms, and treatment areas that provide access and accommodate the needs of the disabled.

Ethics

Ethics is defined as sets of moral principles or values indicative of the times. The Standards of Competence espoused by the Federation of State Boards of Physical Therapy assume ethical behavior as an underlying principle for physical therapists. Ethical concerns related to physical therapy include advertising, professional fees and other charges, and the responsibilities and entitlements of the physical therapist relative to the patient. Ethical behavior related to professional fees and charges encourages conformity to local trends, correct billing charges, and fees for items like insurance dealings and missed appointments. Current ethics dictate the physical therapist must not discriminate against seeing a patient on any basis that includes race, religion, financial capabilities, or HIV status.

Jurisprudence Contracts and Torts

Jurisprudence is the legal system set up and enforced at various governmental levels. Laws relating to physical therapy practice would be considered physical therapy jurisprudence. At present, the states of Alabama, Arizona, California, District of Columbia, Florida, Georgia, Nebraska, and Ohio require therapists to take a Jurisprudence Exam under FSBPT [Federation of State Boards of Physical Therapists]. Jurisprudence covers both criminal and civil laws, the latter being more applicable in healthcare settings.

A contract is an enforceable covenant between two or more competent individuals, for example, the physical therapist and patient. It can be an expressed contract, in which terms are established in writing or verbally, or it can be an implied contract, in which necessary actions in effect create the contract.

Torts are wrongful actions that result in injury to the other person. In this context, torts relate primarily to standard of care, potentially resulting in malpractice lawsuits governed by tort laws. On the other hand, criminal laws address crimes recognized as endangering society in general.

Terms Related to Standard of Care

Issues related to standard of care are generally covered by tort laws. Physical therapists are expected to provide due care, which is accepted and judicious care. Malpractice is professional misconduct, resulting in failure to provide due. Most malpractice lawsuits are related to professional negligence, or failure to perform what is deemed standard care. Tort laws also cover what is considered unethical or immoral behavior by the professional, resulting in harm to the patient. Primary examples of these include defamation of character, invasion of privacy, fraud, assault, and battery:

- Defamation of character is harm to another person's character, name, or reputation caused by untrue and malicious statements, either written (libel) or spoken (slander).
- Invasion of privacy refers to unsolicited or unauthorized revelation of patient information.
- Fraud is intentional dishonesty for unfair or illegal gain.
- Assault is the declaration of intent to inappropriately touch a patient.
- Battery is the actual act of inappropriate touching.

HIPAA

HIPAA stands for the Health Insurance Portability and Accountability Act of 1996. It was ratified to institute safeguards related to electronic healthcare communications. These transactions include claims, fund transfers, and correspondence regarding eligibility and claims status. The act also directed the Department of Health and Human Services (HHS) to implement national standards for clerical and financial electronic transmissions related to healthcare.

Healthcare providers, including physical therapists, and health plans must be in compliance. The topics covered in HIPAA that relate to privacy standards include protected health information (PHI), individual rights, current guidelines, parameters related to use and disclosure, enforcement, and preemption. PHI includes any knowledge that could possibly distinguish a patient, such as name or social security number. These must be guarded or encrypted before transmission. HIPAA also grants patients the right to access and copy their own health information.

IDEA

IDEA refers to the Individuals with Disabilities Education Act, a federal law that regulates how states and public agencies afford early intervention, special education, and other services for children with disabilities. IDEA mandates that each state that accepts funding ensures Free Appropriate Public Education (FAPE) to all resident eligible children with disabilities, from preschool through age 21. It requires public schools to provide each of these children with an

Individualized Education Program (IEP) in the least restrictive environment possible. In addition, state and local education agencies are now required to spend a proportionate amount of IDEA federal funds to provide services for parentally placed private school children with disabilities.

FSBPT Standards of Competence

The Federation of State Boards of Physical Therapy (FSBPT) has developed Standards of Competence for physical therapists covering two domains as follows:

1. Domain 1 - Professional Practice: This covers professional accountability, behavior, and development. Accountability refers to use of safe practices; timely and compliant documentation; supervision of assistants; effective communication; and the critical, consistent evaluation, use, and assessment of interventions. Professional behavior involves critical self-assessment, understanding of and adherence to applicable laws and regulations, and the maintenance of professional, sensitive, and unbiased relationships. For professional development, the standards compel the therapist to constantly absorb and apply new information.
2. Domain 2 - Patient/Client Management: Addressing the steps from examination through discharge, these standards direct therapists in the examination, evaluation, and diagnosis of patients safely based on best known practices; dictates that findings are discussed with the patient; and states that appropriate consultations be held prior to development of the care plan. This care plan should use resources wisely and be periodically evaluated and updated. The physical therapist is also responsible for implementation of the plan using legally allowed assistive personnel, education of the patient and others, and coordination of patient discharge.

OSHA Bloodborne Pathogens Standard

OSHA, the Occupational Safety and Health Administration, is part of the U. S. Department of Labor. The OSHA Bloodborne Pathogens Standard covers protection measures for exposure to blood and other potentially infectious materials (OPIMS). It states that every facility where such exposure might occur, such as a physical therapy facility, must review the standard and comply in certain areas. These requirements include development of a written exposure control plan; training of personnel; use of appropriate labels regarding biohazards; provision of hepatitis B vaccine to workers; medical evaluation and exposure follow-up, if needed; maintenance of employee medical and training records; use of universal precautions (discussed elsewhere); management of regulated waste; and housekeeping and contaminated laundry procedures.

Universal vs Standard Precautions

Universal precautions include infection control measures designed to prevent exposure to blood and other bodily fluids of patients, which are treated as potentially infectious. Standard precautions are more inclusive infection control measures that extend to blood; all bodily fluids, such as secretions and excretions (excluding sweat); air droplets; skin that is not intact; and mucous membranes. All of these are considered potentially infectious under standard precautions because even if patients exhibit no symptoms, they can be asymptomatic carriers of disease agents. Wording in the OSHA Bloodborne Pathogens Standard still refers to universal precautions, although the more inclusive standard precautions may be more appropriate. Engineering and workplace practices are considered part of standard precautions; these include measures such as proper hand washing, use and correct disposal of personal protective equipment (PPE), and handling of contaminated sharps. PPE encompasses items like gloves, protective eyewear, and protective clothing.

Proper Body Mechanics and Ergonomics

Proper body mechanics are essential for efficiency and prevention of injury for anyone, but particularly physical therapists, who do a lot of bending and lifting. The therapist should stand with a wide base of support, always preserve a neutral lumbar spine, and use knees and hips (not the waist) to bend down. The therapist should interact with the patient within his base of support, maintaining close body contact. During patient movement, the therapist should widen and stabilize the support base by moving one foot slightly forward. The therapist should stand behind the patient during movement for visualization and assistance.

Ergonomics is the study of good workplace design. Proper ergonomics while seated dictates that feet should be flat on the floor or chair footrest and that knees and hips be bent at 90-degree angles. If using a computer, the screen should be level at eyesight, with head neutral, elbows bent at 90 degrees, and wrist somewhat extended.

How to Teach Proper Body Mechanics

According to good body mechanics, the best way to lift is with the lumbar spine in a neutral position, which provides the greatest stability. However, back injury patients may need to adapt this position for lifting, using either spinal flexion or spinal extension. Neither adaptation is ideal. Spinal flexion utilizes other structures like ligaments, which can be injured, instead of muscles. Spinal extension, in which the spine assumes a lordotic position, does use musculature but increases disk compressive forces. Ideally, patients should be taught to use the load position for lifting or carrying. The therapist should teach the patient to carry and lift objects as close as possible to his center of gravity, which improves balance and control. Additional exercises include having the patient transfer loads to other positions on the side, turn by using legs and hip rotation with minimal trunk rotation, and mimic specific job mechanics. For other types of injuries, good body mechanics should be integrated into functional exercises. Fundamental body mechanics are employed for transitions such as rolling, ambulation, and changing position. Good core strength is integral to optimal body mechanics.

Ergonomic Assessment and Environmental Adaptations

The home and work surroundings of all therapy patients are important. For those undergoing spinal rehabilitation, these are crucial and should be assessed and modified if needed. At home, work, or while driving, seats should have lumbar support, placing the patient in slight lordosis (created with a towel or pillow, if necessary). The chair height should be such that the patient's knees are flexed and feet rest on the floor. Arm rests are suggested. The table or desk should be high enough to prevent leaning on it. Periodic movement should be encouraged for postural change. For sleeping, the patient's mattress should be firm to avert stresses, and the pillow should be high and dense enough for relaxation (foam rubber pillows are discouraged as they cause muscle tension). The ideal sleep position differs, with the primary consideration being avoidance of stress on supporting structures.

Fall Prevention in the Elderly

The elderly are at particular risk for falling and its consequences. Increased age, particularly greater than 80 years, is by itself a risk factor. In many instances, this is because the individual has one or more additional risk factors that include deficits of balance, gait, vision, or cognition; muscle weakness; arthritis; depression; a history of falls; impaired activities of daily living; and utilization of an assistive device. Older adults tend to make postural adjustments more slowly and exhibit balance problems. Those who have experienced falls generally acquire a fear of falling, which decreases their functional abilities, creates social isolation, and leads to psychological issues, such as depression. Representative tests for fall risk and fear of falling include the Tinetti Performance-

Oriented Mobility Assessment (POMA) and the Falls Efficacy Scale, respectively. Use of many medications, particularly those with neurologic effects, puts these individuals at risk as well, and those who have fallen should have their medications reviewed. There are various evidence-based balance exercise programs that can be used to address fall prevention in the elderly in general, patients with balance deficits, and those with low physical functioning (discussed further elsewhere).

ABCs of Cardiopulmonary Resuscitation

Cardiopulmonary resuscitation (CPR) is an emergency technique used to revive a person whose heart has stopped beating. The process follows an ABC (and often D) pattern.

"A" represents the airway, which must be opened first to allow airflow.

"B" signifies breathing, which the rescuer must observe and establish is or is not occurring.

"C" stands for circulation, which the rescuer must check for using the carotid pulse; if no pulse is felt, then chest compressions interspersed with slow breaths are used to establish one.

"D" refers to the accessory technology of defibrillation, with an automated external defibrillation (AED) unit if available.

Rescue Breathing and CPR on an Adult

The first step in an emergency situation, where an adult patient is orally unresponsive, is to call emergency medical services (generally 911). The rescuer should place the individual in a supine position, if possible, and don gloves. He should then observe, listen to, and feel the person for evidence of breathing. If there is none, he should open the patient's airway by inclining the head back and raising the chin. A resuscitation mouthpiece should be placed in the individual's mouth (a standard precaution) and the nose pinched closed. The rescuer applies two breaths, observes the chest rise, and then tests the carotid artery for a pulse for approximately 15 seconds. Rescue breathing—cycles of one slow breath every five seconds for a minute, followed by checking of pulse and breathing—is done if a pulse is felt. If no pulse is present, four cycles of chest compression, followed by two slow breaths are carried out. The chest compressions are performed kneeling at the patient's side, using one hand on top of the other, and compressing down on the breastbone 15 times rapidly. After each set of four cycles, the carotid pulse is rechecked. This sequence is continued until revival, rescuer substitution, or automated external defibrillation (AED) is ready to be performed.

Automated External Defibrillation (AED) Unit

An AED, or automated external defibrillation unit, is used to revive a person in cardiac arrest. Cardiopulmonary resuscitation (CPR) is carried out until the unit is ready. The "analyze" button on the AED is pressed first, and a sequence of steps must ensue before the unit can be used. The electrodes of the AED are then connected to the patient as illustrated on the unit. The rescuer announces that everyone stay clear of the patient while he determines whether an electric shocking is needed, which is established by pushing the analysis button to get a readout. If a shocking is contraindicated, CPR is reinstituted. Otherwise the AED unit will have an audible or visual means of indicating when it is ready to shock the patient. The AED shows when shocking is occurring, and the pulse should be checked after the third shock. If a pulse is found, the airway, breathing, and vital signs are checked. If no pulse is found, additional CPR is done for a minute, after which the pulse is rechecked. If there is still no pulse, defibrillation is repeated using the analysis button up to three more times (maximum nine additional shocks) with interspersed checking and CPR.

OSHA Fire Safety Standard

The OSHA Fire Safety Standard mandates that a fire safety and prevention plan be developed for the office. The components of the fire safety plan can be transmitted verbally in offices with less than 10 employees, but a written plan is required for larger facilities. The written fire safety plan should include, at minimum, an inventory of major fire hazards in the workplace; information about how possible ignition sources are utilized, stored, and disposed of; a list of fire protection equipment in the office; methods by which combustibles and flammables are kept to a minimum; safeguards for heat-producing instruments; responsible parties for equipment; housekeeping duties; and elements of associated employee training. An emergency notification and evacuation plan in case of fire is also mandated, which can be part of the office emergency action plan (discussed further elsewhere). Two or more separated fire exit routes should be identified, and the standard also suggests measures like sprinkler systems.

Office Emergency Action Plan

The OSHA Fire Safety Standard (and the OSHA Hazard Communication Standard, if chemicals are used) requires development of a written emergency action plan (EAP) for offices with at least 10 employees. Similar information can be communicated verbally in smaller offices. The EAP should address, at minimum, the practices for informing authorities about a fire or other emergency, evacuation procedures and escape routes, methods of accounting for all employees after evacuation, employees equipped to perform rescue procedures, and contacts for individuals knowledgeable about the plan. An EAP might include procedures permitting employees to stay longer to shut off equipment or utilities before evacuating. The EAP should be communicated to each new employee and available for ongoing perusal. It should address all potential natural or man-made emergencies, including fires, natural disasters, release of toxic chemicals, radiological and biological accidents, and interpersonal disruptions. It should explain how to contact rescue operations if needed, such as the local fire department and medical facilities. If no medical facility is nearby, personnel should receive formal first aid training. All key responder and employee information should be included.

Evacuation Procedures

The emergency action plan (EAP) should clearly identify the situations that warrant evacuation (fire, chemical spills, certain natural disasters), the emergency plan coordinator and chain of command, and how each type of emergency should be addressed. A map should be posted prominently, delineating evacuation routes and exits. The EAP should detail procedures for alerting employees in the event of an emergency; appropriate measures include distinctive alarm systems, announcement over a public address system, and use of floor wardens to notify and direct employees. Usually fires and other emergencies are reported to authorities by dialing "911", but there may be internal reporting systems, such as coded intercoms, manual pull stations, or alarms that are used in addition or instead. It is suggested the EAP provide for periodic emergency evacuation drills for familiarization.

Reimbursement Procedures for Physical Therapy Services

Most physical therapy services are reimbursed, at least in part, through third-party payers. In the United States, the third-party payer can be the government insurance programs Medicaid or Medicare or a managed care organization. Medicaid only reimburses services performed by individuals they consider to be "providers." A provider is generally defined as a healthcare worker with a medical or related degree (such as a physical therapist), national certification, and a provider number (obtained from the state). The likelihood of reimbursement is largely controlled through the state. Managed care organizations, such as insurance company HMOs or other forms, use similar criteria for reimbursement. State Medicaid agencies are billed using an HFCA form that incorporates information like the International Classification of Diseases ICD-10 code, the Current Procedural Terminology (CPT) code, charges, and patient and provider information.

Documentation

Documentation is any type of entry into the client's record. According to the APTA Guidelines for Physical Therapy Practice, all documentation by a physical therapist or assistant should conform to the certain guidelines. All handwritten documentation should be done in ink, including the therapist's original signature. If errors are made, the only acceptable change method is to put a line through the error and initial and date it. The documentation should include the client's name, identification number, referral source, and informed consent. It should be dated and signed by the therapist, with denotation of his or her designation. If the documentation is recorded by a physical therapy student or graduate, the licensed physical therapist should cosign it. At each physical therapy session, documentation should include an initial evaluation (history, review of bodily systems, tests done, evaluation, diagnosis, prognosis, goals, care plan). Interventions and patient responses during the session should also be documented, and summation and discharge plans should be detailed at the end.

SOAP Method of Charting

The SOAP method of charting is an orderly charting approach that is problem-oriented. The SOAP acronym stands for the first four components of the approach. These components include available subjective data (S) obtained by questioning the patient and/or family objective data (O) that can be observed and measured, such as test results and information on the medical chart; an assessment (A) of the patient's problems and goals based on both types of data; and a care plan (P) developed based on the data, assessment, and goals. In addition, this approach usually has two other components: the intended, or subsequent, interventions (I); and an evaluation (E) of outcomes. Another type of charting is narrative, in which diary-type documentation is kept with dates, times, and progress notes.

Review Video: SOAP
Visit mometrix.com/academy and enter code: 543158

Medical Professionals in a Physical Therapy Practice

A physical therapist is a professional who has completed an appropriate college-level program in physical therapy and been licensed by the state licensing authority. This typically involves, at minimum, passing the National Physical Therapy Exam (NPTE). Physical therapists assess and treat injuries or physical conditions by external means, such as heat, massage, or exercise, to bring about optimal physical functioning. They usually work under a physician licensed in physical medicine. Patients are usually referred to a physical therapist, although some states allow direct access without referral. Other assistive personnel include licensed physical therapist assistants, who can perform certain interventions under a physical therapist's supervision, and unlicensed physical therapy aides or technicians, who provide support services, such as putting orthoses on patients or setting up treatment modalities. Physical therapists also interact with other referring physicians, physician's assistants, nurses, occupational therapists, speech pathologists, athletic trainers, and other professionals.

American Hospital Association's *A Patient's Bill of Rights*

The American Hospital Association (AHA)'s *A Patient's Bill of Rights*, published in 1973 and later revised, lists twelve patient entitlements. Patients have the right to:

- Thoughtful and respectful care
- Access and opportunity to discuss information regarding their diagnosis, treatment, and prognosis
- Decision making regarding their care plan, including the right of refusal of specific treatments as allowed by law and hospital policies
- An advanced directive that will be honored, if necessary, within the scope of law and hospital policies
- Protection of privacy
- Confidentiality of their records, except in cases of suspected abuse (which generally requires mandatory reporting) or public health hazards
- Examination of their own medical records, unless restricted by law
- Reasonable response to healthcare requests or possibility of transfer
- Information about business relationships affecting care
- Ability to consent to or decline research participation and effective care if they choose not to participate
- Continuity of care and information on options after discharge
- Information on institutional policies and practices

Informed Consent and Privacy

Informed consent refers to permission granted by the patient to receive a particular treatment or participate in a research study. It must be based on access and opportunity, before giving informed consent, to discuss with the healthcare provider all intervention options, the risks and benefits of each, and associated information. The consent should be signed by the patient or, in some cases, a family member or other representative. Informed consent is an essential component for participation in research studies. The right to privacy protects patients against revelation of their medical records or information without consent. Both of these rights are inherent in the American Hospital Association's *A Patient's Bill of Rights*. The right to privacy is now enforced by the Office for Civil Rights of the Department of Health and Human Services.

Teaching and Learning

Nagi Disablement Model

The Nagi Disablement Model describes four stages of evolving health status related to functioning:

1. The first condition is disease, which is a pathological state in which there are signs and symptoms of disrupted homeostasis.
2. Impairment is a structural or functional change in anatomy or physiology. Impairments can eventually result in functional limitations on the person's ability to perform routine, everyday activities.
3. Disability occurs when functional limitations are severe enough to prevent the individual from meeting age-specific expectations within societal norms.
4. The term handicap refers to a state of disability that is perceived within the context of society to be debilitating; it is subjective and often offensive.

INTERNATIONAL CLASSIFICATION OF FUNCTIONING DISABILITY AND HEALTH

The International Classification of Functioning, Disability, and Health (ICF) is a relatively recent classification system developed by the World Health Organization (WHO). It basically defines a disability as any impairment, activity limitation, or participation restriction. According to the ICF model, impairment is a structural or functional body deficit. An activity limitation is a limited ability to complete a task, while participation restriction is a situation that impedes the person's involvement in activities.

According to previous WHO models, what the ICF now calls activity limitation and participation restriction were formerly considered disability and handicap, respectively.

THREE SCHOOLS OF LEARNING THEORY

People learn in one of three ways:

1. The first is by association, in which the learner makes a connection between a stimulus and an expected reaction. In other words, the individual develops a conditioned response. Behaviorists endorse this type of learning or behavior modification. Conditioning is part of behavioral theory.
2. Other learning theories stress the cognitive approach, meaning the process of gathering information to make associations and answer questions is considered more important. This approach is more internal for learners because it requires their input and is shaded by their experiences.
3. The third type of learning theory is humanistic, in which the individual's potential for growth is emphasized by making him an active participant in the process.

SOCIAL COGNITIVE AND LOCUS OF CONTROL THEORIES

The social cognitive theory expounds that behavioral change occurs relative to both the outcome of the behavior and the individual's perception of his capacity to perform the new activity (the degree of self-efficacy). According to this theory, outcomes are highly influenced by the person's expectations, the positive or negative reinforcement received, the environment, and personal beliefs.

The locus of control theory (LOC), or attribution model, proposes that how much control a person has over an outcome influences his receptivity to a behavioral change. If he believes he influences the outcome (have internal LOC), he is more likely to implement the change than if he feels his fate is controlled by external forces (external LOC).

HEALTH BELIEF AND TRANSTHEORETICAL MODELS

The health belief model (HBM) proposes that individuals' receptiveness to behavioral change is related to their own probability of having a particular problem, their perception that it is a serious problem, their belief that the benefits to acting are greater than the impediments, their feeling of self-efficacy to institute the change, and a conviction their health will be enhanced by making the change.

The transtheoretical model of change emphasizes an individual's readiness to change. It theorizes that people must go through five stages of change at their own pace to implement a new health or other behavior. These stages are precontemplation, where no change is imminently planned; contemplation, during which they evaluate the pros and cons of change; preparation, where they are planning to shortly implement the change; action, or implementation of the change; and maintenance of the new behavior.

Other behavioral change theories include cognitive dissonance theory, developmental learning theories, and the theory of reasoned action, which relate change, respectively, to degree of discomfort, developmental level, and outside influences, such as the referring doctor.

MOTOR TASKS

MOTOR LEARNING AND MOTOR TASKS

Motor learning is a multifaceted set of internal processes that, through practice, result in reasonably permanent acquisition and retention of skilled movements or tasks. This is different than mere performance of the task, which requires acquisition but not retention of the skill. Motor learning alters the manner in which sensory information is organized and processed in the central nervous system.

Motor tasks are of three main types: discrete, with an identifiable beginning and end; serial, which involve a sequence of discrete tasks; or continuous, which entail repetitive, uninterrupted movements with no decided beginning and end (like walking).

Patients go through three stages of motor learning when mastering tasks. The first is the cognitive stage, in which they ascertain the goals and basic requirements of how to do the exercise or task. Next is the associative stage, in which the patient uses problem solving and feedback to fine-tune performance of the task. Last is the autonomous stage, in which the movement has become automatic.

TAXONOMY OF LEARNING ACTIVITIES OF DAILY LIVING OR OTHER MOTOR TASKS

The taxonomy of motor tasks involves four dimensions:

1. The first is the environment in which the task is carried out, either closed or open. A closed environment is one without other movement or distractions, in which the person can completely focus attention on the task. An open environment is more complex, with other movement going on.
2. The next dimension looks at whether or not there is intertrial variability in the environment. Absent intertrial variability means the conditions of performance are consistent, whereas present intertribal variability indicates some change between attempts, which is more difficult.
3. The third dimension is body stable versus body transport, which refers to whether the task is done with the body stationary or in motion, respectively.
4. The final aspect is determined by whether or not upper-extremity manipulation of objects is absent or present.

VARIABLES THAT AFFECT MOTOR LEARNING DURING EXERCISE INSTRUCTION OR FUNCTIONAL TRAINING

Motor learning is greatly affected by certain pre-practice considerations, practice, and feedback:

- Some pre-practice factors that promote motor learning are the patient's interest in the task and understanding of its purpose, ability to focus attention on the imminent task, prior demonstration, and concise verbal instructions.
- Acquisition and retention of a motor skill is most influenced by the amount, type, and variability of practice. There are a number of valid practice strategies. Part practice is useful in the initial stage of learning a serial task, whereas whole practice is more effective for mastering continuous tasks. During the initial cognitive stage of learning, blocked practice, in which the same task or series is done repeatedly, is appropriate. Retention is encouraged with later random practice, in which minor variations are introduced, or random-blocked practice, with variations and random order but repetition. In addition to physical practice, mental practice, or motor imagery, has been shown to be helpful.
- The other major factor influencing motor learning is feedback, sensory data obtained and processed by the learner during or after the task. Feedback is either intrinsic (internally derived) or extrinsic (provided by others like the therapist, also known as augmented).

FEEDBACK ASSOCIATED WITH MOTOR LEARNING

The source of feedback associated with motor learning is either intrinsic or extrinsic. Intrinsic feedback refers to sensory cues received by the learner during or immediately after performance of a task. Extrinsic, or augmented feedback, includes sensory cues transmitted by an external source and not necessarily inherent to completion of the task. Examples of extrinsic feedback include verbal and tactile cues from the therapist, visual feedback, and various devices. Both intrinsic and extrinsic feedback contribute to the learner's knowledge of performance, the nature or quality of the task, and knowledge of results or outcome. The timing and frequency of augmented feedback is believed to be important. Concurrent feedback is that given during performance while postresponse feedback is that given after completion of the task. Postresponse feedback can be immediate, delayed, or summary. Feedback that is delayed by a certain time interval or summary after several repetitions generally results in slower initial skill acquisition but greater ultimate retention. Feedback can also be given intermittently or continuously during the course of a task, with intermittent feedback resulting in greater promotion of learning.

Research and Evidence-Based Practice

ASSUMPTIONS OF QUANTITATIVE RESEARCH

Quantitative research is conducted under the paradigm, or assumption, that there is a measurable, predictable, and controllable truth that can be determined. Quantitative research studies begin with a hypothesis (or theory), a formal declaration of a perceived relationship between two or more variables, which is tested using data analysis and statistics. Inherent to the conduct of quantitative research is maintenance of a lack of bias between the researcher and subjects. Generally, the sample size is large, the participants are randomly assigned to experimental or control groups, and data collection is carefully controlled. The goal is to establish cause-and-effect relationships that are applicable to other circumstances.

QUANTITATIVE RESEARCH METHODS

Quantitative research is either non-experimental or experimental. There are two approaches to non-experimental research: descriptive or correlational studies. Descriptive studies are generally used to glean information in areas of minimal knowledge. Correlational studies look at the connection between two or more factors and determine whether trends are statistically significant. Data is collected in a very controlled manner in correlational studies.

Experimental studies are even more controlled and designed to determine possible cause and effect between variables, factors that can change or vary. A proper experimental study is characterized by rigorous control of the experimental circumstances, administration of a prescribed experimental intervention by the investigator, and randomization of experimental and control groups. In an experimental study, a population with similar traits (termed the "independent variable") is subjected to different interventions, typically treated versus control groups, to look at differences in the outcome of another defined factor (the "dependent variable").

Sampling Methods

Researchers pick samples or subjects from a larger population group. This sampling can be based on probability or non-probability criteria. Probability sampling is preferable for quantitative studies as it is more representative of the target population. Subjects are randomly chosen from a larger group through simple, systematic, or stratified random sampling. Simple random sampling employs completely unbiased means, such as using a random sampling table, tossing a coin, or picking numbers from a hat. Systematic sampling involves selection of individuals at certain intervals off a completely random list. Stratified random sampling is choosing subjects based on known distributions of subgroups in a populace. Research projects involving humans often cannot identify all appropriate subjects, necessitating non-probability sampling. Types of non-probability sampling include convenience sampling from a readily available source, advertised solicited volunteer sampling, purposeful sampling, theoretical sampling, and network sampling. The latter, also called nominated or snowball sampling, uses people in the study to identify other possible participants.

Assumptions of Qualitative Research

As opposed to quantitative research that strives to prove or disprove a theory under highly controlled conditions, qualitative research operates under the assumption that multiple truths shaded by individual experiences are possible. Qualitative research studies are generally descriptive, rely on non-probability methods of population sampling, and have relatively small numbers of subjects, the number and type of which may be somewhat open ended. Qualitative studies use examination of documents, interviews, field observations, and focus groups to gather information. The process of data analysis is usually continuous and evolving. Unlike quantitative research where data analysis is based on strict measurement and statistics, here the data is looked at in terms of common themes, descriptions of experiences, ethnographically, or, sometimes, in a more structured fashion through coding and categorization.

Reliability and Validity in Data Collection

Reliability and validity are essential components of quantitative research studies. Reliability refers to the exactness and consistency of data collection and assessment tools. There are several aspects of reliability, which can include:

- Intra-rater reliability, the exactness over time for one tester
- Inter-rater reliability, the accurateness and constancy of data collection between testers
- Instrument reliability or accuracy

- Intra-subject reliability, the ability of a subject to duplicate performance on multiple occasions
- Test-test reliability, agreement of measurements at different time points; can change if some event has occurred in the interim

Validity refers to how logical and meaningful the method of data collection is relative to the underlying hypothesis. Aspects of validity include:

- Content validity, the asking of relevant questions
- Concurrent validity, the degree of equivalence between similar assessment tools
- Construct validity, whether the means of assessment actually quantify the intended measurement

Predictive validity (possible), a design that can predict future outcomes based on current measurements

Reliability of Qualitative Research

Qualitative research is inherently less reproducible and reliable than quantitative research. However, qualitative research can be considered relatively reliable if it meets four criteria:

- The first is credibility or believability. Credibility is enhanced by incorporation of certain study design features, such as long periods of data collection, use of several data sources, peer review, and informed participant involvement.
- Another measure of reliability is dependability or trustworthiness, which is enhanced by having another researcher rigorously critique the analysis.
- Another important criterion is confirmability, which means the data can be checked.
- Lastly, the reliability of qualitative research is increased if its observations can be applied to other groups or settings.

Levels of Data Measurement

Quantitative studies require numerical analysis of data. There are four levels of possible measurement. The first is nominal measurement, in which data points are placed into discreet but unordered categories; nominal measurements are only suitable for descriptive studies. Ordinal measurements consign ranked, ordered data categories with disparate intervals. Interval level measurements are ordered and equidistant, such as temperature on the Celsius scale. Ratio level measurements are also ordered and equidistant, but they have a true zero point enabling all mathematical calculations as well. Ordinal and, particularly, interval and ratio measurements are more applicable to correlational and experimental studies.

Parametric and Nonparametric Statistical Methods

Parametric statistical methods are more critical types of analysis than nonparametric procedures. They are only appropriate for correlational, experimental, or quasi-experimental research. They should only be used when there has been random sample selection, a normal distribution of variables between research groups, and quantification of the dependent variable(s) expressed at the interval or ratio level (discussed elsewhere).

Nonparametric statistical methods are those techniques that have no underlying assumptions about distribution. These methods are used for smaller sample populations, with unknown characteristics and the level of quantification at only the nominal or ordinal level. Nonparametric tests can also be used for quantitative studies, for example, descriptive studies that cannot be analyzed using parametric methods.

Statistical Terms for Descriptive Studies

For the most part, data from descriptive studies can only be measured using nonparametric statistical methods at the nominal or ordinal level. If there is only one variable in the study, the most commonly used statistical representations are frequency, the rate of occurrence; percentage, or proportion; mode, the value that occurs most frequently; median, the middle value in a set of ordered values; mean, the average value; and standard deviation (SD), the deviation from the mean. Standard deviation is defined as the square root of the variance, which is the degree of variation of a set of data from the mean. A normal curve is a typical bell-shaped curve that shows the numerical mean and distribution based on standard deviations of data points. These statistical methods can be used for other types of studies as well.

Statistical Parameters in Correlational Studies

Correlational studies are often analyzed in terms of some of the following statistical parameters:

- Correlation coefficient: determines the degree of correlation between two variables, indicating whether or not they have a relationship; values range from +1 (strong positive relationship) to -1 (strong negative relationship), with values near 0 indicating absence of linkage
- Risk ratio (RR, also known as relative risk): used in cohort studies to represent the frequency of disease or condition in the exposed group relative to the rate in the unexposed control group
- Odds ratio (OR): used in case studies; represents the ratio of chance of exposure in the specific case relative to controls; high-risk, or odds ratios greater than 1.0, are suggestive of increased risk in the exposed group

There are also several ordinal level tests that are utilized.

Statistical Parameters in Experimental Studies

Experimental studies are often expressed in terms of some of the following parameters:

- p-value: the probability or mathematical likelihood of an event; used to express statistical significance of results and whether the null hypothesis (no difference between groups) should be rejected; the most common p-value selected is .05, which is a 5 in 100 chance of error
- Multivariate analysis: simultaneous analysis of at least three variables through advanced mathematical techniques, such as multiple regression, analysis of variance, and multivariate analysis of variance
- t-test: an interval parametric test using a relatively small sample to test for distribution in larger populations; two forms include the pooled t-test for two independent groups and the paired t-test for two dependent, or paired, groups
- F test or ANOVA: the analysis of variance, or difference, in outcomes to determine contributing factors; an interval parametric test for two or more experimental groups
- Non-parametric tests: may also be utilized; examples include chi-square

Clinical Research Studies

The most rigorous, reliable, and valid clinical research studies are randomized, controlled clinical trials in which research subjects with a particular characteristic (the independent variable) are randomly assigned to treatment or control groups and the dependent variable is assessed in a controlled environment. Cohort and case-control studies differ from randomized clinical trials in their method of subject selection, making them slightly less reliable and valid. Cohort studies usually pick subjects prospectively, based on the presence of a particular marker or exposure factor, usually on the basis of the risk ratio (RR). Case-control studies generally pick smaller numbers of subjects, often retrospectively, with and without a particular condition, typically on the basis of the odds ratio (OR). A case study describes one case over time; it can provide interesting information but cannot be considered truly experimental.

NPTE Practice Exam

1. A physical therapist is working in an outpatient orthopedic clinic. During the patient's history the patient reports, "I tore 3 of my 4 Rotator cuff muscles in the past." Which of the following muscles cannot be considered as possibly being torn?

a. Teres minor
b. Teres major
c. Supraspinatus
d. Infraspinatus

2. A physical therapist at an outpatient clinic is returning phone calls that have been made to the clinic. Which of the following calls should have the highest priority for medical intervention?

a. A home health patient reports, "I am starting to have breakdown of my heels."
b. A patient that received an upper extremity cast yesterday reports, "I can't feel my fingers in my right hand today."
c. A young female reports, "I think I sprained my ankle about 2 weeks ago."
d. A middle-aged patient reports, "My knee is still hurting from the TKR."

3. A physical therapist working on an ICU unit, notices a patient is experiencing SOB, calf pain, and warmth over the posterior calf. All of these may indicate which of the following medical conditions?

a. Patient may have a DVT.
b. Patient may be exhibiting signs of dermatitis.
c. Patient may be in the late phases of CHF.
d. Patient may be experiencing anxiety after surgery.

4. A physical therapist is performing a screening on a patient that has been casted recently on the left lower extremity. Which of the following statements should the physical therapist be most concerned about?

a. The patient reports, "I didn't keep my extremity elevated like the doctor asked me to."
b. The patient reports, "I have been having pain in my left calf."
c. The patient reports, "My left leg has really been itching."
d. The patient reports, "The arthritis in my wrists is flaring up, when I put weight on my crutches."

5. A 93-year-old female with a history of Alzheimer's disease gets admitted to an Alzheimer's unit. The patient has exhibited signs of increased confusion and limited stability with gait. Moreover, the patient is refusing to use a w/c. Which of the following is the most appropriate course of action for the physical therapist?

a. Recommend the patient remains in her room at all times.
b. Recommend family members bring pictures to the patient's room.
c. Recommend a speech therapy consult to the doctor.
d. Recommend the patient attempt to walk pushing the w/c for safety.

6. A physical therapist is covering a pediatric unit and is responsible for a 15-year-old male patient on the floor. The mother of the child states, "I think my son is sexually interested in girls." The most appropriate course of action of the physical therapist is to respond by stating:

a. "I will talk to the doctor about it."
b. "Has this been going on for a while?"
c. "How do you know this?"
d. "Teenagers often exhibit signs of sexual interest in females."

7. A physical therapist is caring for a patient who has recently been diagnosed with fibromyalgia and COPD. Which of the following tasks should the physical therapist delegate to an aide?

a. Transferring the patient during the third visit.
b. Ambulating the patient for the first time.
c. Taking the patient's vital sign while setting up an exercise program
d. Educating the patient on monitoring fatigue

8. A physical therapist has been instructed to provide wound care for a patient that has active TB and HIV. The physical therapist should wear which of the following safety equipment?

a. Sterile gloves, mask, and goggles
b. Surgical cap, gloves, mask, and proper shoe wear
c. Double gloves, gown, and mask
d. Goggles, mask, gloves, and gown

9. A physical therapist is instructing a person who had a left CVA and right lower extremity hemiparesis to use a quad cane. Which of the following is the most appropriate gait sequence?

a. Place the cane in the patient's left upper extremity, encourage cane, then right lower extremity, then left upper extremity gait sequence.
b. Place the cane in the patient's left upper extremity, encourage cane, then left lower extremity, then right upper extremity gait sequence.
c. Place the cane in the patient's right upper extremity, encourage cane, then right lower extremity, then left upper extremity gait sequence.
d. Place the cane in the patient's right upper extremity, encourage cane, then left lower extremity, then right upper extremity gait sequence.

10. A 64-year-old Alzheimer's patient has exhibited excessive cognitive decline resulting in harmful behaviors. The physician orders restraints to be placed on the patient. Which of the following is the appropriate procedure?

a. Secure the restraints to the bed rails on all extremities.
b. Notify the physician that restraints have been placed properly.
c. Communicate with the patient and family the need for restraints.
d. Position the head of the bed at a 45-degree angle.

11. A 22-year-old patient in a mental health lock-down unit under suicide watch appears happy about being discharged. Which of the following is probably happening?

a. The patient is excited about being around family again.
b. The patient's suicide plan has probably progressed.
c. The patient's plans for the future have been clarified.
d. The patient's mood is improving.

12. A patient that has delivered a 8.2 lb. baby boy 3 days ago via c-section, reports white patches on her breast that aren't going away. Which of the following medications may be necessary?

a. Nystatin
b. Atropine
c. Amoxil
d. Loritab

13. A 64-year-old male who has been diagnosed with COPD, and CHF exhibits an increase in total body weight of 10 lbs. over the last few days during inpatient therapy. The physical therapist should:

a. Contact the patient's physician immediately.
b. Check the intake and output on the patient's flow sheet.
c. Encourage the patient to ambulate to reduce lower extremity edema.
d. Check the patient's vitals every 2 hours.

14. A patient that has TB can be taken off restrictions after which of the following parameters have been met?

a. Negative culture results.
b. After 30 days of isolation.
c. Normal body temperature for 48 hours.
d. Non-productive cough for 72 hours.

15. A physical therapist teaching a patient with COPD pulmonary exercises should do which of the following?

a. Teach purse-lip breathing techniques.
b. Encourage repetitive heavy lifting exercises that will increase strength.
c. Limit exercises based on respiratory acidosis.
d. Take breaks every 10-20 minutes with exercises.

16. A patient asks a physical therapist the following question. Exposure to TB can be identified best with which of the following procedures?

a. Chest x-ray
b. Mantoux test
c. Breath sounds examination
d. Sputum culture for gram-negative bacteria

17. A twenty-one-year-old man suffered a concussion and the MD ordered a MRI. The patient asks, "Will they allow me to sit up during the MRI?" The correct response by the physical therapist should be.

a. "I will have to talk to the doctor about letting you sit upright during the test."
b. "You will be positioned in the reverse Trendelenburg position to maximize the view of the brain."
c. "The radiologist will let you know."
d. "You will have to lie down on your back during the test."

18. A fifty-five-year-old man suffered a left frontal lobe CVA. Which of the following should the physical therapist watch most closely for?

a. Changes in emotion and behavior
b. Monitor loss of hearing
c. Observe appetite and vision deficits
d. Changes in facial muscle control

19. A physical therapist working in a pediatric clinic observes bruises on the body of a four-year-old boy. The parents report the boy fell riding his bike. The bruises are located on his posterior chest wall and gluteal region. The physical therapist should:

a. Suggest a script for counseling for the family to the doctor on duty.
b. Recommend a warm bath for the boy to decrease healing time.
c. Notify the case manager in the clinic about possible child abuse concerns.
d. Recommend ROM to the patient's spine to decrease healing time.

20. A 14-year-old boy has been admitted to a mental health unit for observation and treatment for a broken leg. The boy becomes agitated and starts yelling at staff members. What should the physical therapist first response be?

a. Create an atmosphere of seclusion for the boy according to procedures.
b. Remove other patients from the area via wheelchairs for added speed.
c. Ask the patient, "What is making you mad?"
d. Ask the patient, "Why are you doing this, have you thought about what your parents might say?"

21. A physical therapist is instructing a patient on the order of sensations with the application of an ice water bath for a swollen right ankle. Which of the following is the correct order of sensations experienced with an ice water bath?

a. cold, burning, aching, and numbness
b. burning, aching, cold, and numbness
c. aching, cold, burning and numbness
d. cold, aching, burning and numbness

22. A physical therapist reviewed the arterial blood gas reading of a 25 year-old male as listed below. The physical therapist should be able to conclude the patient is experiencing which of the following conditions?

Bicarbonate ion-24 mEq/l
PH-7.41
PaC02-29 mmHg
Pa02-54 mmHg
(Fi02)-.23

a. metabolic acidosis
b. respiratory acidosis
c. metabolic alkalosis
d. respiratory alkalosis

23. A physical therapist assesses a 83 year-old female's venous ulcer for the second time that is located near the right medial malleolus. The wound is exhibiting purulent drainage and the patient has limited mobility in her home. Which of the options is the best course of action?

a. Encourage warm water soaks to the right foot.
b. Notify the case manager of the purulent drainage.
c. Determine the patient's pulse in the right ankle.
d. Recommend increased activity to reduce the purulent drainage.

24. Tricyclics (Antidepressants) sometimes have which of the following adverse effects on patients that have a diagnosis of depression?

a. Shortness of breath
b. Fainting
c. Large Intestine ulcers
d. Distal muscular weakness

25. A physical therapist is instructing a patient about the warning signs of (Digitalis) side effects. Which of the following side effects should the physical therapist tell the patient are sometimes associated with excessive levels of Digitalis?

a. Seizures
b. Muscle weakness
c. Depression
d. Anxiety

26. A physical therapist is assessing a patient in the ICU. The patient has the following signs: weak pulse, quick respiration, acetone breath, and nausea. Which of the following conditions is most likely occurring?

a. Hypoglycemic patient
b. Hyperglycemic patient
c. Cardiac arrest
d. End-stage renal failure

27. Medical records indicate a patient has developed a condition of respiratory alkalosis. Which of the following clinical signs would not apply to a condition of respiratory alkalosis?

a. Muscle tetany
b. Syncope
c. Numbness
d. Anxiety

28. Which of the following lab values would indicate symptomatic AIDS in the medical chart? (T4 cell count per deciliter)

a. Greater than 1000 cells per deciliter
b. Less than 500 cells per deciliter
c. Greater than 2000 cells per deciliter
d. Less than 200 cells per deciliter

29. A physical therapist is assessing a patient that has undergone a recent CABG. The physical therapist notices a mole with irregular edges with a bluish color. The physical therapist should:

a. Recommend a dermatological consult to the MD.
b. Note the location of the mole and contact the physician via the telephone.
c. Note the location of the mole and follow-up with the attending physician via the medical record and phone call.
d. Remove the mole with a sharp's debridement technique.

30. A physical therapist is assessing a 18 year-old female who has recently suffered a TBI. The physical therapist notes a slower pulse and impaired respiration. The physical therapist should report these findings immediately to the physician, due to the possibility the patient is experiencing which of the following conditions?

a. Increased intracranial pressure
b. Increased function of cranial nerve X
c. Sympathetic response to activity
d. Meningitis

31. A physical therapist taking a patient's history realizes the patient is complaining of SOB and weakness in the lower extremities. The patient has a history of hyperlipidemia, and hypertension. Which of the following may be occurring?

a. The patient is developing CHF
b. The patient may be having a MI
c. The patient may be developing COPD
d. The patient may be having an onset of PVD

32. A physical therapist has been assigned a patient who has recently been diagnosed with Guillain-Barre' Syndrome. Which of the following statements is the most applicable when discussing the impairments with Guillain-Barre' Syndrome with the patient?

a. Guillain-Barre' Syndrome gets better after 5 years in almost all cases.
b. Guillain-Barre' Syndrome causes limited sensation in the abdominal region.
c. Guillain-Barre' Syndrome causes muscle weakness in the legs.
d. Guillain-Barre' Syndrome does not affect breathing in severe cases.

33. A physical therapist is returning phone calls in a pediatric clinic. Which of the following reports most requires the physical therapist's immediate attention and phone call?

a. An 8-year-old boy has been vomiting and appears to have slower movements and has a history of an atrio-ventricular shunt placement.
b. A 10-year-old girl feels a dull pain in her abdomen after doing sit-ups in gym class.
c. A 7-year-old boy has been having a low fever and headache for the past 3 days that has history of an anterior knee wound.
d. A 7-year-old girl that had a cast on her right ankle is complaining of itching.

34. A physical therapist is assessing a patient in the rehab unit. The patient has suffered a TBI 3 weeks ago. Which of the following is the most distinguishing characteristic of a neurological disturbance?

a. LOC (level of consciousness)
b. Short term memory
c. + Babinski sign
d. + Clonus sign

35. A patient is currently having a petit mal seizure in the clinic on the floor. Which of the following criteria has the highest priority in this situation?

a. Provide a safe environment free of obstructions in the immediate area
b. Call a code
c. Contact the patient's physician
d. Prevent excessive movement of the extremities

36. A physical therapist is caring for a patient in the step-down unit. The patient has signs of increased intracranial pressure. Which of the following is not a sign of increased intracranial pressure?

a. Bradycardia
b. Increased pupil size bilaterally
c. Change in LOC
d. Vomiting

37. The charge nurse on a cardiac unit tells you a patient is exhibiting signs of right-sided heart failure. Which of the following would not indicate right-sided heart failure?

a. Nausea
b. Anorexia
c. Rapid weight gain
d. SOB (shortness of breath)

38. A 24-year-old man has been admitted to the hospital due to work-related back injury. The patient's wife would like to see the patient's chart. The physical therapist should:

a. Provide the chart to the patient's wife following verbal approval by the patient.
b. Provide the chart to the patient's wife after consulting with the patient's physician.
c. Get written approval from the patient prior to providing the wife with chart information and call the MD about the patient's request.
d. Tell the patient' wife, a copy of the patient's medical record is on-file with medical records.

39. A 46-year-old has returned from a heart catheterization and wants to get up to start walking 3 hours after the procedure. The physical therapist should:

a. Tell the patient to remain with the leg straight for at least another hour and check the chart for activity orders.
b. Allow the patient to begin limited ambulation with assistance.
c. Recommend a consultation for ambulation.
d. Tell the patient to remain with leg straight for another 6 hours and check the chart for activity orders.

40. A patient has just been prescribed Minipress to control hypertension. The physical therapist should instruct the patient to be observant of the following:

a. Dizziness and light headed sensations
b. Weight gain
c. Sensory changes in the lower extremities
d. Fatigue

41. A 15-year-old high school wrestler has been taking diuretics to lose weight to compete in a lower weight class. Which of the following medical tests is most like to be given?

a. Lab values of Potassium and Sodium
b. Lab values of glucose and hemoglobin
c. ECG
d. CT scan

42. A 55-year-old female asks a physical therapist the following, "Which mineral/vitamin is the most important to prevent progression of osteoporosis. The physical therapist should state:

a. Potassium
b. Magnesium
c. Calcium
d. Vitamin B12

43. A patient has recently been diagnosed with symptomatic bradycardia. Which of the following medications is the most recognized for treatment of symptomatic bradycardia?

a. Questran
b. Digitalis
c. Nitroglycerin
d. Atropine

44. A patient has recently been prescribed Lidocaine Hydrochloride. Which of the following symptoms may occur with over dosage?

a. Memory loss and lack of appetite
b. Confusion and fatigue
c. Heightened reflexes
d. Tinnitus and spasticity

45. Which of the following arterial blood gas values indicates a patient may be experiencing a condition of metabolic acidosis?

a. PaO2 (91%)
b. Bicarbonate 159
c. CO(2) 48 mm Hg
d. pH 7.33

46. A patient has suffered a left CVA and has developed severe hemiparesis resulting in a loss of mobility. The physical therapist notices on assessment that an area over the patient's left elbow appears as non-blanchable erythema and the skin is intact. The physical therapist should score the patient as having which of the following?

a. Stage I pressure ulcer
b. Stage II pressure ulcer
c. Stage III pressure ulcer
d. Stage IV pressure ulcer

47. A newborn baby exhibits a reflex that includes: hand opening, abducted and extended extremities following a jarring motion. Which of the following correctly identifies the reflex?

a. ATNR reflex
b. Startle reflex
c. Grasping reflex
d. Moro reflex

48. A physical therapist suspects a patient is developing Bell's Palsy. The physical therapist wants to test the function of cranial nerve VII. Which of the following would be the most appropriate testing procedures?

a. Test the taste sensation over the back of the tongue and activation of the facial muscles.
b. Test the taste sensation over the front of the tongue and activation of the facial muscles.
c. Test the sensation of the facial muscles and sensation of the back of the tongue.
d. Test the sensation of the facial muscles and sensation of the front of the tongue.

49. A physical therapist is reviewing a patient's serum glucose levels. Which of the following scenarios would indicate abnormal serum glucose values for a 30-year-old male?

a.70 mg/dl
b.55 mg/dl
c.110 mg/dl
d.100 mg/dl

50. A two-year old has been in the hospital for 3 weeks and seldom seen family members due to isolation precautions. Which of the following hospitalization changes is most like to be occurring?

a. Guilt
b. Trust
c. Separation anxiety
d. Shame

51. A physical therapist is working in a pediatric clinic and a 25-year-old mother comes in with a 12-week-old baby for initial evaluation. The mother is stress out about loss of sleep and the baby exhibits signs of colic. Which of the following techniques should the physical therapist teach the mother?

a. Distraction of the infant with a red object
b. Prone positioning techniques
c. Tapping reflex techniques
d. Neural warmth techniques

52. A physical therapist is working in a pediatric clinic and a mother brings in her 13-month-old child who has Down Syndrome. The mother reports, "My child's muscles feel weak and he isn't moving well. My RN friend check his reflexes and she said they are diminished." Which of the following actions should the physical therapist take first?

a. Contact the physician immediately
b. Have the patient go to X-ray for a c-spine work-up.
c. Start an IV on the patient
d. Position the child's neck in a neutral position

53. A physical therapist is reviewing a patient's arterial blood gas values. Which of the following conditions apply under the following values?

pH- 7.49
Bicarbonate ion 24 mEq/dl
PaC02 – 31 mmHg
Pa02 – 52 mmHg
Fi02 - .22

a. respiratory acidosis
b. respiratory alkalosis
c. metabolic acidosis
d. metabolic alkalosis

54. A 29-year-old male has a diagnosis of AIDS. The patient has had a two-year history of AIDS. The most like cognitive deficits include which of the following?

a. Disorientation
b. Sensory changes
c. Inability to produce sound
d. Hearing deficits

55. A patient has been admitted to the hospital with a HNP L4-5 segment diagnosis. After 24 hours the patient is able to ambulate with assistance with reduced muscle spasms. Which of the following medications was the most beneficial in changing the patient's mobility status?

a. Mivacron
b. Atropine
c. Bethanechol
d. Flexeril

56. Which of the following medications is not considered a neuromuscular blocker?

a. Anectine
b. Pavulon
c. Pitressin
d. Mivacron

57. A physical therapist is caring for a 10-year-old boy who has just been diagnosed with a congenital heart defect. Which of the following clinical signs does not indicate CHF?

a. Increased body weight
b. Elevated heart rate
c. Lower extremity edema
d. Compulsive behavior

58. A physical therapist working in a pediatric clinic and observes the following situations. Which of the following may indicate a delayed child to the physical therapist?

a. A 12-month old that does not "cruise".
b. A 8-month old that can sit upright unsupported.
c. A 6-month old that is rolling prone to supine.
d. A 3-month old that does not roll supine to prone.

59. A physical therapist is reviewing a patient's current Lithium levels. Which of the following values is outside the therapeutic range?

a. 1.0 mEq/L
b. 1.1 mEq/L
c. 1.2 mEq/L
d. 1.3 mEq/L

60. A client is going to have an endoscopy performed. Which of the following is not a probable reason for an endoscopy procedure?

a. Aspiration noted on honey thick diet.
b. Pain with a bowel movement
c. Pain felt in the left upper quadrant
d. Right shoulder pain

61. A patient has been ordered to get Klonapin for the first time. Which of the following side effects is not associated with Klonapin?

a. Drowsiness
b. Ataxia
c. Salivation elevated
d. Diplopia

62. A patient has been diagnosed with diabetes mellitus. Which of the following is not a clinical sign of diabetes mellitus?

a. Polyphagia
b. Polyuria
c. Metabolic acidosis
d. Lower extremity edema

63. A patient has fallen off a bicycle and fractured the head of the proximal fibula. A cast was placed on the patient's lower extremity. Which of the following is the most probable result of the fall?

a. Peroneal nerve injury
b. Tibial nerve injury
c. Sciatic nerve injury
d. Femoral nerve injury

64. Which of the following motions is identified with the corresponding action?

(Action- Turning palm of hand over to face in the anterior direction, dorsum of the hand is pointed downward toward the floor.)

a. Pronation
b. Supination
c. Abduction
d. Adduction

65. A physical therapist is caring for a retired MD. The MD asks the question, "What type of cells secrete insulin?" The correct answer is:

a. Alpha cells
b. Beta cells
c. CD4 cells
d. Helper cells

66. Which of the following is not considered one of the main mechanisms of Type II Diabetes treatment?

a. Medications
b. Nutrition
c. Increased activity
d. Continuous Insulin

67. A physical therapist is caring for a retired MD. The MD asks the question, "What type of cells create exocrine secretions?" The correct answer is:

a. Alpha cells
b. Beta cells
c. Acinar cells
d. Plasma cells

68. A physical therapist is caring for a patient who has experienced burns to the right lower extremity. According to the Rule of Nines which of the following percents most accurately describes the severity of the injury?

a. 36%
b. 27%
c. 18%
d. 9%

69. A patient has experienced a severe third degree burn to the trunk in the last 36 hours. Which phase of burn management is the patient in?

a. Shock phase
b. Emergent phase
c. Healing phase
d. Wound proliferation phase

70. A physical therapist is reviewing a patient's medical record. The record indicates the patient has limited shoulder flexion on the left. Which plane of movement is limited?

a. Horizontal
b. Sagittal
c. Frontal
d. Vertical

71. A client is 36 hours post-op a TKR surgery. The physical therapist notices that 270 cc's of sero-sanguinous accumulates in the surgical drains. What action should the physical therapist take?

a. Notify the doctor
b. Empty the drain
c. Do nothing
d. Remove the drain

72. A physical therapist is assigned to do home education teaching to a blind patient who is scheduled for discharge the following morning. What teaching strategy would best fit the situation?

a. Verbal teaching in short sessions throughout the day
b. Pre-operative booklet on the surgery in Braille
c. Provide a tape for the client
d. Have the blind patient's family member instruct the patient.

73. A violation of a patient's confidentiality occurs if two physical therapists are discussing client information in which of the following scenarios?

a. With a physical therapist treating the patient
b. With a social worker planning for discharge
c. With another physical therapist on duty to plan for break time
d. In the hallway outside the patient's room.

74. If your patient is acutely psychotic, which of the following independent interventions would not be appropriate?

a. Conveying calmness with one on one interaction
b. Recognizing and dealing with your own feelings to prevent escalation of the patient's anxiety level
c. Encourage client participation in group therapy
d. Listen and identify causes of their behavior

75. A physical therapist runs into the significant other of a patient with end stage AIDS crying during her smoke break. Which of the following is most appropriate action for the physical therapist to take?

a. Allow her to grieve by herself.
b. Tell her go ahead and cry, after all your husband's pretty bad off.
c. Tell her you realize how upset she is, but you don't want to talk about it now.
d. Approach her, offering tissues and encourage her to verbalize her feelings.

Answer Key and Explanations

Question	Question	Question	Question	Question
1. B	16. B	31. B	46. A	61. D
2. B	17. D	32. C	47. D	62. D
3. A	18. A	33. A	48. B	63. A
4. B	19. C	34. A	49. B	64. B
5. B	20. A	35. A	50. C	65. B
6. D	21. A	36. B	51. D	66. D
7. A	22. D	37. D	52. D	67. C
8. D	23. C	38. C	53. B	68. C
9. A	24. B	39. A	54. A	69. A
10. C	25. B	40. A	55. D	70. B
11. B	26. B	41. A	56. C	71. A
12. A	27. D	42. C	57. D	72. A
13. B	28. D	43. D	58. A	73. D
14. A	29. C	44. B	59. D	74. C
15. A	30. A	45. B	60. B	75. D

1. B: Teres Minor, Infraspinatus, Supraspinatus, and Subscapularis make up the Rotator Cuff.

2. B: The patient experiencing neurovascular changes should have the highest priority. Pain following a TKR is normal, and breakdown over the heels is a gradual process. Moreover, a subacute ankle sprain is almost never a medical emergency.

3. A: All of these factors indicate a DVT.

4. B: Pain may be indicating neurovascular complication.

5. B: Stimulation in the form of pictures may decrease signs of confusion.

6. D: Adolescents exhibiting signs of sexual development and interest are normal.

7. A: Aides should be competent on transfers.

8. D: All protective measures must be worn; it is not required to double glove.

9. A: The cane should be placed in the patient's strong upper extremity, and left arm/right foot go together, for normal gait.

10. C: Both the family and the patient should have the need for restraints explained to them.

11. B: The suicide plan may have been decided.

12. A: Thrush may be occurring and the patient may need Nystatin.

13. B: Check the intake and output prior to making any decisions about patient care.

14. A: Negative culture results would indicate absence of infection.

15. A: Purse lip breathing will help decrease the volume of air expelled by increased bronchial airways.

16. B: The Mantoux is the most accurate test to determine the presence of TB.

17. D: The MRI will require supine positioning.

18. A: The frontal lobe is responsible for behavior and emotions.

19. C: The patient's safety should have the highest priority.

20. A: Seclusion is your best option in this scenario.

21. A: CBAN, cold, burn, ache, numbness

22. D: Respiratory alkalosis-elevated pH, and low carbon dioxide levels, no compensation noted.

23. C: A determination of arterial blood flow should be made, prior to encouraging increased activity, or notifying additional team members.

24. B: Fainting and hypotension can be caused by Tricyclics.

25. B: Palpitations and muscle weakness are found with excessive levels of Digitalis.

26. B: All of the clinical signs indicate a hyperglycemic condition.

27. D: Anxiety is a clinical sign associated with respiratory acidosis.

28. D: <200 T4 cells/deciliter

29. C: Contacting the attending physician via the medical record is appropriate due to the possibility of melanoma.

30. A: The patient is at high risk of developing increased intracranial pressure ICP.

31. B: Myocardial infarction may be associated with SOB and muscle weakness.

32. C: Muscle weakness in the lower extremities is found in acute cases of Guillain-Barre' Syndrome.

33. A: The shunt may be blocked and require immediate medical attention.

34. A: LOC is the most critical indicator of impaired neurological capabilities.

35. A: Patient safety should be the top concern about this patient.

36. B: Unilateral pupil changes indicate changes in ICP.

37. D: Left sided heart failure exhibits signs of pulmonary compromise SOB.

38. C: Some facilities require the physician to be notified about a patient's request and written permission from the husband is required for the wife to view the chart.

39. A: The patient should keep the leg straight for at least 4 hours.

40. A: Hypotension may be result of over correction of a hypertensive condition.

41. A: Diuretics can disturb the sodium and potassium balance resulting in cardiac complications. An ECG is not indicated without evidence of cardiac conditions.

42. C: Calcium is the most recognized osteoporosis treatment.

43. D: Atropine encourages increased rate of conduction in the AV node.

44. B: Lidocaine Hydrochloride can cause fatigue and confusion if an over dosage occurs.

45. B: The bicarbonate value is below normal, indicating a condition of metabolic acidosis.

46. A: Erythema with the skin intact can indicate a Stage I pressure ulcer.

47. D: The moro reflex has all of the listed characteristics.

48. B: The facial nerve VII: is motor to the face and sensory to the anterior tongue.

49. B: 60-115 mg/dl is standard range for serum glucose levels.

50. C: Separation anxiety can easily occur after six months during hospitalization.

51. D: Neural warmth will help to lower the baby's agitation level.

52. D: An atlanto-axial dislocation may have occurred. Position the child in a neutral c-spine posture and then contact the doctor immediately.

53. B: Elevated pH and low CO2 level indicate respiratory alkalosis; no compensation is noted.

54. A: Cognitive changes may include confusion and disorientation.

55. D: Flexeril is a muscle relaxant for acute muscle pain and spasms.

56. C: Pitressin is a hormone replacement medication.

57. D: Compulsive behavior does not indicate CHF.

58. A: At 12 months a child should at least be "cruising" holding on to objects to walk. Cruising is considered pre-walking.

59. D: 1.0-1.2 mEq/L is considered standard therapeutic range for patient care.

60. B: Bowel movement pain should be examined with a colonoscopy not a endoscopy.

61. D: A-C are associated side effects of Klonapin.

62. D: A-C are associated with diabetes mellitus.

63. A: The head of the proximal fibula is in close proximity to the peroneal nerve.

64. B: Supination- "Holding a bowl of soup in your hand."

65. B: Beta cells secrete insulin.

66. D: Insulin is not required in continuous treatment for every Type II diabetic.

67. C: Acinar cells create exocrine secretions.

68. C: Each lower extremity is scored as 18% according to the Rule of Nines.

69. A: The shock phase is considered the first 24-48 hours in wound management.

70. B: Sagittal motion occurs in the midline plane of the body.

71. A: The physician should be notified if excessive drainage is noted from the surgical site.

72. A: Information is smaller amounts is easier to retain. Teaching the day before the discharge is best accomplished in a one on one format.

73. D: Hallway discussions should not occur, because you do not who is listening, even though it may be a professional discussion.

74. C: Acutely psychotic patients will disrupt group activities.

75. D: Being left alone during the grief process, isolates individuals. These individuals need an outlet for their feelings and to talk to someone who is empathetic.

How to Overcome Test Anxiety

Just the thought of taking a test is enough to make most people a little nervous. A test is an important event that can have a long-term impact on your future, so it's important to take it seriously and it's natural to feel anxious about performing well. But just because anxiety is normal, that doesn't mean that it's helpful in test taking, or that you should simply accept it as part of your life. Anxiety can have a variety of effects. These effects can be mild, like making you feel slightly nervous, or severe, like blocking your ability to focus or remember even a simple detail.

If you experience test anxiety—whether severe or mild—it's important to know how to beat it. To discover this, first you need to understand what causes test anxiety.

Causes of Test Anxiety

While we often think of anxiety as an uncontrollable emotional state, it can actually be caused by simple, practical things. One of the most common causes of test anxiety is that a person does not feel adequately prepared for their test. This feeling can be the result of many different issues such as poor study habits or lack of organization, but the most common culprit is time management. Starting to study too late, failing to organize your study time to cover all of the material, or being distracted while you study will mean that you're not well prepared for the test. This may lead to cramming the night before, which will cause you to be physically and mentally exhausted for the test. Poor time management also contributes to feelings of stress, fear, and hopelessness as you realize you are not well prepared but don't know what to do about it.

Other times, test anxiety is not related to your preparation for the test but comes from unresolved fear. This may be a past failure on a test, or poor performance on tests in general. It may come from comparing yourself to others who seem to be performing better or from the stress of living up to expectations. Anxiety may be driven by fears of the future—how failure on this test would affect your educational and career goals. These fears are often completely irrational, but they can still negatively impact your test performance.

Review Video: 3 Reasons You Have Test Anxiety
Visit mometrix.com/academy and enter code: 428468

Elements of Test Anxiety

As mentioned earlier, test anxiety is considered to be an emotional state, but it has physical and mental components as well. Sometimes you may not even realize that you are suffering from test anxiety until you notice the physical symptoms. These can include trembling hands, rapid heartbeat, sweating, nausea, and tense muscles. Extreme anxiety may lead to fainting or vomiting. Obviously, any of these symptoms can have a negative impact on testing. It is important to recognize them as soon as they begin to occur so that you can address the problem before it damages your performance.

Review Video: 3 Ways to Tell You Have Test Anxiety
Visit mometrix.com/academy and enter code: 927847

The mental components of test anxiety include trouble focusing and inability to remember learned information. During a test, your mind is on high alert, which can help you recall information and stay focused for an extended period of time. However, anxiety interferes with your mind's natural processes, causing you to blank out, even on the questions you know well. The strain of testing during anxiety makes it difficult to stay focused, especially on a test that may take several hours. Extreme anxiety can take a huge mental toll, making it difficult not only to recall test information but even to understand the test questions or pull your thoughts together.

Review Video: How Test Anxiety Affects Memory
Visit mometrix.com/academy and enter code: 609003

Effects of Test Anxiety

Test anxiety is like a disease—if left untreated, it will get progressively worse. Anxiety leads to poor performance, and this reinforces the feelings of fear and failure, which in turn lead to poor performances on subsequent tests. It can grow from a mild nervousness to a crippling condition. If allowed to progress, test anxiety can have a big impact on your schooling, and consequently on your future.

Test anxiety can spread to other parts of your life. Anxiety on tests can become anxiety in any stressful situation, and blanking on a test can turn into panicking in a job situation. But fortunately, you don't have to let anxiety rule your testing and determine your grades. There are a number of relatively simple steps you can take to move past anxiety and function normally on a test and in the rest of life.

Review Video: How Test Anxiety Impacts Your Grades
Visit mometrix.com/academy and enter code: 939819

Physical Steps for Beating Test Anxiety

While test anxiety is a serious problem, the good news is that it can be overcome. It doesn't have to control your ability to think and remember information. While it may take time, you can begin taking steps today to beat anxiety.

Just as your first hint that you may be struggling with anxiety comes from the physical symptoms, the first step to treating it is also physical. Rest is crucial for having a clear, strong mind. If you are tired, it is much easier to give in to anxiety. But if you establish good sleep habits, your body and mind will be ready to perform optimally, without the strain of exhaustion. Additionally, sleeping well helps you to retain information better, so you're more likely to recall the answers when you see the test questions.

Getting good sleep means more than going to bed on time. It's important to allow your brain time to relax. Take study breaks from time to time so it doesn't get overworked, and don't study right before bed. Take time to rest your mind before trying to rest your body, or you may find it difficult to fall asleep.

Review Video: The Importance of Sleep for Your Brain
Visit mometrix.com/academy and enter code: 319338

Along with sleep, other aspects of physical health are important in preparing for a test. Good nutrition is vital for good brain function. Sugary foods and drinks may give a burst of energy but this burst is followed by a crash, both physically and emotionally. Instead, fuel your body with protein and vitamin-rich foods.

Also, drink plenty of water. Dehydration can lead to headaches and exhaustion, especially if your brain is already under stress from the rigors of the test. Particularly if your test is a long one, drink water during the breaks. And if possible, take an energy-boosting snack to eat between sections.

Review Video: How Diet Can Affect your Mood
Visit mometrix.com/academy and enter code: 624317

Along with sleep and diet, a third important part of physical health is exercise. Maintaining a steady workout schedule is helpful, but even taking 5-minute study breaks to walk can help get your blood pumping faster and clear your head. Exercise also releases endorphins, which contribute to a positive feeling and can help combat test anxiety.

When you nurture your physical health, you are also contributing to your mental health. If your body is healthy, your mind is much more likely to be healthy as well. So take time to rest, nourish your body with healthy food and water, and get moving as much as possible. Taking these physical steps will make you stronger and more able to take the mental steps necessary to overcome test anxiety.

Mental Steps for Beating Test Anxiety

Working on the mental side of test anxiety can be more challenging, but as with the physical side, there are clear steps you can take to overcome it. As mentioned earlier, test anxiety often stems from lack of preparation, so the obvious solution is to prepare for the test. Effective studying may be the most important weapon you have for beating test anxiety, but you can and should employ several other mental tools to combat fear.

First, boost your confidence by reminding yourself of past success—tests or projects that you aced. If you're putting as much effort into preparing for this test as you did for those, there's no reason you should expect to fail here. Work hard to prepare; then trust your preparation.

Second, surround yourself with encouraging people. It can be helpful to find a study group, but be sure that the people you're around will encourage a positive attitude. If you spend time with others who are anxious or cynical, this will only contribute to your own anxiety. Look for others who are motivated to study hard from a desire to succeed, not from a fear of failure.

Third, reward yourself. A test is physically and mentally tiring, even without anxiety, and it can be helpful to have something to look forward to. Plan an activity following the test, regardless of the outcome, such as going to a movie or getting ice cream.

When you are taking the test, if you find yourself beginning to feel anxious, remind yourself that you know the material. Visualize successfully completing the test. Then take a few deep, relaxing breaths and return to it. Work through the questions carefully but with confidence, knowing that you are capable of succeeding.

Developing a healthy mental approach to test taking will also aid in other areas of life. Test anxiety affects more than just the actual test—it can be damaging to your mental health and even contribute to depression. It's important to beat test anxiety before it becomes a problem for more than testing.

Review Video: Test Anxiety and Depression
Visit mometrix.com/academy and enter code: 904704

Study Strategy

Being prepared for the test is necessary to combat anxiety, but what does being prepared look like? You may study for hours on end and still not feel prepared. What you need is a strategy for test prep. The next few pages outline our recommended steps to help you plan out and conquer the challenge of preparation.

Step 1: Scope Out the Test

Learn everything you can about the format (multiple choice, essay, etc.) and what will be on the test. Gather any study materials, course outlines, or sample exams that may be available. Not only will this help you to prepare, but knowing what to expect can help to alleviate test anxiety.

Step 2: Map Out the Material

Look through the textbook or study guide and make note of how many chapters or sections it has. Then divide these over the time you have. For example, if a book has 15 chapters and you have five days to study, you need to cover three chapters each day. Even better, if you have the time, leave an extra day at the end for overall review after you have gone through the material in depth.

If time is limited, you may need to prioritize the material. Look through it and make note of which sections you think you already have a good grasp on, and which need review. While you are studying, skim quickly through the familiar sections and take more time on the challenging parts. Write out your plan so you don't get lost as you go. Having a written plan also helps you feel more in control of the study, so anxiety is less likely to arise from feeling overwhelmed at the amount to cover.

Step 3: Gather Your Tools

Decide what study method works best for you. Do you prefer to highlight in the book as you study and then go back over the highlighted portions? Or do you type out notes of the important information? Or is it helpful to make flashcards that you can carry with you? Assemble the pens, index cards, highlighters, post-it notes, and any other materials you may need so you won't be distracted by getting up to find things while you study.

If you're having a hard time retaining the information or organizing your notes, experiment with different methods. For example, try color-coding by subject with colored pens, highlighters, or post-it notes. If you learn better by hearing, try recording yourself reading your notes so you can listen while in the car, working out, or simply sitting at your desk. Ask a friend to quiz you from your flashcards, or try teaching someone the material to solidify it in your mind.

Step 4: Create Your Environment

It's important to avoid distractions while you study. This includes both the obvious distractions like visitors and the subtle distractions like an uncomfortable chair (or a too-comfortable couch that makes you want to fall asleep). Set up the best study environment possible: good lighting and a comfortable work area. If background music helps you focus, you may want to turn it on, but otherwise keep the room quiet. If you are using a computer to take notes, be sure you don't have any other windows open, especially applications like social media, games, or anything else that could distract you. Silence your phone and turn off notifications. Be sure to keep water close by so you stay hydrated while you study (but avoid unhealthy drinks and snacks).

Also, take into account the best time of day to study. Are you freshest first thing in the morning? Try to set aside some time then to work through the material. Is your mind clearer in the afternoon or evening? Schedule your study session then. Another method is to study at the same time of day that you will take the test, so that your brain gets used to working on the material at that time and will be ready to focus at test time.

STEP 5: STUDY!

Once you have done all the study preparation, it's time to settle into the actual studying. Sit down, take a few moments to settle your mind so you can focus, and begin to follow your study plan. Don't give in to distractions or let yourself procrastinate. This is your time to prepare so you'll be ready to fearlessly approach the test. Make the most of the time and stay focused.

Of course, you don't want to burn out. If you study too long you may find that you're not retaining the information very well. Take regular study breaks. For example, taking five minutes out of every hour to walk briskly, breathing deeply and swinging your arms, can help your mind stay fresh.

As you get to the end of each chapter or section, it's a good idea to do a quick review. Remind yourself of what you learned and work on any difficult parts. When you feel that you've mastered the material, move on to the next part. At the end of your study session, briefly skim through your notes again.

But while review is helpful, cramming last minute is NOT. If at all possible, work ahead so that you won't need to fit all your study into the last day. Cramming overloads your brain with more information than it can process and retain, and your tired mind may struggle to recall even previously learned information when it is overwhelmed with last-minute study. Also, the urgent nature of cramming and the stress placed on your brain contribute to anxiety. You'll be more likely to go to the test feeling unprepared and having trouble thinking clearly.

So don't cram, and don't stay up late before the test, even just to review your notes at a leisurely pace. Your brain needs rest more than it needs to go over the information again. In fact, plan to finish your studies by noon or early afternoon the day before the test. Give your brain the rest of the day to relax or focus on other things, and get a good night's sleep. Then you will be fresh for the test and better able to recall what you've studied.

STEP 6: TAKE A PRACTICE TEST

Many courses offer sample tests, either online or in the study materials. This is an excellent resource to check whether you have mastered the material, as well as to prepare for the test format and environment.

Check the test format ahead of time: the number of questions, the type (multiple choice, free response, etc.), and the time limit. Then create a plan for working through them. For example, if you have 30 minutes to take a 60-question test, your limit is 30 seconds per question. Spend less time on the questions you know well so that you can take more time on the difficult ones.

If you have time to take several practice tests, take the first one open book, with no time limit. Work through the questions at your own pace and make sure you fully understand them. Gradually work up to taking a test under test conditions: sit at a desk with all study materials put away and set a timer. Pace yourself to make sure you finish the test with time to spare and go back to check your answers if you have time.

After each test, check your answers. On the questions you missed, be sure you understand why you missed them. Did you misread the question (tests can use tricky wording)? Did you forget the information? Or was it something you hadn't learned? Go back and study any shaky areas that the practice tests reveal.

Taking these tests not only helps with your grade, but also aids in combating test anxiety. If you're already used to the test conditions, you're less likely to worry about it, and working through tests until you're scoring well gives you a confidence boost. Go through the practice tests until you feel comfortable, and then you can go into the test knowing that you're ready for it.

Test Tips

On test day, you should be confident, knowing that you've prepared well and are ready to answer the questions. But aside from preparation, there are several test day strategies you can employ to maximize your performance.

First, as stated before, get a good night's sleep the night before the test (and for several nights before that, if possible). Go into the test with a fresh, alert mind rather than staying up late to study.

Try not to change too much about your normal routine on the day of the test. It's important to eat a nutritious breakfast, but if you normally don't eat breakfast at all, consider eating just a protein bar. If you're a coffee drinker, go ahead and have your normal coffee. Just make sure you time it so that the caffeine doesn't wear off right in the middle of your test. Avoid sugary beverages, and drink enough water to stay hydrated but not so much that you need a restroom break 10 minutes into the test. If your test isn't first thing in the morning, consider going for a walk or doing a light workout before the test to get your blood flowing.

Allow yourself enough time to get ready, and leave for the test with plenty of time to spare so you won't have the anxiety of scrambling to arrive in time. Another reason to be early is to select a good seat. It's helpful to sit away from doors and windows, which can be distracting. Find a good seat, get out your supplies, and settle your mind before the test begins.

When the test begins, start by going over the instructions carefully, even if you already know what to expect. Make sure you avoid any careless mistakes by following the directions.

Then begin working through the questions, pacing yourself as you've practiced. If you're not sure on an answer, don't spend too much time on it, and don't let it shake your confidence. Either skip it and come back later, or eliminate as many wrong answers as possible and guess among the remaining ones. Don't dwell on these questions as you continue—put them out of your mind and focus on what lies ahead.

Be sure to read all of the answer choices, even if you're sure the first one is the right answer. Sometimes you'll find a better one if you keep reading. But don't second-guess yourself if you do immediately know the answer. Your gut instinct is usually right. Don't let test anxiety rob you of the information you know.

If you have time at the end of the test (and if the test format allows), go back and review your answers. Be cautious about changing any, since your first instinct tends to be correct, but make sure you didn't misread any of the questions or accidentally mark the wrong answer choice. Look over any you skipped and make an educated guess.

At the end, leave the test feeling confident. You've done your best, so don't waste time worrying about your performance or wishing you could change anything. Instead, celebrate the successful completion of this test. And finally, use this test to learn how to deal with anxiety even better next time.

Review Video: 5 Tips to Beat Test Anxiety
Visit mometrix.com/academy and enter code: 570656

Important Qualification

Not all anxiety is created equal. If your test anxiety is causing major issues in your life beyond the classroom or testing center, or if you are experiencing troubling physical symptoms related to your anxiety, it may be a sign of a serious physiological or psychological condition. If this sounds like your situation, we strongly encourage you to seek professional help.

Tell Us Your Story

We at Mometrix would like to extend our heartfelt thanks to you for letting us be a part of your journey. It is an honor to serve people from all walks of life, people like you, who are committed to building the best future they can for themselves.

We know that each person's situation is unique. But we also know that, whether you are a young student or a mother of four, you care about working to make your own life and the lives of those around you better.

That's why we want to hear your story.

We want to know why you're taking this test. We want to know about the trials you've gone through to get here. And we want to know about the successes you've experienced after taking and passing your test.

In addition to your story, which can be an inspiration both to us and to others, we value your feedback. We want to know both what you loved about our book and what you think we can improve on.

The team at Mometrix would be absolutely thrilled to hear from you! So please, send us an email at tellusyourstory@mometrix.com or visit us at mometrix.com/tellusyourstory.php and let's stay in touch.

Additional Bonus Material

Due to our efforts to try to keep this book to a manageable length, we've created a link that will give you access to all of your additional bonus material.

Please visit https://www.mometrix.com/bonus948/npte to access the information.

CPSIA information can be obtained
at www.ICGtesting.com
Printed in the USA
LVHW061653200422
716707LV00005B/46